PEDIATRIC NURSE
CERTIFICATION REVIEW

Maureen Fitzgerald, EdD, MSN, CPN, RNC-NIC, is an assistant professor and program director of the postgraduate certificate program (PGCP) in academic nursing for Jefferson College of Nursing at Thomas Jefferson University, Center City campus in Philadelphia, Pennsylvania. She has been a neonatal and pediatric nurse for 21 years, certified in neonatal intensive care nursing and pediatric nursing. Dr. Fitzgerald has taught all levels of nursing, interacting with students over the past 11 years. Dr. Fitzgerald received her BSN and MSN degrees from Thomas Jefferson University's accelerated nursing program and has a graduate certificate in nursing education from Mount Carmel College of Nursing in Columbus, Ohio. She completed her EdD in higher education administration at Northeastern University, Boston, Massachusetts, and her dissertation focused on nursing students' readiness for professional practice. Currently, Dr. Fitzgerald teaches obstetrics, pediatrics, and research to baccalaureate students and educates students in the PGCP in academic nursing. She received the Excellence in Teaching Award in Baccalaureate Programs in 2017 and the Scholarly Achievement Award 2013 from Jefferson College of Nursing. She is a member of Delta Rho, Jefferson's Chapter of Sigma Theta Tau International Nursing Honor Society, as well as the National League of Nurses and the Society of Pediatric Nurses.

David Jack, PhD, RN, CPN, is an assistant professor of nursing at Jefferson College of Nursing, Thomas Jefferson University, Center City campus in Philadelphia, Pennsylvania. He has been a pediatric nurse for more than 25 years and is certified in pediatric nursing. Dr. Jack has taught both didactic and clinical nursing in various undergraduate and graduate nursing programs. Dr. Jack is a graduate of Helene Fuld School of Nursing program in Camden County, New Jersey. He later received his BSN from La Salle University in Philadelphia, Pennsylvania, and an MSN degree in Nursing Education from Villanova University in Villanova, Pennsylvania. In 2009, he earned his PhD in nursing from Widener University in Chester, Pennsylvania, and was awarded the Widener University PhD Dean's Award for Excellence. This Dean's Award is the recognition of a doctoral dissertation that is exceptional and exemplifies the high standards of scholarship and knowledge development. Dr. Jack's interests include family-centered care, early aggression management strategies, and health promotion and education. Currently, Dr. Jack teaches health assessment and pediatrics to undergraduate students and a nursing theory course to graduate students. He has participated in numerous PhD and DNP projects as both a committee member and chair lead. He received the Excellence in Teaching Award in Baccalaureate Programs in 2013 and Excellence in Teaching Award in the Graduate Program in 2018. He is a board member of Delta Rho, Jefferson's Chapter of Sigma Theta Tau International Nursing Honor Society, as well as the National League of Nurses and the Society of Pediatric Nurses.

PEDIATRIC NURSE CERTIFICATION REVIEW

MAUREEN FITZGERALD, EdD, MSN, CPN, RNC-NIC

DAVID JACK, PhD, RN, CPN

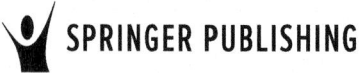

Copyright © 2023 Springer Publishing Company, LLC
All rights reserved.

No part of this publication may be reproduced, stored in a retrieval system, or transmitted in any form or by any means, electronic, mechanical, photocopying, recording, or otherwise, without the prior permission of Springer Publishing Company, LLC, or authorization through payment of the appropriate fees to the Copyright Clearance Center, Inc., 222 Rosewood Drive, Danvers, MA 01923, 978-750-8400, fax 978-646-8600, info@copyright.com or on the Web at www.copyright.com.

Springer Publishing Company, LLC
11 West 42nd Street, New York, NY 10036
www.springerpub.com
connect.springerpub.com/

Acquisitions Editor: Jaclyn Koshofer
Senior Content Development Editor: Lucia Gunzel
Compositor: diacriTech

ISBN: 978-0-8261-7944-9
ebook ISBN: 978-0-8261-7945-6
DOI: 10.1891/9780826179456

22 23 24 25 26 / 5 4 3 2 1

The author and the publisher of this Work have made every effort to use sources believed to be reliable to provide information that is accurate and compatible with the standards generally accepted at the time of publication. Because medical science is continually advancing, our knowledge base continues to expand. Therefore, as new information becomes available, changes in procedures become necessary. We recommend that the reader always consult current research and specific institutional policies before performing any clinical procedure or delivering any medication. The author and publisher shall not be liable for any special, consequential, or exemplary damages resulting, in whole or in part, from the readers' use of, or reliance on, the information contained in this book. The publisher has no responsibility for the persistence or accuracy of URLs for external or third-party Internet websites referred to in this publication and does not guarantee that any content on such websites is, or will remain, accurate or appropriate.

Library of Congress Control Number: 2021918635

Maureen Fitzgerald: https://orcid.org/0000-0003-4113-9343
David Jack: https://orcid.org/0000-0002-5381-6236

Publisher's Note: **New and used products purchased from third-party sellers are not guaranteed for quality, authenticity, or access to any included digital components.**

Printed in the United States of America.

CPN® is a registered service mark of Pediatric Nursing Certification Board (PNCB®). PNCB® does not sponsor or endorse this resource, nor does it have a proprietary relationship with Springer Publishing.

PED-BC™ is a registered service mark of American Nurses Credentialing Center (ANCC). ANCC does not sponsor or endorse this resource, nor does it have a proprietary relationship with Springer Publishing.

Maureen Fitzgerald dedicates this book to her children, Gabrielle Elizabeth Revaitis, Mackenzie Colleen Revaitis, and Jack Christopher Revaitis, for their patience, and also to Ron Obermeier for his support and continued positive outlook on life.

David Jack dedicates this book to his inspiration and muse, Leighann Sell, BSN, RN, pediatric nurse at Children's Hospital of Philadelphia, and all her nurse colleagues who make such a positive impact on the lives of children and their families daily. Thank you to all of you for your great work and dedication to pediatric healthcare.

CONTENTS

Contributors ix
Preface xi
Acknowledgments xv

PART I: EXAM OVERVIEW

Chapter 1: Exam Overview   *3*
Maureen Fitzgerald and David Jack

PART II: ASSESSMENT AND HEALTH PROMOTION

Chapter 2: Growth and Development of Infants, Toddlers, and Preschoolers   *11*
Laura Roettger

Chapter 3: Growth and Development of School-Aged Children and Adolescents   *25*
Allison C. Munn and Tracy P. George

PART III: MANAGEMENT

Chapter 4: Eyes, Ears, Nose, and Throat Conditions   *41*
Terri Giordano

Chapter 5: Neurologic Conditions   *57*
Gina Galosi

Chapter 6: Respiratory Conditions   *79*
Barbara Butynskyi

Chapter 7: Cardiovascular Conditions   *101*
Kevin J. Nusspickel

Chapter 8: Hematologic and Oncologic Conditions   *123*
Terri Giordano

Chapter 9: Gastrointestinal and Nutritional Conditions   *141*
Maureen Fitzgerald

Chapter 10: Genitourinary, Renal, and Reproductive Conditions   *167*
Maureen Fitzgerald and David Jack

Chapter 11: Musculoskeletal Conditions   *191*
David Jack and Maureen Fitzgerald

Chapter 12: Endocrine and Metabolic Conditions   *209*
Joseph Cipriano and Molly Powell

Chapter 13: Wounds, Burns, and Dermatologic Conditions   *233*
DiAnn Ecret

Chapter 14: Infectious Diseases and Immunizations *255*
Jessica L. Peck and Mary Koslap-Petraco

Chapter 15: Immunology and Allergies *275*
Maureen Fitzgerald

Chapter 16: Behavioral and Psychosocial Conditions *287*
Stephen DiDonato and David Jack

Chapter 17: Special Developmental Needs *313*
Maryanne Halligan

Chapter 18: Child Maltreatment and Neglect *327*
Angela Karakachian and Maryanne Halligan

Chapter 19: Emergencies, Trauma, and Poisonings *343*
Genevieve Turner and David Jack

Chapter 20: Palliative and End-of-Life Care *355*
Maryann Godshall

Chapter 21: Professional Responsibilities and Ethics *369*
DiAnn Ecret

PART IV: PRACTICE EXAM

Chapter 22: Practice Exam *381*
Denise R. Brown and Gina Galosi

Chapter 23: Practice Exam Answers and Rationales *409*
Denise R. Brown and Gina Galosi

Index 435

CONTRIBUTORS

Denise R. Brown, MSN, RNC-OB, C-EFM Adjunct Faculty—Clinical, Jefferson College of Nursing, Thomas Jefferson University, Philadelphia, Pennsylvania

Barbara Butynskyi, MSN, RN, CPN Instructor, Undergraduate Nursing Program, Jefferson College of Nursing, Thomas Jefferson University, Philadelphia, Pennsylvania

Joseph Cipriano, DNP, APN, FNP-BC Rutgers University—School of Nursing, Camden, New Jersey

Stephen DiDonato, PhD, LPC, NCC Associate Professor, Jefferson College of Nursing, Thomas Jefferson University, Philadelphia, Pennsylvania

DiAnn Ecret, PhD, MSN, RN, MA cert Ethics Assistant Professor, Jefferson College of Nursing, Thomas Jefferson University, Philadelphia, Pennsylvania; Nurse Ethicist, National Catholic Bioethics Center, Philadelphia, Pennsylvania; Ethics Consultant, "Be Not Afraid" Comprehensive Case Management, Charlotte, North Carolina (serving parents nationally)

Maureen Fitzgerald, EdD, MSN, CPN, RNC-NIC Program Director, Postgraduate Certificate Program—Academic Nursing, Assistant Professor, Jefferson College of Nursing, Thomas Jefferson University, Philadelphia, Pennsylvania

Gina Galosi, DNP, RNC-OB, CNE Assistant Professor, Jefferson College of Nursing, Thomas Jefferson University, Philadelphia, Pennsylvania

Tracy P. George, DNP, APRN-BC, CNE Assistant Professor of Nursing, School of Health Sciences, Francis Marion University, Florence, South Carolina

Terri Giordano, DNP, CRNP, CORLN Clinical Outcomes Research Administrator, Children's Hospital of Philadelphia, Division of Otolaryngology, Philadelphia, Pennsylvania

Maryann Godshall, PhD, CCRN, CPN, CNE Associate Professor, College of Nursing and Health Professions, Drexel University, Philadelphia, Pennsylvania

Maryanne Halligan, DNP, RN, CCRN-K, CHSE, CNML Assistant Professor, Coordinator Simulation and Clinical Skills, Jefferson College of Nursing, Thomas Jefferson University, Philadelphia, Pennsylvania

David Jack, PhD, RN, CPN Assistant Professor, Jefferson College of Nursing, Thomas Jefferson University, Philadelphia, Pennsylvania

Angela Karakachian, PhD, RN Assistant Professor, Duquesne University Nursing School, Pittsburgh, Pennsylvania

Mary Koslap-Petraco, DNP, PPCNP-BC, CPNP, FAANP Clinical Assistant Professor, Primary Care Pediatric Nurse Practitioner Program, MS Program, Stony Brook University School of Nursing, Stony Brook, New York; Nurse Consultant Immunization Action Coalition, Pediatric Nurse Practitioner, House Calls—CEO/Nurse Practitioner

Allison C. Munn, PhD, RN Assistant Professor of Nursing, School of Health Sciences, Francis Marion University, Florence, South Carolina

Kevin J. Nusspickel, MSN, RN, CPNP-AC, CCRN Clinical Nurse Educator for the Cardiac Center, Nursing Professional Development Team Member, Nemours/Alfred I. duPont Hospital for Children, Wilmington, Delaware

Jessica L. Peck, DNP, APRN, CPNP-PC, CNE, CNL, FAANP, FAAN Clinical Professor, Louise Herrington School of Nursing, Baylor University, Dallas, Texas; President, National Association of Pediatric Nurse Practitioners, New York, New York

Molly Powell, DNP, APN, FNP-BC Rutgers University—School of Nursing, Camden, New Jersey

Laura Roettger, PhD, APRN, CPNP-PC Assistant Professor, Program Director—Pediatric Nurse Practitioner, Jefferson College of Nursing, Thomas Jefferson University, Philadelphia, Pennsylvania

Genevieve Turner, DNP, RN Associate Professor, Nursing and Health Professions Division, Rowan College South Jersey, Gloucester, New Jersey

PREFACE

"Life isn't about finding yourself, Life is about creating yourself."—George Bernard Shaw

Congratulations! By purchasing this review book, you have taken one of the first steps toward your certification in pediatric nursing and demonstrating your competence and achievement in this area of practice. We applaud you as you begin the journey of creating yourself as a certified pediatric nurse.

Why Certification?

As healthcare delivery continues to become more evidenced-based, quality driven, and transparent, hospitals and other healthcare agencies have encouraged and promoted certification in their nursing staff. These institutions are finally acknowledging and recognizing nurses for their specialized knowledge and caring techniques. The ability of pediatric nurses to earn their credentialing has been a major focus of professional organizations, hospitals, and healthcare delivery agencies as well. Specifically speaking, the Society of Pediatric Nursing (SPN) encourages and supports nursing certification by providing educational resources and information about certification. The SPN advocates and endorses certification at the clinical and advance practice roles. Additionally, hospitals and agency settings, especially those seeking magnet designation, promote and encourage certification in their staff as well. Finally, certification in pediatric nursing may be personally rewarding and satisfying as the individual's accomplishment of attaining a level of expertise within the pediatric patient population. Once certified, this designation identifies that the nurse has a degree of proficiency in pediatric nursing and is among the growing numbers of expert clinicians.

Pediatric Nurse Certification Review is intended for pediatric nurses who are motivated to achieve an expertise in the specialty of pediatric nursing and to let their colleagues, employers, families, and children they care for know that they have specialized knowledge in the care of infants, children, and adolescents. The book is designed to provide an interesting and gratifying way to obtain valuable information about caring for the child and family from infancy through adolescence.

It is important for you to have a comprehensive review guide that contains the essential components of the certification exam and practice questions all in one resource. This review book incorporates the content areas from the test blueprints on the certification examinations in pediatric nursing: health promotion, assessment, and management. It contains two chapters on wellness or health promotion taking a close look into growth and development of each age group. Each chapter lists essential assessments and nursing interventions in the management of priority clinical problems.

This resource provides:

- An overview of each of the priority clinical problems listed in the detailed content outlines for the certification exam
- Special considerations to analyze as you study
- "Pediatric Pearls," skills, and procedures emphasized for your preparation
- End-of-chapter questions to test your knowledge as you move through the book
- A 175-item practice exam at the end of the book with comprehensive rationales

Each priority clinical problem is in a specific format:

- Overview/Introduction
- Description
- Assessment
- Diagnostics

- Nursing Interventions
- Special Considerations
- Discharge Planning; Patient and Family Education

Some topics may list "Pediatric Pearls," which are essential areas highlighted in this book that the authors consider key knowledge for a pediatric nurse and that may be tested on examinations.

Goals of This Review Book

The overall goal of this book is to provide a comprehensive review of key concepts in pediatric nursing that can appear on both the Pediatric Nursing Certification Board (PNCB®) and the American Nurses Credentialing Center (ANCC) certification pediatric specialty exam.

Concurrent goals include:

1. Develop a plan of study for the successful completion of the pediatric certification through either the PNCB as a Certified Pediatric Nurse (CPN®) or ANCC with the credential Pediatric Nurse - Board Certified (PED-BC™).
2. Discuss the certification process for both the CPN and PED-BC examination and the application processes.
3. Outline essential nursing information regarding pediatric nursing knowledge and skills that will appear on either the CPN or PED-BC examination.
4. Evaluate your level of understanding and proficiency with presented nursing concepts and skills.

Distinguishing Features to Support Student Learning

Pediatric Nurse Certification Review will play a vital role in preparation for certification. This unique book will effectively assist readers in attaining key concepts and skill competencies in a body-system systematic manner. The distinctive format outlines essential knowledge and has end-of-the-chapter knowledge assessment questions. The chapters were authored by identified experts in their field of pediatric care and have shared their insights, wisdom, and pearls (essential knowledge gained) to assist you on your journey of certification. Unique to other pediatric review manuals, this book offers pictorial representation of pediatric concepts that include disease processes and assessment techniques and tables that assist you in organizing, clarifying, and applying this information. Websites have been added to some chapters to assist you in exploring subject matter beyond this review book.

In addition to chapter review questions, *Pediatric Nurse Certification Review* also includes a comprehensive practice exam so you can determine your level of expertise with the given content. Used together with independent review of concepts not adequately understood, this book will be a valuable asset in acquiring the knowledge you need to prepare for the certification exam.

Intended Audience

The manual convers the realm of well-child care through the highly complex care of the critically ill child. Although not meant to be a comprehensive manual covering all pediatric concepts, this review text is a valuable resource for any nurse working exclusively with the pediatric patient population or interacting with the pediatric patient/family in the emergency department, perioperative environment, and/or school settings.

Content Organization

Part I: EXAM OVERVIEW

Our certification review manual begins with a chapter on the two pediatric nurse certification exams and recommendations for study preparation.

Part II: ASSESSMENT AND HEALTH PROMOTION

Chapters 2 and 3 focus on the growth and development of infants, toddlers, and preschoolers and the growth and development of school-aged children and adolescents, respectively.

Specific milestones, anticipatory guidance, and the timetable for expected screening measures that promote health and wellness are identified and discussed. Specific health promotion behaviors are provided.

Part III: MANAGEMENT

Chapters 4–19 provide a full overview of nursing concepts as they relate to knowledge and skills used in primary, secondary, and tertiary pediatric care settings.

Chapters 20–21 describe in detail important concepts of palliative and end-of-life care and ethics and professional responsibilities that the pediatric nurse should possess. Below is a listing of body systems found on the test blueprints in regard to their chapter designation:

4	Eyes, Ears, Nose, and Throat Conditions
5	Neurologic Conditions
6	Respiratory Conditions
7	Cardiovascular Conditions
8	Hematologic and Oncologic Conditions
9	Gastrointestinal and Nutritional Conditions
10	Genitourinary, Renal, and Reproductive Conditions
11	Musculoskeletal Conditions
12	Endocrine and Metabolic Conditions
13	Wounds, Burns, and Dermatologic Conditions
14	Infectious Diseases and Immunizations
15	Immunology and Allergies
16	Behavioral and Psychosocial Conditions
17	Special Developmental Needs
18	Child Maltreatment and Neglect
19	Emergencies, Trauma, and Poisoning
20	Palliative and End-of-Life Care
21	Professional Responsibilities and Ethics

Part IV: PRACTICE EXAM

Part IV includes a 175-question practice exam with items that address the concepts on the blueprints for the certification exams. Answers and complete rationales are presented separately. You can simulate the testing environment by timing yourself for 3 hours when taking the practice exam.

The authors, editors, and publisher of this book hope you find it to be helpful and instrumental to your certification journey. Thank you for taking the necessary step of promoting pediatric nursing and being proud to care for this most vulnerable population.

Thanks and best wishes with your certification examination,
Maureen Fitzgerald and David Jack

ACKNOWLEDGMENTS

The Editors would like to acknowledge our colleagues who have so graciously contributed to this review book, imparting their knowledge, insights, and clinical experiences so that other nurses can benefit from their shared wisdom. In addition, we give a special acknowledgement to Ruth Wittmann-Price, PhD, RN, CNS, CNE, CNEcl, CHSE, ANEF, FAAN, our mentor throughout this scholarship journey who recognized something in us. Lastly, thank you to all neonatal and pediatric nurses who are passionate in their care of a vulnerable population.

PART I
Exam Overview

CHAPTER 1

Exam Overview

Maureen Fitzgerald and David Jack

INTRODUCTION

Certification in a nursing specialty recognizes a registered nurse (RN) in achieving a high standard of education and experience for a particular population or area of expertise. This milestone in a nurse's career offers several benefits to showcase specialized knowledge, skills, abilities, and clinical judgment. A nurse is considered an expert in their field and someone patients and families may feel a great sense of confidence in their nursing care. Certification helps with nurse retention and additional employee benefits at their organization such as bonuses or pay increases, job advancement, to name a few.

Pediatric nurses care for children in all age groups from newborn infants to adolescents (0–18 years of age) in any setting where these vulnerable population groups seek and need care. You may care for these patients at the bedside in a medical–surgical pediatric unit or pediatric ICU, during home care sessions, in pediatric rehabilitation programs, schools, and/or urgent care clinics (Society of Pediatric Nurses, 2006). No matter your experienced role as a direct caregiver, educator, or manager in the specialty of pediatric nursing, if you meet the eligibility requirements, you can take the certification exam.

A key component of the pediatric nurse is their knowledge of growth and development and in applying this knowledge to the care settings and in patient/family teaching where family-centered care is essential to pediatric nursing. In addition, pediatric nurses may care for children in areas of wellness or health promotion or care for acute and chronic (usually occurs over at least 6 months) illnesses in a variety of settings and in a critical period during palliative or end of life. You can build your confidence by holding a certification in your specialty nursing practice.

This comprehensive review manual contains two chapters on wellness or health promotion, taking a close look into growth and development of each age group. Essential components of pediatric nursing are discussed such as anticipatory guidance, family-centered care, nutrition, and safety. There is a separate chapter on immunizations and those related childhood illnesses. Pediatric nurses must always keep in mind growth and development that can be affected during acute and chronic illnesses. The earlier these conditions are identified, the better outcomes will result, especially in less morbidity. If limitations occur due to chronic illnesses such as congenital conditions or cancer, then it is important for pediatric nurses to foster the child's autonomy and provide support in focusing on their strengths and opportunities for positive outcomes. Consider what you can do to encourage a "normal" environment for the child to promote growth and development. The last two chapters review palliative and end-of-life care and professional responsibilities including ethics. Key concepts are advocacy, legal considerations, professional communication, and ethical behavior.

It is important for you to have a comprehensive review guide that contains the essential components of the certification exam and practice questions all in one resource. This review manual provides an overview of each topic on the certification exam blueprints, special considerations to analyze as you study, *Pediatric Pearls* and *Pediatric Skills* to pay close attention to, end-of-chapter questions, and a practice exam. Each exemplar overview is in a specific format: overview, assessment, diagnostics, nursing interventions, special considerations, discharge planning/patient and family teaching. Some chapters may include "Pediatric Pearls," which are essential areas highlighted in this manual that the authors consider key knowledge for a pediatric nurse and that may be tested on examinations. Also, specific pediatric skills are emphasized to prepare you for the certification exam.

There are two nationally recognized certification exams that nurses specializing in pediatrics can sit for: the Certified Pediatric Nurse (CPN®) through the Pediatric Nursing Certification Board (PNCB®) and the Pediatric Nurse-Board Certified (PED-BC™) exam through the American Nurses Credentialing Center (ANCC). Both exams follow the same format. There are a total of 175 test items (multiple choice questions). One hundred and fifty are scored while 25 items are pretested. You have 3 hours to complete the exam. Information about each one is listed later in this chapter, and one of the first steps in this process is to determine your qualifications and requirements for certification. The websites also contain recommendations for study preparation. The certification exam is considered pass/fail, where the test taker must achieve a benchmarked minimum score to pass. This review manual is comprehensive and is a resource for both certification exams.

Continued education in the specialty is required to maintain certification and more information can be found on the organizations' websites that support the valid and reliable certifying exams.

BLUEPRINT/TEST PLAN

As you study for the exam, it is imperative that you review the blueprints. An exam blueprint is basically an outline of the content on the exam. It will show the number of questions and the percentage of each tested category to focus your studying. The questions are multiple choice, and you must select one answer, the best answer.

The Certified Pediatric Nurse Exam Offered by the Pediatric Nursing Certification Board

The PNCB offers a certification in pediatric nursing called "the CPN Exam." Review the eligibility requirements on the PNCB website to see if you meet all of the requirements before taking the exam: www.pncb.org/certified-pediatric-nurse.

The certification exam assesses your expertise in four categories of pediatric nursing: health promotion; physical assessment including psychosocial assessment; management of clinical situations, palliative, and end-of-life care; and responsibilities related to the role of the pediatric nurse. Table 1.1

TABLE 1.1: Certified Pediatric Nurse Test Blueprint

Content Areas	Number of Questions	Percentage of Test
Health promotion • Identify factors that influence the health of the child, family, and/or community • Provide anticipatory guidance and education • Refer child and family to community resources	21	14%
Assessment • Physical • Psychosocial	57	38%
Management • Acute and chronic illness • Psychosocial/behavioral • Palliative and end-of-life care • Professional responsibilities	72	48%
Total	150	100%

Source: Adapted from Pediatric Nursing Certification Board. (2021, April). *Certified Pediatric Nurse Certification Exam detailed content outline.* https://www.pncb.org/sites/default/files/resources/CPN_Content_Outline_Final.pdf

shows the number of questions on the exam and the percentage of the test for each content area. You can find the blueprint for this exam at www.pncb.org/cpn-exam-resources.

The tested clinical problems are listed in priority order by volume as follows:

1. Respiratory
2. Gastrointestinal/nutritional
3. Infectious disease
4. Emergencies/trauma/poisoning
5. Neurology
6. Hematology/oncology
7. Cardiovascular
8. Special developmental needs
9. Eye, ear, nose, and throat
10. Musculoskeletal
11. Endocrine/metabolic
12. Child maltreatment and neglect
13. Behavioral/mental health
14. Genitourinary/renal/reproductive
15. Skin/wound/burns
16. Allergy/immunology/immunizations

Pediatric nurses must be competent in skills, procedures, and interventions that affect the child, family, and/or community. The ones listed here are on the content outline of the CPN exam:

- Blood product administration
- Body temperature regulation
- Fluid and electrolytes administration
- Safety precautions
- Line and tube maintenance
- Medication administration
- Nutrition support
- Physiologic monitoring
- Positioning
- Procedural sedation and monitoring
- Restrictive intervention
- Skin and wound care
- Specimen collection and point-of-care testing
- Suctioning

The American Nurses Credentialing Center Exam Offered by American Nurses Credentialing Center

The ANCC offers a certification in pediatric nursing in which nurses can become certified as a PED-BC. The name of the exam is the Pediatric Nursing Certification (PED-BC), which is a competency-based examination that provides a valid and reliable assessment of the clinical knowledge and skills of the registered nurse in the pediatric specialty. There is an online process for applying for and renewing certification. Once initiating the application process, the organization will collect the following information from you:

- Demographic data
- Education history
- RN license number
- Any memberships of collaborating organizations used to discount the cost of the exam if you are a member of collaborating organizations (e.g., Society for Vascular Nursing); no specific pediatric-related affiliations are noted
- Optional section for employer demographics
- Attestation statement of integrity

Eligibility requirements include (a) practice as a RN for the equivalent of at least 2 years, full time, and (b) completion of a minimum of 2,000 hours of clinical practice within the last 3 years. Additionally, you will need to provide documented evidence of 30 continuing education hours in the pediatric specialty, which have been received within the 3 years prior to making an application for the certification. There is a cost of $395.00 if you are a nonmember of the American Nurses Association ($295.00 for validated members) with additional discounts as mentioned earlier if you are a member of a collaborating organization. In the exam cost, there is a $140.00 nonrefundable fee, and discounts can be claimed up to a maximum of 5 days following your application to ANCC. Individuals seeking this certification can access ANCC's website at: www.nursingworld.org/our-certifications/pediatric-nurse/

As previously mentioned, and similar to the CPN exam, the ANCC exam consists of 150 examination questions in which 125 are scored and 25 questions are used for pretesting and validation purposes. The pretest questions will not be distinguished from those that will be scored, so it is imperative you answer all of the questions. In this testing, you are not penalized for guessing but are penalized if you leave a question unanswered. As of October 24, 2019, no recent test blueprint has been posted (Table 1.2).

Under the content domain, there are the following identified knowledge and skills:

Domain I: Assessment and Diagnosis

A. Knowledge
- Assessment tools and techniques (e.g., pain scale, fall risk, pressure injury risk)
- Growth and development (e.g., developmental stages and milestones, growth charts)
- Pathophysiology (e.g., childhood diseases, congenital/genetic abnormalities)
- Pharmacology (e.g., immunization, side effects)
- Complementary and alternative therapies (e.g., essential oils, cupping, herbal supplements)
- Diagnostic tests and screenings (e.g., indications, normal ranges)

B. Skill
- Physical and psychosocial assessments (e.g., vital sign parameters, body systems)
- Medication and treatment reconciliation (e.g., allergies, over-the-counter medications)
- Diagnostic specimen collection (e.g., venipuncture, nasal swab, urine specimen)

Domain II: Planning and Implementation

A. Knowledge
- Evidence-based quality improvement measures (e.g., bundles, clinical pathways)
- Treatment interactions (e.g., food–medication, herbal–medication, end-stage renal disease-fluid resuscitation)
- Expected responses to interventions

B. Skill
- Coordination of individualized care (e.g., consultations, case management)
- Formulation of realistic and measurable outcomes
- Evidence-based interventions (e.g., therapeutic holding, chlorhexidine baths, oral sucrose)

TABLE 1.2: Pediatric Nurse - Board Certified Test Blueprint

Category	Content domain	Number of questions	Percentage
I	Assessment and diagnosis	43	34%
II	Planning and implementation	37	30%
III	Evaluation	45	36%
Total		125	100%

Source: Adapted from American Nurses Credentialing Center. (2019). *Test content outline: Pediatric Nursing Board Certification Examination*. https://www.nursingworld.org/~4996e1/globalassets/certification/certification-specialty-pages/resources/test-content-outlines/pediatricnursing-tco-after.pdf

- Patient safety and risk-reduction measures (e.g., restraints, elopement prevention, de-escalation strategies)
- Medication administration (e.g., oral, parenteral, enteral)

Domain III: Evaluation

A. Knowledge
- Family structure and dynamics (e.g., multiple caregivers, Health Insurance Portability and Accountability Act compliance)
- Patient response to illness and hospitalization (e.g., coping, regression)
- Culture, religion, socioeconomic status, and health practices of diverse groups (e.g., treatment refusal, dietary restrictions, financial constraints)
- Legal and ethical considerations (e.g., age of consent, advanced directives, professional role)
- Chronic disease management (e.g., asthma, diabetes, obesity)
- High-risk behaviors (e.g., substance use disorders, unprotected sex)
- Health promotion (e.g., physical activity, nutrition)

B. Skill
- Therapeutic communication techniques (e.g., open-ended questions, active listening)
- Teaching methods (e.g., teach-back, learning environment)
- Learning evaluation (e.g., reinforcement, return demonstration)

This credential is valid for 5 years. ANCC's website (www.nursingworld.org/our-certifications/pediatric-nurse/) provides links to the following areas:

- Test reference list
- Sample test questions and answers
- 2018 role delineation study results
- Prometric test centers link; here you will schedule when you will take your certification examination
- Renewal information and additional supportive content

Table 1.3 shows a comparison between the CPN and PED-BC exams.

TABLE 1.3: Certified Pediatric Nurse Versus Pediatric Nurse - Board Certified Test Comparison Table

Category	PNCB	ANCC	Editor's Comments
Certifications	As of 12/19, the PNCB boasts there are more than 50,000 actively certified nurses, of which 32,174 hold the CPN (2019 stats)	RN-BC: 2,345	PNCB offers a nice video that promotes certification: www.youtube.com/watch?v=z-Gs7s7jE7M PNCB offers remote testing options
Exam Pass Rate	79.53% in 2019 with 4,442 candidates testing	84% in 2019 with 248 candidates testing	
Cost	$300 for initial exam • $255 for SPN members • For initial exam not using No Pass, No Pay there is a $245 for retest • Expedited 5-day application processing: Free	$395 $295 for ANA members; • $270 for retest • Expedited 5-day application processing: $200	

ANA, American Nurses Association; ANCC, American Nurses Credentialing Center; CPN, Certified Pediatric Nurse; PNCB, Pediatric Nursing Certification Board; RN-BC, Registered Nurse - Board Certified; SPN, Society of Pediatric Nurses.

Source: Adapted from Pediatric Nursing Certification Board. (n.d.). *CPN and RN-BC: What's the difference?* https://www.pncb.org/compare-rn-certifications

STUDY PLAN AND PRACTICE QUESTIONS

Nurses seeking certification in a specialty should develop an individualized study plan and use practice questions to determine their strengths and opportunities for deeper knowledge. Suggestions include: add to your calendar study days and times with each content from the blueprints, use highlighters or color codes or a prioritization rubric in your study plan to reinforce the areas for further review. Preparation will help with some anxiety test takers have before and during examinations. Your plan may include a schedule (usually at least 3 months before the exam) of each content area listed on the blueprint. This review guide contains *Knowledge Checks* at the end of each chapter with practice questions and rationales to help in this process. Also, you can familiarize yourself with the testing environment by taking the 175-item practice exam at the end of this book; timing yourself, keeping the 3-hour time limit in mind. The certification exam is taken on a computer, and the test taker is able to highlight areas in the question stem, strike out answers that you think are incorrect, and can flag items to return to review again within the timeframe of the exam.

We congratulate you ahead of time on your success in achieving certification in pediatric nursing, going above and beyond, showing a mastery . . . you are now an expert in your specialty!

BIBLIOGRAPHY

American Nurses Credentialing Center. *Pediatric Nursing Certification (PED-BC™) application portal.* https://www.nursingworld.org/our-certifications/pediatric-nurse/

American Nurses Credentialing Center. *Pediatric Nursing Certification (PED-BC™) test blueprint.* https://www.nursingworld.org/~4acbba/globalassets/certification/certification-specialty-pages/resources/test-content-outlines/pediatricnursing-tco.pdf

Institute of Pediatric Nursing. (n.d.). *Pediatric nursing workforce data.* https://ipedsnursing.org/pediatric-nursing-workforce-data

Pediatric Nursing Certification Board. (n.d.). *CPN® exam resources.* https://www.pncb.org/cpn-exam-resources

Society of Pediatric Nurses. (2006, July). *Becoming a pediatric nurse.* http://www.pedsnurses.org/becominganurse

Straka, K. L., Ambrose, H. L., Burkett, M., Capan, M., Flook, D., Evangelista, T., Houck, P., Lukanski, A., Schenkel, K., & Thornton, M. (2014). The impact and perception of nursing certification in pediatric nursing. *Journal of Pediatric Nursing, 29*(3), 205–211. https://doi.org/10.1016/j.pedn.2013.10.010

PART II
Assessment and Health Promotion

CHAPTER 2

Growth and Development of Infants, Toddlers, and Preschoolers

Laura Roettger

INTRODUCTION

Understanding child developmental principles is the basis for history focus and physical examination. This section focuses on growth and development principles and considerations for infants, toddlers, and preschoolers.

Description

Infancy is the period from birth through 12 months old. A toddler is a child between the ages of 12 months old and 24 months old. The preschool period is between the ages of 24 months old and 5 years old.

Assessment

- Assess reason for visit from parent/admission onto the pediatric unit.
- Assess an interval history (e.g., previous episodic visits/admissions).
- Assess past medical history.
  - Prenatal/birth/neonatal history
  - Illness/injury
  - Hospitalization/surgery/procedures
  - Allergies
  - Immunization
  - Medications
- Assess family history.
  - Medical history
  - Family structure
  - Cultural/ethnic practices
  - Social and family history
    - Health literacy
    - Family health habits (e.g., smoking, firearms)
    - Safety (e.g., injury, car seats, adverse childhood experiences, social determinants of health, housing, food security, smoke/carbon monoxide alarms)
    - **Newborns:** Parent and sibling adjustment to new infant
    - Childcare (e.g., in-home, center, family member, preschool)
    - Parent employment status

- Assess nutrition (e.g., breast milk and/or formula).
  - **Infancy:** Minutes per feeding, ounces per feeding, hours between feedings, type and brand of formula, source of water, vitamin D supplementation, problems with feeding
    - 110 to 120 kcal/kg/d; doubles birth weight at 4 to 6 months, triples birth weight by 1 year
  - For full-term infants, breast milk from a well-nourished mother offers enough vitamins and minerals, with the exception of vitamin D, during the first 6 months. Iron supplementation should begin at age 4 months.
    - Immediately after birth, infants lose approximately 10% of their body weight because of fluid loss and some breakdown of tissue.
    - They usually regain their birth weight within 10 to 14 days.
  - **Toddlers:** Rituals, food refusals
    - Toddlers need between 1,000 and 1,400 calories a day, depending on their age, size, and physical activity level. A child's birth weight quadruples by age 2.
    - The toddler years are a time of transition, especially between 12 and 24 months when they are learning to eat table food and accepting new tastes and textures.
    - As the growth rate declines during early childhood, a child's appetite decreases, and the amount of food consumed may become unpredictable.
    - Children should be offered foods at scheduled mealtimes (three daily) and snack times (two to three daily).
  - **Preschoolers:** Preschoolers need between 1,200 and 2,000 calories a day, depending on their age, size, and physical activity level.
- Assess elimination.
  - Stooling frequency, characteristics
  - Urinary frequency, characteristics, normal stream
- Assess sleep.
  - **Infants:** Back to sleep, safe sleep surface
- **Milestones:** Assess
  - Newborn to 1 month old
    - Physical (e.g., primitive reflexes present [rooting, Moro, Babinski reflex, sucking, grasp, stepping])
    - Social language/self-help (e.g., makes brief eye contact on objects 20 to 25 cm away [8–10 inches])
    - Verbal language (e.g., cries in response to discomfort, calms to voice)
    - Gross motor (e.g., head lag present, turns head when prone, asymmetric tonic neck reflex present, reflexively moves arms and legs)
    - Fine motor (e.g., hold fingers clenched, grasps reflexively)
  - 2 months old
    - Physical (e.g., posterior fontanel closes)
    - Social language/self-help (e.g., social smile, turns head to sounds, follows objects side to side when supine)
    - Verbal language (e.g., coos)
    - Gross motor (e.g., lifts head and chest while prone, symmetric tonic neck position, exhibits head lag when pulled to sit)
    - Fine motor (e.g., opens and closes hands, fading grasp reflex)

CHAPTER 2 GROWTH AND DEVELOPMENT OF INFANTS, TODDLERS, AND PRESCHOOLERS

- 3 months old
  - Physical (e.g., primitive reflexes fading)
  - Social language/self-help (e.g., social smile, turns head to sounds, follows objects side to side when supine, recognizes familiar objects and faces)
  - Verbal language (e.g., coos, vocalizes when spoken to)
  - Gross motor (e.g., holds head erect when sitting briefly, exhibits head lag when pulled to sit, lifts head and shoulders to 45- to 90-degree angle when prone, bears weight when standing, Landau reflex emerges)
  - Fine motor (e.g., grasp reflex disappears, holds objects, hands held open)
- 4 months old
  - Physical (e.g., Moro and tonic neck reflexes disappear)
  - Social language/self-help (e.g., laughs, recognizes familiar objects and faces, focuses on objects 1.25 cm [0.5 in] from face)
  - Verbal language (e.g., laughs; makes b, g, k, n, and p sounds)
  - Gross motor (e.g., rolls from prone to supine position, sits upright if propped, minimal to no head lag, raises head and chest to 90-degree angle when prone)
  - Fine motor (e.g., grasps objects, keeps hands open)
- 5 months old
  - Social language/self-help (e.g., smiles at self in the mirror, follows dropped object)
  - Verbal language (e.g., squeals when excited, vocalizes discontent when objects are removed)
  - Gross motor (e.g., rolls supine to prone, no head lag when pulled to sit)
  - Fine motor (e.g., plays with toes, holds one cube, pats bottle or breast with hands)
- 6 months old
  - Social language/self-help (e.g., fears strangers)
  - Verbal language (e.g., babbles, imitates sounds, makes one-syllable vocalizations)
  - Gross motor (e.g., sits up with support)
  - Fine motor (e.g., reaches [Figure 2.1], bangs and rakes small objects, transfers objects hand to hand)
- 7 months old
  - Social language/self-help (e.g., responds to name when called, plays peek-a-boo, imitates acts and noises)
  - Verbal language (e.g., babbles, imitates sounds, makes one-syllable vocalizations)
  - Gross motor (e.g., tripod sits)
  - Fine motor (e.g., holds two objects)
- 8 months old
  - Physical (e.g., parachute reflex appears at 6–8 months: infant extends arms, hands, and fingers—response is symmetric and "protective")
  - Social language/self-help (e.g., fears strangers, understands the word "no")
  - Verbal language (e.g., makes t and w sounds)
  - Gross motor (e.g., bears weight on legs when standing)
  - Fine motor (e.g., shakes objects, pincer grasp [Figure 2.2])
- 9 months old
  - Social language/self-help (e.g., waves bye-bye, holds arms up to be picked up)
  - Verbal language (e.g., says "dada" and "mama" unintentionally, responds to simple commands)
  - Gross motor (e.g., pulls to stand, sits without support, crawls)
  - Fine motor (e.g., shakes objects, pincer grasp)

14 PART II ASSESSMENT AND HEALTH PROMOTION

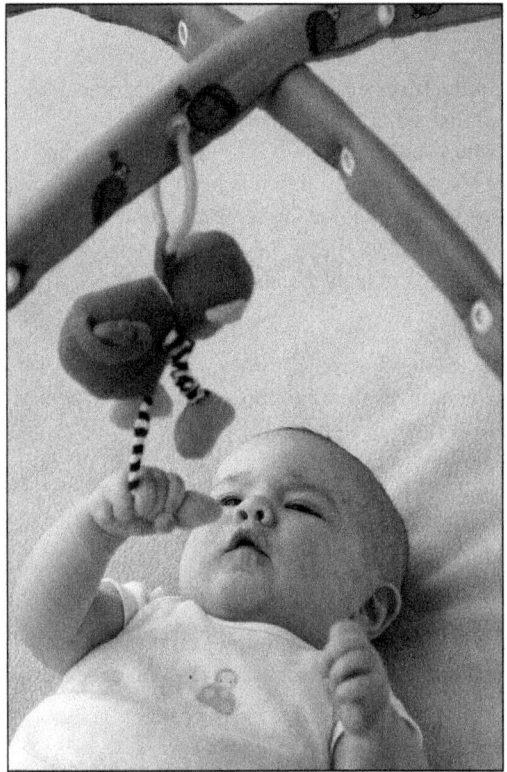

FIGURE 2.1: Reaches (palmar grasp)

Source: Shutterstock. Reprinted from Chiocca, E. M. (2021). *Advanced pediatric assessment* (3rd ed.). Springer Publishing Company.

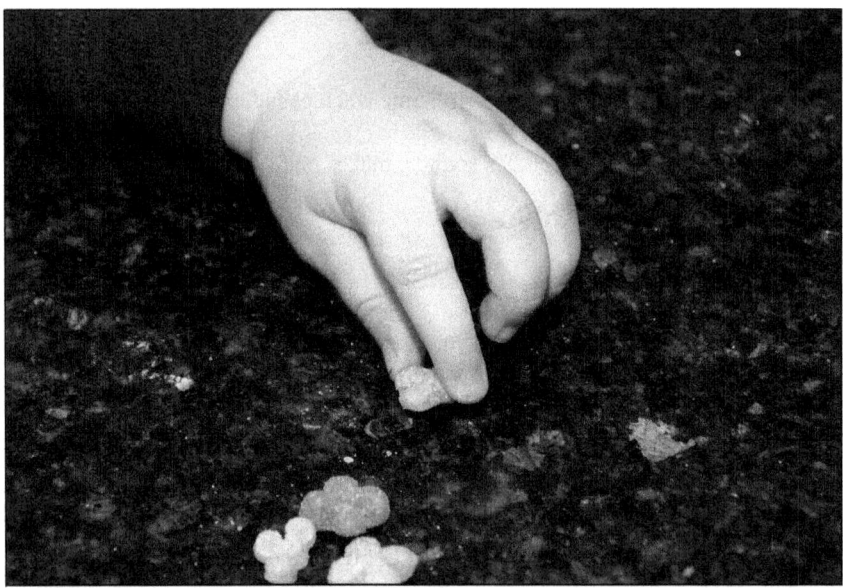

FIGURE 2.2: Fine pincer grasp

Source: Reprinted from Chiocca, E. M. (2021). *Advanced pediatric assessment* (3rd ed.). Springer Publishing Company.

CHAPTER 2 GROWTH AND DEVELOPMENT OF INFANTS, TODDLERS, AND PRESCHOOLERS

- 10 months old
  - Social language/self-help (e.g., develops object permanence, plays pat-a-cake, looks and follows along in books, helps to dress, reacts to the word "no")
  - Verbal language (e.g., says "dada" and "mama" intentionally, may say one-syllable words like "hi" and "bye")
  - Gross motor (e.g., stands and walks holding onto furniture)
  - Fine motor (e.g., feeds self by picking up with fingers)
- 11 months old
  - Physical (e.g., eruption of lower central incisor may occur)
  - Social language/self-help (e.g., shakes head to indicate "no," plays peek-a-boo)
  - Verbal language (e.g., imitates speech sounds)
  - Gross motor (e.g., walks with hands held, pivots while sitting)
  - Fine motor (e.g., manipulates objects into and out of containers)
- 12 months old
  - Physical (e.g., Landau reflex starts to fade, Babinski reflex fades)
  - Social language/self-help (e.g., looks for hidden objects, imitates gestures, follows one-step commands)
  - Verbal language (e.g., uses one word in addition to "mom" and "dad")
  - Gross motor (e.g., takes first steps independently, stands without assistance, rolls ball, moves from standing to sitting without difficulty)
  - Fine motor (e.g., stacks two blocks, claps hands, points at objects)
- 15 months old
  - Social language/self-help (e.g., scribbles, drinks from a cup with no spilling, points to an object, or asks for help)
  - Verbal language (e.g., uses three words other than names)
  - Gross motor (e.g., pulls a pull toy, walks forward and backward, walks upstairs with two feet per step)
  - Fine motor (e.g., holds utensils and attempts to use them)
- 18 months old
  - Social language/self-help (e.g., turns to adult during unfamiliar situations, identifies pictures in a book, helps dress and undress)
  - Verbal language (e.g., uses 6–10 words other than names, identifies two body parts)
  - Gross motor (e.g., walks well, pushes and pulls toys, throws a ball)
  - Fine motor (e.g., builds four-block tower)
- 24 months old
  - Social language/self-help (e.g., engages in parallel play)
  - Verbal language (e.g., uses 50 words, uses two-word phrases, follows two-step commands, speech is 50% intelligible to strangers, names self)
  - Gross motor (e.g., throws ball overhand, runs well, jumps, kicks ball, climbs up ladder)
  - Fine motor (e.g., builds seven-block tower, turns doorknob/lids/toys, turns pages in a book, unbuttons and unzips clothes)
- 30 months old
  - Social language/self-help (e.g., engages in pretend play, uses fork to pick up food)
  - Verbal language (e.g., names one color, uses pronouns correctly)
  - Gross motor (e.g., climbs stairs with alternating feet, tip toes, stands on one foot for 1 second, catches a ball)
  - Fine motor (e.g., copies a circle, copies a vertical line, builds nine-block tower)

- 36 months old
  - Social language/self-help (e.g., eats independently, uses bathroom independently)
  - Verbal language (e.g., uses three-word phrases; speech is 75% intelligible to strangers; understands prepositions [e.g., under, on]; retells story from book or television; understands bigger, shorter, and genders)
  - Gross motor (e.g., uses tricycle, jumps forward)
  - Fine motor (e.g., draws a circle, draws person with head and one other body part, uses children's scissors)
- 48 months old
  - Social language/self-help (e.g., hand preference emerges, responds to three step commands)
  - Verbal language (e.g., uses four-word sentences, speech is 100% intelligible to strangers, answers questions)
  - Gross motor (e.g., walks downstairs with alternating feet, throws ball underhand, skips)
  - Fine motor (e.g., draws person with three body parts, draws cross, grasps pencil with thumb and finger)

Diagnostics

Routine screenings are recommended at specific ages.

- Newborn screen
  - Verify completed in newborn nursery.
  - Verify results are documented.
  - Flag abnormal results.

- Hearing screen
  - Verify newborn hearing screen results are documented, and flag abnormal results.
  - Obtain evaluation if patient has positive risk factor identified.
  - **Risk factors:** Family history of hearing loss, neonatal ICU stay greater than 5 days during newborn period, infection with herpes varicella, meningitis, treatment with aminoglycosides, cranial-facial anomalies, skull trauma/fracture, treatment with chemotherapy.

- Conduct maternal depression screen at infant well visits from 1 month through 6 months old.
  - Utilize the Edinburgh Postnatal Depression Scale (EPDS)

- Blood pressure measurement
  - Obtain blood pressure measurement if patient has a positive risk identified—routine screening starting at age 3.
  - **Risk factors:** Prematurity, very low birth weight, congenital heart disease, recurrent urinary tract infections, hematuria or proteinuria, kidney disease, urologic malformations, family history of congenital kidney disease, solid-organ transplant, malignancy or bone marrow transplant, signs of increased intracranial pressure, children with underlying conditions associated with hypertension (e.g., tuberous sclerosis, neurofibromatosis)

- Lead
  - Obtain lead blood test if patient has a positive risk identified.
  - **Risk factors:** Child lives in or visits a home or child care center where lead is present at hazardous levels, lives in a home built before 1960, or lives in a home that was renovated in the past 6 months; refugee children 6 months to 16 years old.

- Anemia
  - Obtain hematocrit or hemoglobin if patient has a positive risk identified.
  - **Risk factors:** Preterm and low birth weight infants and formula fed infants not on iron-fortified formula.

CHAPTER 2 GROWTH AND DEVELOPMENT OF INFANTS, TODDLERS, AND PRESCHOOLERS

- Tuberculosis
  - Obtain tuberculosis test if patient has a positive risk identified.
  - **Risk factors:** History of HIV, child or household member born in or traveled to country where tuberculosis is endemic (e.g., Africa, Asia, Latin America, and Eastern Europe), exposure to person with tuberculosis or who has a positive test result.
- Oral health (6 months to 16 years old)
  - Anticipate oral fluoride supplementation.
  - **Risk factors:** Drinking water supply deficient in fluoride.
- Vision
  - Anticipate ophthalmology referral.
  - **Risk factors:** Family history of early childhood eye disorders, parental concern.

Nursing Interventions

- Expected growth patterns: assess and identify abnormal
  - **Newborn**
    - **Weight:** Gains 5 to 7 ounces/wk, loses about 8% to 10% of birth weight in first 5 to 7 days of life, regains birth weight by 10 to 14 days of age
    - **Length:** Grows by 2.5 cm (1 inch)/mo
    - **Head circumference:** Increases by 2 cm (0.8 inch)/mo
    - **Temperature:** 97.7°F to 99.3°F (36.5°C–37.4°C)
    - **Respiratory rate:** 30 to 60 breaths/min
    - **Heart rate:** 100 to 190 beats/min
  - **Infancy through 6 months old**
    - **Weight:** Gains 5 to 7 ounces/wk; doubles at 6 months old
    - **Length:** Grows by 2.5 cm (1 inch)/mo
    - **Head circumference:** Increases by 1.5 cm (0.6 inch)/mo; slows to 0.5 cm (0.2 inches)/mo during second half of first year
    - **Temperature:** 97.7°F to 99.3°F (36.5°C–37.4°C)
    - **Respiratory rate:** 30 to 60 breaths/min
    - **Heart rate:** 80 to 160 beats/min
  - **Infancy through 12 months old**
    - **Weight:** Gains 3 to 5 ounces/wk; triples at 12 months old
    - **Length:** Grows by 1.25 cm (0.5 inch)/mo; 50% increase from birth at 12 months old
    - **Head circumference:** Increases by 0.5 cm (0.6 inch)/mo
    - **Temperature:** 97.7°F to 99.3°F (36.5°C–37.4°C)
    - **Respiratory rate:** 30 to 60 breaths/min
    - **Heart rate:** 80 to 160 beats/min
  - **Toddler and preschool**
    - **Weight:** Gain 2 kg (4.4 pounds)/y
    - Linear growth
      - **12 to 24 months old:** Gains 4 inches (10 cm)/y
      - **24 to 36 months old:** Gains 3 inches (7.5 cm)/y
      - **35 to 48 months old:** Gains 3 inches (7.5 cm)/y
    - **Temperature:** 96.7°F to 99.3°F (36.5°C–37.4°C)
    - **Respiratory rate:** 20 to 30 breaths/min
    - **Heart rate:** 70 to 110 beats/min

Discharge Planning; Patient and Family Education

- Age-appropriate preventative care guidelines
  - Instruct on feeding practices.
    - Breastfeeding (ideally up to 6 months old) or iron-fortified formula up to 12 months old.
      - **Breastfeed:** Newborn 8 to 12 times daily, and give vitamin D drops (400 IU daily); infants every 1 to 3 hours during day, and every 3 hours at night, and give vitamin D drops (400 IU daily). Vitamin D supplementation is recommended for infants receiving less than 1 L (32 ounces) of formula per day.
      - **Formula feed:** Newborn offer 2 ounces every 2 to 3 hours, and offer more if baby looks hungry (e.g., follow feeding cues); infants up to 4 months old feed 24 to 27 ounces daily; infants 4 months and up to 12 months old feed 30 to 32 ounces daily.
      - Know feeding cues (e.g., sucking or rooting, fussiness).
      - Refrain from bottle propping.
    - Monitor elimination.
      - Five wet diapers and three stools diapers daily, along with good weight gain, indicate baby is getting enough.
    - Introduce solid foods at 6 months old.
      - Introduce iron-rich food and zinc-fortified cereals two to three times daily.
        - Examples of iron-rich foods are pureed red meat, beef, or lamb.
      - Foods containing eggs and peanut butter should be encouraged.
      - Avoid raw honey and large chunks of food that increase risk for choking (e.g., popcorn; hotdogs; grapes; nuts; hard, raw vegetables).
      - Introduce one new food at a time, space 3 days between new foods.
      - Introduce baby to a cup at 6 months old.
    - Introduce whole cow's milk at 12 months old.
      - 16 to 24 ounces daily
    - Provide three meals and two to three snacks spaced evenly throughout the day (12 months old through 48 months old).
    - Limit juice to 4 ounces daily.
  - Instruct parents on circumcision care (newborn).
    - Cleanse penis daily with tap water and apply dime-sized amount of petroleum jelly to the tip of penis for the first 3 days after procedure with each diaper change.
  - Instruct parents on bathing.
    - Sponge bath newborn until umbilical cord separates and naval is healed.
    - Daily baths are not necessary; use mild cleansing soaps and unscented lotions for dry skin.
    - Never leave an infant alone in bath.
  - Developmental
    - Set routines for feeding, sleep, and play.
    - Sing, talk, and read to baby.
    - Refrain from providing digital media or screen time.
    - Never leave an infant alone on tummy.
    - Brush baby's teeth and gums with first tooth eruption two times per day with soft cloth or small smear of fluoride toothpaste. Visit dentist with first tooth eruption or by 12 months old.

CHAPTER 2 GROWTH AND DEVELOPMENT OF INFANTS, TODDLERS, AND PRESCHOOLERS

- Keep small objects away from baby.
- Instruct on toilet training (18 months old to 48 months old).
  - Toilet training readiness:
    - Physical skills
      - Has voluntary sphincter control
      - Stays dry for 2 hours, may wake from naps still dry
      - Is able to sit, walk, and squat
      - Assists in dressing self
    - Cognitive skills
      - Recognizes urge to urinate or defecate
      - Understands meaning of words used by family in toileting
      - Understands what the toilet is for
      - Understands connection between dry pants and toilet
      - Is able to follow directions
      - Is able to communicate their needs
  - Once child shows signs of readiness, educate on reinforcement strategies (e.g., reading books about toilet training, praising with accomplishment).
  - Toilet training management:
    - Use training pants or underwear when child stays dry for several hours during the day; use diapers at night.
    - Praise child for asking to have diaper changed.
    - Provide a potty chair or portable toilet seat.
    - Encourage child to use potty chair when parent uses regular toilet.
    - Have child sit on potty chair without diapers for 5 to 10 minutes at a time.
    - Practice at times the child usually urinates or defecates.
- Encourage playtime with peers once child reaches preschool years.
- Psychosocial issues
  - Food insecurity and poor living situations
    - Refer to community agencies and programs such as Women, Infant, and Children (WIC) and Supplemental Nutrition Assistance Program (SNAP).
  - Encourage smoke-free and drug-free spaces.
    - Keep car and home tobacco smoke-free.
    - Refrain from use of e-cigarettes.
    - Refrain from use of drugs and alcohol.
    - Encourage self-care.
    - Contact primary care clinician with feelings of sadness or tiredness.
- Age-related safety issues
  - Instruct parents on safe sleep environment.
    - Place infants on back to sleep until at least 6 months old.
    - Use firm mattress and do not place bumper pads/comforters/stuffed toys/blankets/toys in the crib.
    - Avoid bed sharing/co-sleeping.
  - Instruct parents on healthy coping with a fussy or crying baby.
    - Placing baby in a safe place during a moment of stress and calling a support person to help.

- Instruct on car safety restraints.
  - Instruct on rear-facing car seat in the back seat of vehicles until child reaches height and weight limit under manufacturer guidelines.
  - Instruct on forward-facing car seat or belt-positioning booster seat until child reaches height and weight limit under manufacturer guidelines.
  - Back seat is safest position for children younger than 13 years old.
- Instruct on water safety.
  - Prevent water burns: Set the home water heater to 120°F (49°C) or lower.
  - Encourage swim lessons.
  - Never leave a child unattended near or in water.
- Instruct on sun exposure.
  - Newborn to 6 months old: Use a wide brimmed hat and umbrellas, and cover trunk and extremities.
  - 6 months old and older: Use a wide brimmed hat, and sunscreen with SPF (sun protection factor) 15 or higher.
- Instruct on infection prevention.
  - Avoid crowds.
  - Wash hands frequently.
  - Call your primary care clinician if the baby has a rectal temperature of 100.4°F (38.0°C) or higher.
- Instruct on safe home environment.
  - Keep poison, medications, and cleaning supplies out of reach of children.
  - Keep poison control phone number in visible place and saved on all phones.
  - Ensure working smoke and carbon monoxide alarms on every floor in home; test every month and replace batteries annually.
  - Store unloaded guns and ammunition separately and in locked location.
- Instruct safe community environment.
  - Use a helmet that fits properly.
  - Educate parents on how to speak to children (4 years and older) about sexual health.
    - Use correct terms for private parts when child inquires about the difference between boys and girls.
    - Inform child that it is not OK for adults to ask to see their private parts.
    - Inform child that it is not OK for adults to ask children to help with their private parts.
    - Inform child that it is not OK for adults to tell child to keep a secret from their parents.

BIBLIOGRAPHY

American Academy of Pediatrics. (2018). *Early childhood medical screening reference table*. https://brightfutures.aap.org/Bright%20Futures%20Documents/MSRTable_ECVisits_BF4.pdf

American Academy of Pediatrics. (2018). *Infancy medical screening reference table*. https://brightfutures.aap.org/Bright%20Futures%20Documents/MSRTable_InfancyVisits_BF4.pdf

Hagan, J. F., Shaw, J. S., & Duncan, P. M. (2017). *Bright futures: Guidelines for health supervision of infants, children and adolescents* (4th ed.). American Academy of Pediatrics.

Maaks, D. L., Starr, N. B., Brady, M. A., Gaylord, N. M, Driessnack, M., & Duderstadt, K. (2019). *Burns' pediatric primary care* (7th ed.). Elsevier.

CHAPTER 2 GROWTH AND DEVELOPMENT OF INFANTS, TODDLERS, AND PRESCHOOLERS

KNOWLEDGE CHECK

1. The pediatric nurse performs a developmental assessment on a child whose parent reports that 75% of the child's speech is intelligible to strangers. The pediatric nurse expects to observe this in a child who is what age?

   A. 18 months old
   B. 24 months old
   C. 36 months old
   D. 48 months old

2. When providing anticipatory guidance about toilet training to parents of a 24-month-old who is routinely telling parents that she feels the urge to urinate, the pediatric nurse provides which of the following recommendations?

   A. Read books about toilet training
   B. Assess for signs of toilet readiness
   C. Have child sit on potty chair for 5 to 10 minutes when urge is felt
   D. Make a rewards chart with child

3. The pediatric nurse is providing care to a 7-day-old infant who is breastfeeding. The infant weighed 3,500 g at birth. The infant weighs 3,200 g at this visit. The nurse understands which of the following to be true about newborn growth?

   A. Infants lose 8% to 10% of birth weight in first 7 days of life
   B. Infants regain birth weight by 28 days old
   C. Neonates gain 0.25 to 0.5 ounces per day
   D. Low birth weight infants require fortified milk

4. The pediatric nurse is providing anticipatory guidance to the parents of a 4-month-old infant. Which of the following is an appropriate recommendation?

   A. Apply sunscreen with at least 15 SPF to the infant's skin daily
   B. Introduce cubed fruits and vegetables in the infant's daily diet
   C. Discontinue feeding the infant iron-fortified formula
   D. Feed the infant 30 to 32 ounce of iron-fortified formula daily

5. The mother of a 9-month-old infant asks at what age can she offer her baby cow's milk. The pediatric nurse tells the mother that cow's milk is introduced once an infant reaches what age?

   A. 9 months old
   B. 12 months old
   C. 15 months old
   D. 18 months old

6. The pediatric nurse understands that the newborn infant who is exclusively breast feeding should be prescribed which of the following supplements?

   A. 200 IU vitamin D
   B. 400 IU vitamin D
   C. 0.25 mg fluoride
   D. 0.50 mg fluoride

1. **Correct Answer: C) 36 months old.** Speech is 75% intelligible to strangers in a child who is 36 months old. Speech is 100% intelligible to strangers in a child who is 48 months old. Speech is 50% intelligible to strangers in a 24-month-old.

2. **Correct Answer: C) Have child sit on potty chair for 5 to 10 minutes when urge is felt.** The child is exhibiting signs of toilet readiness by verbalizing voluntary sphincter control. While reading books about toilet training is helpful, this is the primary focus for interventions prior to a child showing toilet readiness signs. Making a rewards chart with a child is recommended once the child has urinated in the toilet.

3. **Correct Answer: A) Infants lose 8% to 10% of birth weight in first 7 days of life.** Infants lose about 8% to 10% of their birth weight in the first 7 days of life. Infants regain their birth weight by 10 to 14 days of life. Neonates gain 0.5 to 1.0 ounce per day. Low-birth-weight infants have an individualized nutrition plan that varies in vitamin, minerals, and caloric content. Additionally, the question is focused on growth, not nutrition requirements.

4. **Correct Answer: D) Feed the infant 30 to 32 ounce of iron-fortified formula daily.** 30 to 32 ounces of iron-fortified formula is recommended from birth through 12 months of age. Sunscreen is recommended for application to infants who are 6 months or older. Pureed fruits and vegetables, not cube-cut foods, are introduced at 6 months old.

5. **Correct Answer: B) 12 months old.** Cow's milk is introduced at 12 months old. Breast milk or iron-fortified formula is recommended for neonates to 12 months old.

6. **Correct Answer: B) 400 IU vitamin D.** Infants who are exclusively breastfeeding or receiving less than 1 L (32 ounces) of formula should receive 400 IU vitamin D daily.

CHAPTER 2 GROWTH AND DEVELOPMENT OF INFANTS, TODDLERS, AND PRESCHOOLERS

7. As the pediatric nurse, which question is important to ask the parent when gathering a history on a 6-month-old infant?

    A. Does the infant's water supply have sufficient fluoride?
    B. Was the home the infant lives in built after 1980?
    C. Does the infant fit well in a forward-facing car seat?
    D. What words does your infant vocalize?

8. As the pediatric nurse, which of the following foods is appropriate to recommend for feeding a 9-month-old infant?

    A. Raw honey
    B. Grapes
    C. Popcorn
    D. Eggs

9. At what age would the pediatric nurse expect a child to make two-word phrases, turn pages in a book, and build a tower of seven blocks?

    A. 12 months old
    B. 15 months old
    C. 18 months old
    D. 24 months old

10. At what age does the pediatric nurse expect to observe the parachute reflex?

    A. 2 months old
    B. 4 months old
    C. 6 months old
    D. 9 months old

7. **Correct Answer: A) Does the infant's water supply have sufficient fluoride?** Beginning at 6 months old it is recommended that children are assessed for the need for fluoride supplementation. If the child's primary source of water is deficient in fluoride, fluoride supplementation is recommended. Considering the increasing mobility of a 6-month-old and their developmental oral fixation, infants at this age should be screened for lead ingestion. Lead has been found in homes built prior to 1980, not after 1980. Children younger than 2 years of age should be placed in a rear-facing car seat. Infants form words closer to 12 months old. Infants at 6 months old babble, imitate sounds, and make one-syllable vocalizations.

8. **Correct Answer: D) Eggs.** At 9 months old children should be offered soft foods that are not associated with being a high choking hazard. Foods that are associated with a high choking hazard include grapes and popcorn. Due to the risk of botulism, raw honey is to be avoided in children younger than 1 year of age. A toxin from *Clostridium botulinum* bacteria, which causes infant botulism, can contaminate honey.

9. **Correct Answer: D) 24 months old.** A 12-month-old, 15-month-old, and 18-month-old make one-word phrases. A 12-month-old stacks two-block towers. An 18-month-old toddler stacks four-block towers. A 24-month-old toddler makes two-word phrases, turns pages in a book, and builds a tower of seven blocks.

10. **Correct Answer: D) 9 months old.** The parachute reflex emerges at 9 months of age. This reflex is elicited while the clinician holds the infant tilted down toward the examination table, and the infant outstretches their arms toward the mat. In a younger infant, when the reflex is not present, the infant will pull their arms back to the plane of the body.

CHAPTER 3

Growth and Development of School-Aged Children and Adolescents

Allison C. Munn and Tracy P. George

INTRODUCTION

Understanding child developmental principles is the basis for history focus and physical examination. This section focuses on growth and development principles and considerations for school-aged children and adolescents.

Description

- The school-age years include middle and late childhood, which are ages 6 through 12 years. Adolescence is between 11 years and 21 years.
  - Adolescence is divided into three phases: early adolescence (ages 11–14), middle adolescence (ages 15–17), and late adolescence (ages 18–21).

ASSESSMENT: SCHOOL-AGED CHILDREN

Physical Assessment

- It is important to involve the school-aged child in the physical assessment process. Speak and ask questions directly to the child and have the parent/caregiver fill in the information gaps.
  - Ask the younger child simple questions.
  - Ask the older child more open and complex questions to encourage sharing of information.
- School-aged children should feel comfortable sitting on an exam table and having the exam proceed in a head-to-toe manner.
  - If a genitalia exam is necessary, perform this exam last.
  - The caregiver should remain in the room for the entirety of the exam.
- Explain each portion of the physical assessment to the child in concrete terms. Describe what will happen during the exam and why it is needed. For example, "I am going to listen to your lungs to make sure they sound clear and full of air."
- Most school-aged children grow 2 inches and gain about 5 to 7 pounds per year.
  - Identify trends in height and weight, determine growth percentiles, and calculate the child's body mass index (BMI) to determine if the child has proper growth or is at risk for overweight or obesity status.

Head, Eyes, Ears, Nose, and Throat

- There are several important changes to note in the school-aged child's growth that can be identified within the head, eyes, ears, nose, and throat (HEENT) assessment.
    - Ask about any concerns with hearing or vision, history of illnesses and infections of the HEENT system, and whether the child has seen a dentist.
    - Frontal sinuses completely develop by seven years of age. Thus, school-aged children may begin to develop sinus infections. Palpate the sinuses for tenderness.
    - School-aged children are able to use the traditional Snellen chart for eye exams. They typically know the letters of the alphabet and are beginning to read.
    - School-aged children will have most of their primary teeth and some permanent teeth. Children usually lose their first primary tooth around 6 years of age. Once a primary tooth is lost, it is soon replaced by a permanent tooth. See Table 3.1 for ages of permanent teeth eruption.
- Observe tonsils for size, redness, or exudate. Tonsils hypertrophy during the school-age years and are graded on a scale of 0–4+.
    - Assess for history of tonsillitis or strep infections, depending on the size of the tonsils within the oropharynx.
    - Chronic tonsil hypertrophy may interfere with normal breathing during sleep and can cause sleep apnea.
    - Frequent strep infections or chronic tonsil hypertrophy may require surgical intervention.
- Assess for orientation to person, place, and time. School-aged children should be able to tell you the day of the week, and they should know their address and phone number.
- Assess cranial nerve function; fine motor function, and sharp/dull sensation. School-aged children can follow commands.
    - Assess each of these tasks (e.g., Romberg fine motor testing—finger-to-nose test, cranial nerve [CN] testing—6 cardinal fields of gaze: CN 3 [oculomotor], CN 4 [trochlear], and CN 6 [abducens]).

TABLE 3.1: Ages of Permanent Teeth Eruption

Lower Tooth	Age of Eruption	Upper Tooth	Age of Eruption
Central incisor	6–7 years	Central incisor	7–8 years
Lateral incisor	7–8 years	Lateral incisor	8–9 years
Canine (cuspid)	9–10 years	Canine (cuspid)	11–12 years
First premolar (first biscuspid)	10–12 years	First premolar (first biscuspid)	10–11 years
Second premolar (second bicuspid)	11–12 years	Second premolar (second bicuspid)	10–12 years
First molar	6–7 years	First molar	6–7 years
Second molar[1]	11–13 years	Second molar[1]	12–13 years
Third molar (wisdom tooth)[2]	17–21 years	Third molar (wisdom tooth)[2]	17–21 years

Note: [1]May erupt during adolescence.
[2]Erupt during adolescence or young adulthood.
Source: Adapted from Kyle, T., and Carman, S. (2016). *Essentials of pediatric nursing* (3rd ed.). Wolters Kluwer.

Respiratory Assessment

- Normal respiratory rate for school-aged children is 16–22 breaths per minute.
- Alveoli reach full development in number and functioning between ages 8–10 years.
- Inquire about a history of asthma or other respiratory disorders and assess respiratory effort.
- Auscultate in all lung fields and listen for adventitious lung sounds.

Cardiovascular Assessment

- Inquire about any history of congenital heart disease, surgery, or infection.
- In school-aged children, after seven years of age, the point of maximal impulse (PMI) moves from the fourth intercostal space to the fifth intercostal space at the midclavicular line.
- Normal heart rate ranges from 70 to 110 beats per minute. Normal blood pressure (BP) ranges from 95 to 120 mm Hg (systolic) and from 60 to 76 mm Hg (diastolic).
- Assess for uniformity of pulses and capillary refill in all extremities. Note any differences in BP or pulses between the arms and legs.
- Auscultate for regular heart sounds, rhythm, and listen for murmurs.
- Screen all children for hyperlipidemia (total cholesterol and triglycerides) at 10 years of age. Screen those with a family history of high cholesterol by the early school-age years.
    - Refer to https://downloads.aap.org/AAP/PDF/periodicity_schedule.pdf

Gastrointestinal Assessment

- Determine history of gastrointestinal (GI) surgeries, illness, or injury.
- Inquire about regularity of bowel movements or issues with constipation or diarrhea.
- Inspect the abdomen for a flat (not sunken or protruding) appearance.
- Palpate the abdomen and note any bloating, firm areas (stool or masses), tenderness, or presence of hepatosplenomegaly.

Genitourinary Assessment

- Bladder capacity increases and children should have the ability to remain dry at night. Inquire about nighttime bedwetting to determine if further measures are needed.
- Inquire about a history of recurrent urinary tract infections.
    - A clean catch urine specimen may be obtained to screen for blood, glucose, or white blood cells in the urine.
    - This screening tool can help to evaluate genitourinary (GU) system and overall health.
- Older school-aged children will enter prepubescence and will begin to experience development of secondary sexual characteristics due to hormonal changes.
- Many factors influence the age of entrance into puberty.
    - Females typically enter into puberty earlier than males.
    - Genetics, environment, and nutrition may contribute to the age and timing of development.
        - Obese females typically enter into puberty earlier than normal-weight females.
        - However, obese males usually enter into puberty later than normal-weight males.
- Tanner Stages to determine progression of secondary sexual characteristics development are outlined in the adolescent physical exam section.
- Evaluate whether parents/caregivers have talked to their child about upcoming physical and emotional changes associated with puberty.
    - Ask whether the child or parent has any questions about these changes, and offer educational resources for how to manage the physical, social, and cognitive transitions.

Musculoskeletal Assessment

- Muscle strength and coordination increase in the school-age years, but children are still at an increased risk for injuries because their bones are not completely ossified.
- Full skeletal maturation aligns with puberty, the appearance of secondary sexual characteristics, and the associated prepubertal/pubertal growth spurts. Bones are not fully ossified until mid to late adolescence.
- Inquire about past musculoskeletal injuries and test for muscle strength using push/pull testing against the examiner's hands. Assess for range of motion in all extremities.
- Have the child bend forward and touch their toes and assess for spinal curvature. Observation of symmetric hip height (standing) or shoulder symmetry (sitting) can also indicate spinal curvature.

Psychosocial Assessment

- During the school-age years, children begin to think concretely, are able to understand the viewpoints of others, and become physically stronger and more coordinated.
- While physical growth is slow and steady, considerable cognitive and psychosocial changes become apparent during the school-age years.

PEDIATRIC PEARLS

- Learning to read is a substantial development milestone for younger school-aged kids. Inquire about their ability to read and establish rapport by allowing them an opportunity to share things about things that they have accomplished and are proud of.

- **Cognitive Development**
    - School-aged children are in the concrete operational stages of logical thought and reasoning as defined by Piaget.
    - Their emerging ability to organize thoughts leads to a better understanding of cause and effect than those of younger children.
    - While school-aged children are able to think logically, they are unable to work through abstract thoughts, ideas, and concepts until adolescence.
    - Concrete thinking enables school-aged children to understand how things work when observing or manipulating the individual parts. Thus, school-age children like to build things and take things apart to obtain a better understanding of the objects' functional ability.
        - School-aged children may like to play with advanced building block sets, build or take apart motors or computers, or play with coding games or devices to develop their cognitive abilities.
    - The concept of conservation is developed in the early school-age years. Conservation includes the ability to determine differences in number, volume, matter, and length when the materials are redistributed.
        - The classic example of this includes redistributing an equal amount of liquid (volume) into two containers in front of a child. One container is short and wide. The other container is tall and narrow. The child who has not mastered conservation and concrete thought will believe that the taller, narrow container has more water because the water level is higher than that of the wide container. A child who has mastered conservation will understand that the container shapes are different, but the amount of water within those containers remains the same.
    - School and learning become very important to a school-aged child. They are rapidly developing cognitive understanding and their personal knowledge becomes important to their mental health and sense of self-worth.

- It is important that a school-aged child receive positive reinforcement from parents and teachers when learning to master knowledge and new tasks.

■ **Psychosocial Development**
- According to Erikson's theory of psychosocial development, school-aged children are in the developmental stage of industry versus inferiority.
- This means that school-aged children develop confidence and positive self-esteem through the successful completion of tasks, completion and achievement of goals, and the sense of independence gained when doing more things on their own without parental assistance.
- If children are unable to successfully learn, perform, and achieve their goals, they are at risk for developing a sense of inadequacy and negative self-image.
- Same-sex peers become increasingly important to school-aged children. They enjoy cooperative play through team sports and organized activities.
- School-aged children understand how to follow the rules of the game and how to work together as a team to achieve a common goal or to score a goal.
  - Accomplishing these tasks in groups builds both a sense of individual self-worth and peer group bonding.
- Increased levels of independence and sports participation increase the risk for injury in school-aged children.
  - Parents and clinicians should remind school-aged children about road safety and the importance of wearing safety equipment such as helmets and elbow pads when riding bikes and skateboards or playing sports.
    - Other dangers include the following:
      - Water—Teach school-aged children how to swim, never allow children to swim alone, always wear life jackets in bodies of water other than a swimming pool (e.g., oceans, lakes, or rivers).
      - Automobiles—Children less than 4 ft. 9 in. should be in a booster seat with a regular car safety belt. Children should be in the back seat until 12 years of age.
      - Sports—Wear proper safety equipment, maintain hydration with exercise, recognize the signs of concussion, contusions, muscle strains or sprains, or broken bones.
      - Household—Keep dangerous tools and firearms in a locked cabinet. Warn children of the dangers of power tool and firearms.
      - Fire—Have a fire safety escape plan for the home. Teach children the danger of fire and burns with cooking and with campfire activities.
- The successful completion of schoolwork and school activities is important to a school-aged child's sense of self-worth.
  - It is important for a child to have positive parental support when learning to read and when completing homework. This helps the child to have a positive view of school.
  - It is also important for parents to have good communication with teachers to ensure that children are learning and socializing well in school.
- Being in school gives school-aged children opportunities to play cooperatively, follow rules, adapt to challenges and new situations, and grow socially through interactions with teachers, administrators, and peers.
- Being in school also puts the child at risk for negative peer interactions such as bullying.
  - With the increased use of social media in school-aged children, cyberbullying is an additional risk.
  - Parents should recognize the signs of bullying in children such as changes in sleep and eating behaviors, loss of interest in normal activities, reluctance or refusal to go to

school, anxiety, sadness or depression, or psychosomatic health complaints like frequent stomach aches or headaches.
- Some children may have limitations or disabilities that require special accommodations for them to be successful in the school-learning environment.
  - If a child requires special medical services, they will need an individualized health plan (IHP) with instructions for medications or treatments that will be needed during school hours. Children with chronic medical conditions such as type I diabetes mellitus, asthma, or seizure disorders will need an IHP.
  - If a child requires special educational services, they will need an individualized education plan (IEP) with instructions for learning and testing procedures to ensure academic success. Children with learning disabilities, attention deficit hyperactivity disorder, or autism may need an IEP.
  - Children with disabilities may need an IHP, IEP, or both to be successful in the school environment.

Diagnostics

- Routine screenings are recommended at specific ages.
  - Height/weight/BMI, Blood Pressure (BP) screening—annually
  - Hearing and vision screening—annually till age 6, then at age 8, 10, and 12 years old
  - Developmental surveillance, psychosocial/behavioral and physical examination assessment—annually
  - Depression screening at age 12 years of age, then annually
  - Tuberculosis (TB) screening or anemia—if at risk
  - Cholesterol screening at age 10
  - Provide anticipatory guidance—annually

Nursing Interventions

- Provide education and teaching pamphlets as needed; review with child.
- Administer age-appropriate immunizations (see Chapter 14).

ASSESSMENT: ADOLESCENTS

Physical Assessment

- Privacy is important to adolescents during a physical exam.
  - Younger adolescents usually have a parent/caregiver present than can help to answer questions about the child's history or present health.
  - Older adolescents may drive and come alone to health appointments.
- Ask the parent/caregiver if they have concerns about the child's behavior or health.
  - However, it is important to ask the adolescent about some behaviors without a parent present. It may be helpful to ask the parent to leave the room and then to question the child about substance use, smoking, or sexual activity.
  - Tell the adolescent that what they disclose is confidential unless they reveal an intention to do harm to themselves or others or if they are experiencing any form of abuse (physical, emotional, sexual, neglect).
- Adolescents experience a growth spurt and sexual maturation in puberty that results in adult size and reproductive ability.
- The average female adolescent in the United States gains about 38 pounds and grows 9 inches between ages 10 and 14 years of age.
- The average male adolescent gains 42 pounds and grows 9 inches between 12 and 16 years of age.

ASSESSMENT: ADOLESCENTS

- It is important for the nurse to encourage exercise, healthy nutrition, adequate sleep patterns, and sports participation.
- The use of helmets and seat belts, as well as safe driving, should be discussed with adolescents.

Head, Eyes, Ears, Nose, and Throat

- Inquire about hearing and vision and conduct screening as appropriate. Ask whether the child wears contacts or glasses or has had a recent eye exam.
- Assess for history of head injuries or concussions.
  - Determine if the child plays contact sports where helmets and safety equipment are important to maintaining health.
- Not any nose, ear, or facial piercings.
  - Educate the adolescent on having piercings or tattoos done at reputable establishments. Improper sterilization techniques and needle reuse can result in skin/tissue infections or viral infections like hepatitis C and HIV.
- Inspect teeth for braces and gum redness or swelling. Some adolescents have poor hygiene or mouth lesions associated with rubbing of braces' wires and brackets.

Respiratory Assessment

- Lung volume and capacity increase to adult levels and the respiratory rate is that of an adult between 12 and 20 breaths per minute.
- Inquire about substance use of tobacco, marijuana, or vaping that may affect lung functioning and health.

Cardiovascular Assessment

- Adolescents' heart rate and strength reach adult levels. A normal heart rate is 60 to 100 beats/minute.
- BP parameters are equal to that of adults. Normal systolic BP is 110 to 120 mm Hg, and normal diastolic BP is 64 to 80 mm Hg.

Genitourinary Assessment

- The Sexual Maturity Rating is divided into five stages for males and females, known as Tanner Stages (Tables 3.2 and 3.3).

TABLE 3.2: Tanner Stages in Females

Tanner Stage	Characteristics
1	Prepuberty No secondary sexual characteristics
2	Breast buds with papilla elevated, downy pigmented pubic hair along labia majora
3	Breast mound enlarges, darker, coarse curling pubic hair on mons and labia majora Onset of growth spurt
4	Areola and papilla become elevated to form a second mound above the level of the rest of the breast Adult type pubic hair appears with no spread to medial surface of thighs Menarche
5	Full adult genitalia Recession of areola into mound of the breast Pubic hair extends to the medial thigh

TABLE 3.3: Tanner Stages in Males

Tanner Stage	Characteristics
1	Prepuberty No secondary sexual characteristics
2	Testes enlarge, scrotal skin reddening along with change in texture Sparse growth of long, slightly pigmented pubic hair at the base of penis
3	Increase penile length, no change in width, further scrotal development Pubic hair becomes more dark, coarse, and covers a greater area Onset of growth spurt
4	Increase in penile length and width, development of glans, further darkening of scrotal skin Adult type pubic hair with no spread to medial surface of thighs
5	Full adult genitalia Adult-type pubic hair with spread to medial surface of thighs

PEDIATRIC PEARLS

- Stage 1 is prepuberty, and Stage 5 is adult genitalia for both males and females. So just focus on learning Tanner Stages 2 to 4.

- Puberty usually begins at 9 to 10 years of age in females. The average age of menarche is 12 years.
  - Puberty is considered to be delayed in a female if it starts after age 13.
  - Precocious puberty is puberty that occurs prior to age 8 in a female.
  - Adolescent females may have anovulatory menstrual cycles during the first 2 years.
- In males, the average start of puberty is 11 to 12 years of age.
  - Puberty is usually considered to be delayed if it starts after age 14 in a male.
  - Precocious puberty is puberty that begins before age 9 in a male.
- It is important for the nurse to ask the adolescent how they feel about changes in their body. If the adolescent voices concerns about their body, it is important to follow up with questions about eating disorders, body dysmorphia, and gender dysphoria.

Integumentary Assessment

- Puberty hormones and thickening of the skin lead to increased activity of the sebaceous glands. Thus, many adolescents develop acne on the face and back. Inspect the skin for lesions, ask the adolescent about skin cleansing routines, and ask if they have questions about skin care.

Psychosocial Assessment

Developmental tasks of adolescents focus on identity development, forming a moral code/base, and developing abstract thinking. Accomplishing these tasks is important as the adolescent transitions to adulthood.

- **Cognitive Development**
  - Adolescents in early adolescents (Tanner Stages 1–2) are concrete in their thoughts. There is a movement toward abstract thinking in Tanner Stages 3 to 5 in middle adolescence. By late adolescence, they are future-oriented and can see the perspectives of others.

- In early adolescence (Tanner Stages 1–2), most adolescents cannot perceive long-term consequences of their decisions. As they progress into Tanner Stages 3 to 5 in middle adolescence, they may start to understand future implications of their decisions, but they may have difficulty applying it to their decisions. By late adolescence, they are able to think through decisions and consequences independently. By late adolescence, they may begin to consider future choices, such as careers, college, marriage, and jobs.
- When assessing adolescents, it is important for the nurse to ask adolescents about school performance and attendance, and educational and career goals.
- Adolescents are at risk for substance use disorders because of changes in the brain. It is important for the nurse to ask about drugs, alcohol, and smoking/vaping. Encourage adolescents to resist peer pressure.
- The nurse should also assess for violence and weapon use.
- Screen time and technology use is also an issue that the nurse should ask about.
- Adolescents may question values during this time.

Psychosocial Development

- Adolescents often spend more time with peers than with adults, and peers are their primary influence.
- In early adolescence, same-sex peer friendships are important, often with a best friend. In middle adolescence, there is increased involvement in peer groups and their values. In middle adolescence, there may be more interest in attracting a partner of the opposite gender, same gender, or both. By late adolescence, the peer group becomes less important. Late adolescents may become committed to a partner.
- There may be adolescent-parent conflict. Adolescents may request more privacy. Adolescents often use "slang" terms, jargon, or text to communicate with one another. This creates tension with parents/adults who do not understand the teenage language. It is important for the nurse to ask about these family and peer relationships.
- It is important for the nurse to discuss sexuality, including responsible sexual choices, sexually transmitted infections, contraception, and sexual orientation.
- The adolescent brain is not fully developed. Thus, adolescents lack a degree of impulse control and recognition of consequences for various actions. The lack of impulse control may lead to risky behavior, unintended consequences, and impact mental and physical health.
- Mental health is a growing area of concern among adolescents. It is important for the nurse to ask about mental health issues, such as depression, anger, self-harm behaviors such as cutting, and suicidal ideations. In addition, the nurse should explore gang involvement and bullying.

- Routine screenings are recommended at specific ages.
  - Height/weight/BMI, BP screening—annually
  - Vision screening—at age 12 and 15 years old
  - Hearing screening—at age 13, 16, and 20 years old
  - Developmental surveillance, psychosocial/behavioral and physical examination assessment—annually
  - Depression screening at age 12 years of age, then annually
  - TB screening or anemia—if at risk
  - Cholesterol screening at age 20
  - Provide anticipatory guidance—annually—consider hepatitis C and HIV for high-risk individuals

Nursing Interventions

- Provide education and teaching pamphlets as needed; review with child.
- Administer age-appropriate immunizations (see Chapter 14).

BIBLIOGRAPHY

Drutz, J. E. (2020). The pediatric physical examination: General principles and standard measurements. *UpToDate*. Retrieved March 16, 2021, from https://www.uptodate.com/contents/the-pediatric-physical-examination-general-principles-and-standard-measurements

Erikson, E. H. (1963). *Childhood and society*. W.W. Norton and Company.

Hagan, J. F., Shaw, J. S., & Duncan, P. (Eds.). (2017). *Bright futures: Guidelines for health supervision of infants, children and adolescents* (4th ed.). https://brightfutures.aap.org/materials-and-tools/guidelines-and-pocket-guide/Pages/default.aspx

Kyle, T., & Carman, S. (2016). *Essentials of pediatric nursing* (3rd ed.). Wolters Kluwer.

London, M. L., Ladewig, P. W., Davidson, M., Ball, J. W., Binder, R. C., & Cowen, K. (2017). *Maternal and child nursing care* (5th ed.). Pearson.

Maaks, D. L. G., Starr, N. B., Brady, M. A., Gaylord, N. M., Driessnack, M., & Duderstadt, K. (2020). *Burns' pediatric primary care* (7th ed.). Elsevier.

Piaget, J. (1930). *The child's conception of physical causality*. Routledge & Kegan Paul Ltd.

Silbert-Flagg, J., & Sloand, E. D. (2020). *Pediatric nurse practitioner certification review guide: Primary care* (7th ed.). Jones & Bartlett Publishers.

Tagher, G., & Knapp, L. (2019). *Pediatric nursing: A case-based approach*. Wolters Kluwer.

KNOWLEDGE CHECK

1. A female has breast buds and a small amount of downy pubic hair. Which Tanner Stage is this?

   A. Stage 1
   B. Stage 2
   C. Stage 3
   D. Stage 4

2. What is not a priority in an 11- to 14-year-old well-child visit for the nurse to discuss?

   A. Physical activity
   B. Prevention of sexually transmitted infections
   C. School performance
   D. Apply fluoride varnish every 6 months

3. A parent is concerned because her 16-year-old daughter is not as interested in family activities and is more interested in activities with friends. What statement by the nurse is most appropriate?

   A. You should require your daughter to attend all family activities
   B. Continue to involve your teenager in family activities, and you can offer to allow a friend to come when it's appropriate
   C. Your daughter may have mental health issues and should see a psychologist
   D. Stop inviting your daughter to family outings while she is a teenager

4. The nurse is caring for a patient who is unable to think about the consequences of experimenting with marijuana, is not future-oriented, and exhibits concrete thought processes. What is the most likely age for this patient?

   A. 9
   B. 13
   C. 16
   D. 19

5. John is a 13-year-old male who is concerned that he has not started his growth spurt yet. He is shorter than many of his friends. His testes have enlarged, and he has a sparse growth of long, slightly pigmented pubic hair. How should the nurse respond?

   A. You should begin your growth spurt soon
   B. You may need to see a pediatric endocrinologist because your growth spurt is late
   C. Delayed puberty may be associated with Klinefelter syndrome, so you may need genetic testing
   D. If you are highly physically active, that could delay your growth spurt

6. The nurse is caring for a Natalie, a 7-year-old female, in the pediatric clinic. What would be appropriate to discuss at this visit?

   A. Use of fluoride varnish every six months.
   B. School performance
   C. Autism screening
   D. Naps

KNOWLEDGE CHECK

1. **Correct Answer: B) Stage 2.** Stage 1 is prepuberty. Stage 2 includes breast buds. Stage 3 includes the growth spurt, and menarche occurs in Stage 4.

2. **Correct Answer: D) Apply fluoride varnish every 6 months.** Applying fluoride varnish is not applicable to this age group and should not be prioritized on a well-child visit. According to Bright Futures, exercise, prevention of sexually transmitted infections, and school performance should be discussed by the nurse at 11- to 14-year-old visits.

3. **Correct Answer: B) Continue to involve your teenager in family activities, and you can offer to allow a friend to come when it's appropriate.** Adolescents may be more interested in friends and peer social events than in family activities. It is important for parents to continue to include adolescents in family activities. Allowing the teen to invite a friend to certain events may be a useful strategy.

4. **Correct Answer: B) 13.** Early adolescence is ages 10 to 14. This stage is associated with concrete operations, the inability to perceive the long-term outcomes of decisions, and a lack of future orientation. In middle adolescence (ages 15–17), there is the emergence of abstract thoughts, and teens may perceive some implications for their actions. In late adolescence (ages 18–21), patients are more future-oriented with abstract reasoning.

5. **Correct Answer: A) You should begin your growth spurt soon.** John is in Tanner Stage 2, so he should begin his growth spurt in Tanner Stage 3. The nurse should let him know that his growth spurt should begin soon. Physical activity is not known to delay an adolescent's growth spurt. John has already shown signs of puberty; puberty is not considered delayed until a male adolescent has reached 14 years of age.

6. **Correct Answer: B) School performance.** School performance is an appropriate topic at the 7-year-old well-child visit. Autism screening, naps, and fluoride varnish should be discussed at an earlier age.

7. A nurse is preparing to perform a physical assessment on a 10-year-old girl. Which of these actions would be most appropriate for the nurse to take?

   A. Explain each part of the examination to child before performing it
   B. Ask the mother to hold the child down for invasive procedures
   C. Leave intrusive procedures such as examination of the eyes and ears until the end
   D. Ask the mother to tell the child to not be afraid

8. Which nursing actions are developmentally appropriate when caring for a hospitalized school-aged child? Select all that apply.

   A. Knocking on the school-aged child's hospital room door prior to entering
   B. Singing the ABCs while taking vital signs
   C. Asking parent or caregiver to leave room prior to administering care
   D. Using toys for distraction during a painful procedure

9. Which of the following is an expected physical exam finding on a 7-year-old child?

   A. Presence of frontal sinuses
   B. Axillary and pubic hair growth
   C. Eruption of 5 permanent teeth
   D. Rapid weight gain

10. The nurse is taking the history of a 9-year-old child. During the interview, the parents admit to owning firearms. What is the most appropriate safety measure for the nurse to suggest?

    A. Keep the guns on the top shelf of a closet
    B. Take the child to a shooting range for lessons on how to use the gun properly
    C. Store the guns and ammunition in the same cabinet
    D. Keep all firearms in a locked safe or case

7. **Correct Answer: A) Explain each part of the examination to child before performing it.** For a 10-year-old child, it is appropriate for the nurse to explain each part of the exam first. Asking the mother to hold the child down, prolonging the eyes and ears exam, and asking them other to tell the girl to not be fearful are not appropriate with this age of child.

8. **Correct Answer: A) Knocking on the school-aged child's hospital room door prior to entering.** Knocking on the school-aged child's room provides privacy to the patient, which is important at this age. Singing to a child or using toys for distraction is appropriate with younger-aged children but is not appropriate for the school-aged patient. It is not necessary for the parent or caregiver to be absent from the room when administering care.

9. **Correct Answer: A) Presence of frontal sinuses.** Most 7-year-old children have frontal sinuses. Axillary and pubic hair growth, having more than one to three permanent teeth erupt, and rapid weight gain are abnormal findings on a child at age seven.

10. **Correct Answer: D) Keep all firearms in a locked safe or case.** Firearms should be in a locked location so that school-aged children cannot reach them. It is not advised to store guns on a shelf or to store guns and ammunition in the same place. Additionally, it is not suggested to take school-aged children to a shooting range to learn how to shoot the guns.

PART III
Management

CHAPTER 4

Eyes, Ears, Nose, and Throat Conditions

Terri Giordano

INTRODUCTION TO PEDIATRIC EYES, EARS, NOSE, AND THROAT

- The ear can be divided into the following three anatomic compartments:
  - **Outer ear:** Auricle, external auditory canal, and lateral surface of tympanic membrane
  - **Middle ear:** Space between tympanic membrane and inner ear
  - **Inner ear:** Vestibular apparatus and cochlea
- The eustachian tube connects the middle ear and nasopharynx; it is shorter, wider, and more horizontal in infants and young children.
- Hearing loss is classified as conductive or sensorineural.
- The high position of the larynx in neonates and the opposition of the epiglottis to the soft palate forces the neonate to breathe through the nose and nasopharynx.

ALLERGIC RHINITIS

Description

- Inflammatory disorder of nasal mucosa with nasal congestion, rhinorrhea, itching, sneezing, and conjunctival inflammation; can be seasonal or perennial.
- Children often perform allergic salute, an upward rubbing of the nose with an open palm that forms a transverse nasal crease on the nose.

Assessment

- Observe for presence of nasal congestion, clear rhinorrhea, itching, allergic shiners (dark circles under the eyes).
- Assess for loss of sense of smell and/or taste.

Diagnostics

Allergy testing to diagnose

Nursing Interventions

- Refer to pediatric allergist for allergy testing.
- Avoid allergens.
- Administer antihistamines, nasal sprays/washes as ordered.

Discharge Planning; Patient and Family Education

- Educate caregivers on how to encase child's mattress and pillow in allergen proof coverings; the importance of washing bed linens and blankets weekly; removal of pet if patient allergic to animal dander; if possible, use air conditioning and keep windows and doors closed to reduce pollen exposure; avoid exposure to secondhand smoke.

CONJUNCTIVITIS

Description

- Inflammation/infection of palpebral (eyelid lining) and bulbar (tissue layer over sclera) conjunctiva.
- Red appearing eye, common in childhood, can be infectious or noninfectious; bacterial type very contagious, especially in day-care and school environments.
    - **Viral conjunctivitis:** Watery discharge from eyes, seen more often during the summertime and in children over 5 years of age
    - **Bacterial conjunctivitis:** Mucopurulent unilateral or bilateral discharge from eyes; highly contagious
    - **Allergic conjunctivitis:** Clear, watery discharge with intense itching and conjunctival edema, often seen in spring and summer

Assessment

- Assess for recent upper respiratory infection.
- Assess conjunctiva for redness and edema.
- Assess for excessive tearing/discharge, pruritus, eye discomfort.

Nursing Interventions

- Keep eye clean; apply warm compress to affected eye to loosen crusted drainage; if allergic rhinitis, use cool compresses to relieve itching and wash face and hands with cool water after outdoor playing.
- Administer antibiotic ophthalmic drops as ordered for bacterial conjunctivitis.
- Avoid known allergens.

Discharge Planning; Patient and Family Education

- Educate patient and caregivers on topical instillation of antibiotic ophthalmic drops and importance of not touching the tip of the container on any surface and not sharing the bottle with other family members; keep child's washcloth and towels separate; wiping from inner canthus outward.
- Avoid day care and school until antibiotics are given for 24 hours for bacterial conjunctivitis.
- Instruct patient and caregivers to apply warm compress to eye but not to keep compress on eye as occlusive covering promotes bacterial growth.
- No contact lenses until eye infection resolves.
- Discard any eye makeup used during infection.

PEDIATRIC SKILL 4.1: OPHTHALMIC DROPS ADMINISTRATION

- Verify the order with child's medical record.
- Perform hand hygiene and don gloves.
- Position the child supine in bed looking up, rest the dominant hand against child's forehead; with other hand pull down the lower eyelid exposing conjunctival sac; instill the ordered amount of drops into the conjunctival sac being careful not to touch the dropper to the eye; remove gloves and perform hand hygiene.

DACRYOSTENOSIS (CONGENITAL NASOLACRIMAL DUCT OBSTRUCTION)

Description
- "Blocked tear ducts"
- Complete or partial obstruction of the nasolacrimal duct
- Occurs in up to 20% to 30% of all newborns; can involve one or both eyes

Assessment
- Assess for excessive watery eyes or mucopurulent discharge.
- Assess for erythema and/or maceration of skin around eyes from irritation and rubbing produced from dripping of tears and discharge; conjunctive clear without redness or edema.

Diagnostics
Gentle pressure over nasolacrimal sac produces mucopurulent discharge.

Nursing Interventions
- Refer to pediatric ophthalmologist if not resolved by 12 months of age.
- Nasolacrimal massage two to three times daily.

Special Considerations
Children with Trisomy 21, CHARGE syndrome, and Goldenhar syndrome have an increased risk of congenital nasolacrimal duct obstruction.

Discharge Planning; Patient and Family Education
- Educate caregivers on the importance of handwashing before touching infant's eyes.
- Teach caregivers nasolacrimal massage by placing index finger over lacrimal sac with gently downward pressure toward the infant's mouth; educate caregivers if not resolved by 1 year of age, may require surgical intervention.

EPISTAXIS (NOSEBLEED)

Description
Most common site of bleeding is the Kiesselbach plexus (area in the anterior nasal septum); thin mucosa in the area makes it prone to exposure to dry air and digital trauma (nose picking).

Assessment
- Inspect nose for signs of blood clot or crusty debris; assess for any family history of bleeding disorder.
- Assess for tarry stools with frequent bleeding.

Nursing Interventions
Administer moisture therapy to nose; refer to pediatric otolaryngology if not improved with moisture therapy; postoperative care of nasal cautery-surgical treatment to cauterize bleeding vessels.

Special Considerations
Recurrent epistaxis should be evaluated for bleeding or platelet disorders.

Discharge Planning; Patient and Family Education

- Discourage digital trauma and vigorous nose blowing; educate parents and caregivers on preventive measures for epistaxis with use of humidity in home, and teach how to use moisture therapy with nasal saline and gels.
- Teach proper technique of how to stop nosebleed by leaning forward and pinching the soft part of the nose for at least 5 minutes; if nosebleed continues, hold for a full 15 minutes.

HEARING LOSS

Description

- Deficit in hearing; mild indicated at 15 to 30 dB (configuration or decibel [dB] loss); with a sensory stimulus, child and infant should turn head; born able to hear.
- Impacts speech and ability to communicate clearly with linguistic sounds and intellectual function.
- Ears and kidneys develop simultaneously in utero. Suspected condition in ears or hearing suggests assessment of kidney function.
- Conductive (conductive hearing loss [CHL])
  - Due to dysfunction in transmission of sound through external or middle ear
  - Middle ear fluid (otitis media with effusion [OME]) most common cause; other causes include impacted cerumen (wax), perforation of the tympanic membrane, aural atresia or stenosis, foreign body
- Sensorineural (sensorineural hearing loss [SNHL])
  - Due to damage to structures in the inner ear from disease, ototoxic agents, hair cell destruction from exposure to noise, cochlear malformations
  - Most common infectious cause of congenital SNHL is cytomegalovirus (CMV)
- **Mixed:** Combination of CHL and SNHL
- Can be unilateral or bilateral, mild, moderate, severe, profound, sudden or gradual onset, stable, progressive, or fluctuating.

Assessment

- If newborn, determine if universal newborn hearing screen was completed after birth.
- Assess for hearing loss before 3 months of age with intervention no later than 6 months of age to facilitate language development: Lack of babbling/vocalization by 7 months; prolonged babbling stage of development; decreased babbling noted by caregivers; observe response to stimulus such as sound, assess from various locations: front, next to, behind, child. Lack of startle reflex; communicate with child with speaker's lips not visible (behind paper or object); call child's name at different speaking levels and with back turned toward child; assess ability to follow simple directions without nonverbal gestures.
- Assess outer ear for presence of any deformity; assess for family history of hearing loss.

Diagnostics

Audiologic evaluation by newborn hearing screen or auditory brainstem evoked responses (ABRs); visual reinforcement audiometry from 6 months to 2½ years; play audiometry 2½ years to 4 years; behavioral observation audiometry 4 years and older to evaluate for hearing loss

Nursing Interventions

- Refer to pediatric otolaryngology and/or audiology.
- Face the child for communication; educate parent and child about lip reading and alternate forms of communication: cued speech (hand gestures with verbal communication), sign language, electronics, whiteboards, and verbal communication as appropriate.

Special Considerations

- **Syndromes associated with SNHL:** Waardenburg, Branchiootorenal, CHARGE, Goldenhar, Pendred, Alport, and Usher.
- **Sensorineural loss:** Surgical treatment = cochlear implant for extensive hearing loss, sends impulses to nerve (extremely sensitive to magnets).
- **Conductive loss:** Hearing aids (appliances require care; store batteries in safe place; turn down volume or readjust for whistling sounds).
- Consultations with audiologists, speech, occupational therapy, any interprofessional referrals are necessary for early identification and decrease delays in growth and development.

Discharge Planning; Patient and Family Education

- Provide emotional support to patient and family; if child is under 3 years of age, refer patient and family to early intervention.
- For infants and children fitted for hearing aids, educate caregivers on the importance of storing hearing aid batteries in a safe location, out of reach of children; hearing aid battery ingestion requires immediate emergency management.
- Educate families that school-aged children should sit in front of the classroom; use hearing protection by avoiding exposure to environmental noise; wear ear protection when engaging in activities associated with high intensity noise such as model airplane flying, target shooting, or snowmobiling.

INFECTIOUS RHINITIS (COMMON COLD)

Description

- Most common pathogen is human rhinovirus but can also be influenza, adenovirus, human metapneumovirus, human coronavirus, and nonpolio enterovirus
- Occurs year round with highest incidence early fall through late spring
- **Risk factors:** Day care, secondhand smoke exposure

Assessment

Observe for presence of nasal discharge, fever, sore throat, cough, headache, irritability, decreased appetite.

Nursing Interventions

Assess for fever, nasal discharge, sore throat.

Discharge Planning; Patient and Family Education

Encourage fluid intake and rest; educate patient and caregivers on the use of saline nasal spray; spray bottle should only be used on one child and with one illness because bottle becomes easily contaminated.

LARYNGOMALACIA

Description

- Congenital softening of tissues of larynx (voice box)
- Most common cause of stridor during infancy; intermittent inspiratory stridor develops within the first 2 weeks of life, increases severity for up to 6 months with gradual improvement; median age to resolution is 7 to 9 months of age with majority having no stridor by 18 months of age
- Inspiratory stridor exacerbated by crying, feeding, or agitation

Assessment

- Assess for dysphagia (feeding difficulty) and failure to thrive.
- Assess for increased work of breathing, apnea, or cyanosis.
- Assess for gastroesophageal reflux.

Diagnostics

Primarily based on symptoms; flexible laryngoscopy to evaluate collapse of arytenoids (cartilage) and folding of epiglottis during inspiration

Nursing Interventions

- Referral to pediatric otolaryngology for severe symptoms of apnea, cyanosis, aspiration
- **Supraglottoplasty:** Surgical treatment for severe cases of laryngomalacia

Discharge Planning; Patient and Family Education

Educate caregivers that stridor will resolve spontaneously and may sound louder or worse before it decreases or resolves; educate caregivers on postoperative supraglottoplasty care.

OBSTRUCTIVE SLEEP APNEA SYNDROME

Description

- Repeated episodes of prolonged upper airway obstruction during sleep despite continued or increased respiratory effort, resulting in complete apnea or partial apnea (hypopnea), decreased airflow at the nose and/or mouth, and disrupted sleep
- Apnea defined as a pause in breathing lasting >20 seconds or a brief respiratory pause along with cyanosis, bradycardia, marked pallor, or hypotonia

Assessment

Assess for presence of snoring, mouth breathing, restless sleep, hyponasal speech, difficulty swallowing, enuresis.

Diagnostics

Overnight polysomnography (sleep study) to evaluate if sleep apnea is present

Nursing Interventions

- Refer to pediatric otolaryngology if adenotonsillectomy (first-line treatment) indicated or pediatric sleep medicine if initiation of CPAP (continuous positive airway pressure) is required.
- Tonsillectomy is a surgical procedure to remove the tonsils; performed with or without adenoidectomy.
- **Postoperative tonsillectomy care:** Maintain normal diet as tolerated, encourage fluid intake, encourage fruit snacks, popsicles, pudding, yogurt, or ice cream but avoid citrus juice and brown or red-colored foods; monitor for excessive swallowing and frequent throat clearing to indicate early bleeding; assess for pain and administer pain medication as prescribed; apply cold or hot pack to neck and/or ears.

Special Considerations

- Conditions that predispose children to obstructive sleep apnea syndrome (OSAS) include adenotonsillar hypertrophy, micrognathia, Trisomy 21, Crouzon disease, Apert syndrome, Pierre Robin, Treacher Collins, and achondroplasia.

OTITIS EXTERNA (OUTER EAR INFECTION)

- Decision on whether and how to treat OSAS in children varies with severity of symptoms, duration of disease, and presence of comorbid conditions.

Discharge Planning; Patient and Family Education

- **Postoperative tonsillectomy care:** Avoid coughing, clearing of throat, blowing nose, and use of straws to prevent trauma to throat.
- Educate caregivers that tonsillectomy can improve sleep outcomes in majority of children, but additional interventions may be recommended.

OTITIS EXTERNA (OUTER EAR INFECTION)

Description

- Inflammation of outer ear and ear canal
- Chronic irritation from excessive moisture in the ear canal
- Referred to as "swimmer's ear"

Assessment

Assess for pain, swelling, redness, exudate, itching of the ear and/or ear canal; assess for any hearing loss.

Nursing Interventions

- Administer topical antibiotic otic drops as prescribed; medication needs to absorb within ear canal wall for effectiveness.
- Administer analgesics for pain; apply warm compress to affected ear.
- Refer to pediatric otolaryngologist if ear canal swells and unable to instill ear drops.

Special Considerations

May require placement of cotton ear wick soaked with antibiotics to reduce edema

Discharge Planning; Patient and Family Education

- Educate caregivers on how to instill otic drops and the importance of completing antibiotic drops as instructed; educate on the importance of keeping ear dry.
- Avoid swimming for about 10 days; discuss use of 50:50 solution of acetic acid (white vinegar) and rubbing alcohol, instill into ear canals in the morning, at bedtime, and at the end of a swimming session to restore pH and prevent recurrence; instruct caregivers to contact clinician if unable to instill drops.
- Wear ear plugs while swimming for prevention.

PEDIATRIC SKILL 4.2: INSTILL OTIC DROPS

- Verify order with child's medical record; perform hand hygiene and don gloves; have child lie in a supine position with their head turned to the appropriate side.
- For children younger than 3 years of age, pull the pinna down and back.
- For children older than 3 years, pull the pinna up and back.
- Administer the ordered number of drops into the ear canal, holding the dropper ½ inch above the ear canal being careful not to contaminate the ear dropper. Gently massage the tragus (area anterior to ear canal), have child remain in supine position with head turned for 3 to 5 minutes. Repeat with other ear if prescribed, remove gloves and perform hand hygiene.

OTITIS MEDIA (EAR INFECTION)

Description

- Inflammation of the middle ear; one of the most common illnesses in children
- *Streptococcus pneumonia*, *Haemophilus influenza*, and *Moraxella catarrhalis* most common causative organisms
- **Risk factors:** Young age, attending day care, exposure to secondhand smoke, use of a pacifier, having older siblings, supine bottle feeding (bottle propping), craniofacial anomaly, and family history

Assessment

- Monitor for fever.
- Assess for pain or discomfort by child crying at night laying down, and/or infant pulling on ears.
- Assess for poor feeding or loss of appetite, irritable/fussy.

Diagnostics

Pneumatic otoscopy to check tympanic membrane for mobility and signs of bulging, redness (Figure 4.1)

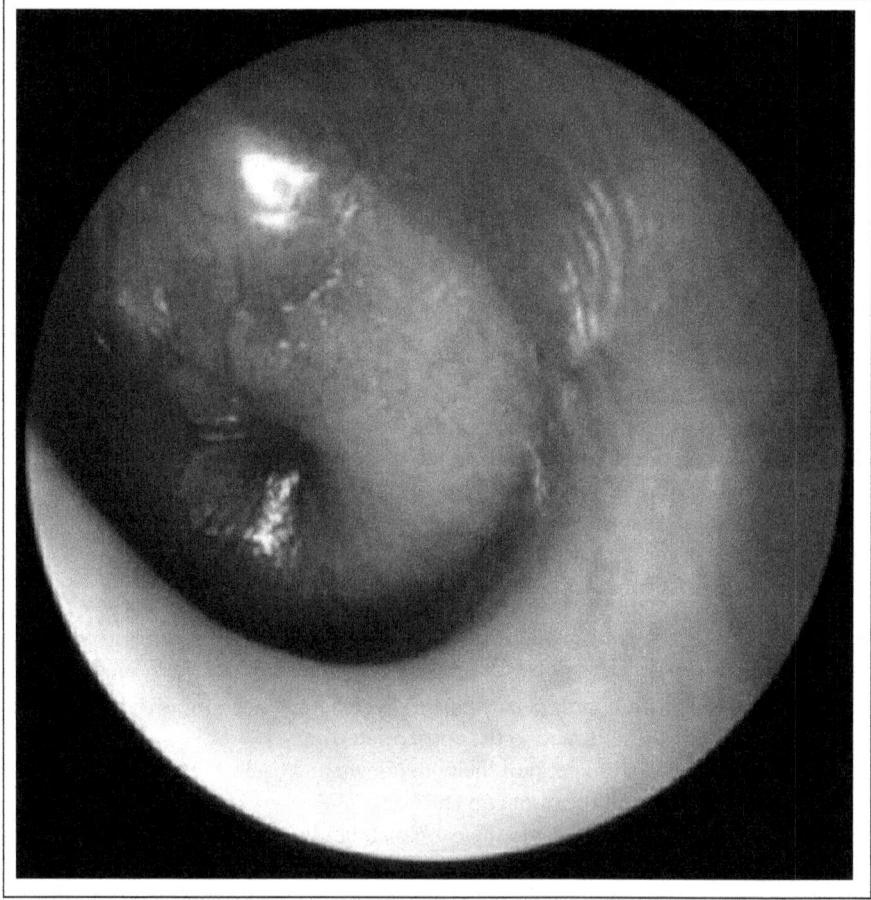

FIGURE 4.1: Serous otitis media

Source: Reprinted from Myrick, K., and Karosas, L. (2019). *Advanced health assessment and differential diagnosis* (1st ed.). Springer Publishing Company.

Nursing Interventions

- Administer antibiotics as prescribed, antipyretics as needed for fever.
- Refer to pediatric otolaryngology for recurrent infections.
- **Bilateral myringotomies and tympanostomy tubes:** Surgical treatment for recurrent ear infections to prevent hearing loss; tubes allow infection to drain from ears, treated with topical antibiotic otic drops; postoperative care after tympanostomy tubes includes positioning on affected side for drainage and avoid water in ears.

Special Considerations

Complications of otitis media (OM): mastoiditis, meningitis, facial nerve palsy

Discharge Planning; Patient and Family Education

- Provide emotional support; educate caregivers on postop care after tympanostomy tubes; educate caregivers that the tubes allow the infection or ear drainage (otorrhea) to drain from one or both ears, it can be any color and is treated with antibiotic otic (ear) drops.
- Instruct caregivers on instillation of ear drops.
- **Prevention:** Teach the importance of hand hygiene to prevent common cold and completing course of antibiotics; avoid exposure to tobacco smoke; encourage breastfeeding, upright positioning for infant feedings, and removal of pacifier; offer support in routine vaccinations including annual influenza vaccine for children 6 months of age and older.

OTITIS MEDIA WITH EFFUSION

Description

- Inflammation and presence of fluid in the middle ear mainly due to eustachian tube dysfunction
- Not associated with signs and symptoms of acute infection
- Main symptom CHL

Assessment

- Observe for decreased hearing or speech delay.
- May have a sense of fullness in ear.

Diagnostics

Pneumatic otoscopy to check tympanic membrane for the presence of fluid in the middle ear

Nursing Interventions

- Usually asymptomatic.
- Monitor for hearing loss.
- Refer to audiologist for audiogram and tympanogram if persists longer than 3 months or has hearing loss; may need myringotomy with tympanostomy for chronic OME.
- Refer to early intervention if hearing loss or speech delay present.

Discharge Planning; Patient and Family Education

- Important to educate families that most fluid resolves on its own in weeks or months
- Prevention similar to OM

PERIORBITAL CELLULITIS

Description

- Infection and inflammation of eyelids and periorbital tissue; usually unilateral
- Red, painful swelling around eye, proptosis, chemosis, decreased visual acuity, eye pain

Assessment

- Assess for recent upper respiratory infection.
- Assess eye movements and visual acuity.
- Monitor for fever.
- Assess the periorbital area for erythema, edema, pain, warmth.

Diagnostics

- Complete blood count and blood culture to assess for infection
- Head CT scan to evaluate extent of infection

Nursing Interventions

- Administer antibiotics as ordered.
- Refer to pediatric ophthalmology.
- Monitor for visual changes or loss of vision.

Discharge Planning; Patient and Family Education

Educate caregivers and child on the importance of frequent handwashing and avoiding touching the eyes; educate caregivers on the importance of completing antibiotics as instructed; contact clinician if symptoms worsen.

PHARYNGITIS

Description

- Inflammation of the pharynx (throat)
- Viral due to influenza, parainfluenza, adenovirus, coronavirus, Epstein–Barr virus
- **Bacterial:** Group A *Streptococcus* most common bacterial cause; most prevalent in winter and spring; more common in children 5 to 15 years of age; can occur due to exposure to tobacco smoke, vaping

Assessment

- Assess for fever, exudate in back of throat, headache, cough, hoarseness, laryngitis, conjunctivitis, abdominal pain, vomiting, diarrhea, dehydration.
- Assess for difficulty swallowing.
- Monitor wet diapers, presence of tears, skin turgor.

Diagnostics

Obtain throat culture and sensitivity.

Nursing Interventions

- Monitor intake and output (I&O), signs of infection.
- Offer saline gargles and/or throat lozenges; administer analgesics.
- Administer antibiotics as ordered for bacterial cause.

SINUSITIS

Discharge Planning; Patient and Family Education

Educate caregivers and patients on the importance of avoiding smoke exposure and not vaping; encourage child to drink plenty of fluids.

SINUSITIS

Description

- Inflammation of mucosal lining of paranasal sinus cavities around nasal passages
- Nonspecific complaints such as nasal congestion, purulent nasal discharge, fever, cough, halitosis, hyposmia (decreased sense of smell), headache, facial, and/or dental pain
  - **Acute:** Symptoms usually last 7 to 10 days but can be up to 4 weeks
  - **Chronic:** Symptoms last more than 12 weeks
  - **Recurrent:** Greater than 4 episodes within 1 year
  - **Fungal:** Rare, occurs in immunocompromised children

Assessment

- Assess for nasal congestion, purulent rhinorrhea, fever, and cough.
- Assess for pain in area of sinuses, headache.

Diagnostics

If symptoms persist, sinus x-rays or CT of sinuses

Nursing Interventions

- Instruct child and caregivers on frequent handwashing.
- Administer antibiotics and nasal steroids as ordered.
- Encourage increasing fluid intake to stay hydrated.
- Provide comfort measures such as analgesics, humidified environment.

Discharge Planning; Patient and Family Education

- Educate child and family how to do saline nasal washes, encourage using two times per day.
- Avoid swimming during infection.
- Refer to otolaryngologist and/or allergist if symptoms persist.

STREPTOCOCCUS TONSILLITIS GROUP A (STREP THROAT)

Description

- Inflammation of tonsillar tissue in back of throat
- Group A beta-hemolytic *Streptococcus* (GABHS) most common bacterial pathogen
- Enlarged, erythematous tonsils, fever, odynophagia (painful swallowing), malaise, halitosis

Assessment

- Assess for fever, difficulty swallowing, dehydration.
- **Assess for signs of scarlet fever:** Fever; abdominal pain; halitosis; fine, sandpaper-like bright red ("scarlet-colored") rash ("scarlatina rash") more intense in folds of joints; "strawberry tongue."

Diagnostics

Obtain throat culture and sensitivity.

Nursing Interventions

- Refer to pediatric otolaryngology for recurrent infections.
- Monitor I&O, encourage fluid intake and warm saltwater gargles, administer antibiotics and antipyretics as ordered.
- Administer antibiotics as ordered; first line should be oral penicillin.
- **Tonsillectomy:** Surgical procedure to remove the tonsils, performed with or without adenoidectomy.
- Postoperative tonsillectomy care: maintain normal diet as tolerated, encourage fluid intake, encourage fruit snacks, popsicles, pudding, yogurt, or ice cream but avoid citrus juice and brown or red-colored foods; monitor for excessive swallowing and frequent throat clearing to indicate early bleeding; assess for pain and administer pain medication as prescribed, apply cold or hot pack to neck and/or ears; prevent trauma to back of throat such as no suctioning, avoiding straws.

Discharge Planning; Patient and Family Education

- Provide emotional support to patient and caregivers; encourage fluid intake and warm saltwater gargling; avoid sharing drinking and eating items; educate patient and caregivers to discard toothbrush and replace with a new one after they have taken antibiotics for 24 hours to prevent reinfection; provide postoperative tonsillectomy education.
- **Postoperative tonsillectomy care:** Avoid coughing, clearing of throat, blowing nose, and use of straws to prevent trauma to throat.
- Avoid day care and school until afebrile and started antibiotics for 24 hours.

BIBLIOGRAPHY

Bowden, V. R., & Greenberg, C. S. (Eds.). (2016). *Pediatric nursing procedures*. Lippincott Williams and Wilkins.

Burns, C., Dunn, A., Brady, M., Starr, N., Blosser, C., & Garzon, D. (2017). *Pediatric primary care* (6th ed.). Elsevier Health Sciences.

Flint, P. W., Francis, H. W., Haughey, B. H., Lesperance, M. M., Lund, V. J., Robbins, K. T., & Thomas, J. R. (Eds.). (2021). *Cummings otolaryngology-head and neck surgery* (7th ed.). Elsevier Inc.

Hockenberry, M. J., Wilson, D., & Rodgers, C. C. (2019). *Wong's nursing care of infants and children* (11th ed.). Elsevier Inc.

Kliegman, R. M., St. Geme, J. W., Blum, N. J., Shah, S. S., Tasker, R. C., & Wilson, K. M. (Eds.). (2020). *Nelson textbook of pediatrics* (21st ed.). Elsevier Inc.

Mitchell, R. B., Archer, S. M., Ishman, S. L., Rosenfeld, R. M., Coles, S., Finestone, S. A., Friedman, N. R., Giordano, T., Hildrew, D. M., Kim, T. W., Lloyd, R. M., Parikh, S. R., Shulman, S. T., Walner, D. L., Walsh, S. A., & Nnacheta, L. C. (2019). Clinical practice guideline: Tonsillectomy in children (update). *Otolaryngology–Head and Neck Surgery*, *160*(1S), S1–S42. https://doi.org/10.1177/0194599818801757

Richardson, B. (2017). *Pediatric primary care* (3rd ed.). Jones & Bartlett Learning.

KNOWLEDGE CHECK

1. A nurse is caring for a 16-month-old with recurrent OM. When providing teaching with caregivers, the nurse should include all the following as risk factors for OM except:

   A. Attending day care
   B. Upright bottle feeding
   C. Being an only child
   D. Breastfeeding

2. A nurse is caring for an infant with nasolacrimal duct obstruction. The nurse should perform nasolacrimal massage by:

   A. Placing index finger over lacrimal sac and gently massage using downward pressure toward infant's mouth
   B. Nasolacrimal massage should not be attempted
   C. Firmly massage lacrimal sac using downward pressure
   D. Place index finger in mouth and massage

3. A nurse is providing discharge instructions to a family with a child diagnosed with otitis externa. Which statement by the caregivers indicates the need for further teaching?

   A. "I should call the doctor if the ear drops do not go into the ear."
   B. "I can put solution of ½ white vinegar and ½ rubbing alcohol into the ear canal to help prevent this."
   C. "Since it is summer, they can swim in our pool."
   D. "We will be sure to complete the entire course of antibiotic ear drops."

4. A nurse is caring for an 8-year-old with scarlet fever due to recurrent streptococcus tonsillitis. What would the nurse most likely expect to assess for in this child?

   A. Stridor
   B. Vesicle surrounded by erythematous base rash on trunk
   C. Irritability
   D. Bright red rash with sandpaper texture of skin

5. A nurse is caring for a 2-year-old child with ear drainage after tympanostomy tube insertion. What technique should the nurse use to instill the otic antibiotic drops?

   A. Have the child sit on caregiver's lap and instill drops
   B. Have the child lie supine, with head turned, pull pinna down and back, and instill drops
   C. Two-year-old children do not require otic drops
   D. Have child lie supine, with head turned, pull pinna up and back, and instill drops

6. A nurse is caring for a child with streptococcus tonsillitis. To prevent reinfection, patient and family teaching should include to:

   A. Replace child's toothbrush after 10 days of antibiotics
   B. Soak child's toothbrush in warm salt water after use
   C. Replace child's toothbrush after 24 hours of antibiotics
   D. Allow child's toothbrush to air dry

KNOWLEDGE CHECK

1. **Correct Answer: D) Breastfeeding.** Breastfeeding is considered a preventative measure. Young age, attending day care, exposure to secondhand smoke, use of a pacifier, having older siblings, supine bottle feeding (bottle propping), craniofacial anomaly, and family history are all risk factors of OM.

2. **Correct Answer: A) Placing index finger over lacrimal sac and gently massage using downward pressure toward infant's mouth.** Placing index finger over lacrimal sac and gently massage using downward pressure toward infant's mouth is the proper technique to help unblock obstruction.

3. **Correct Answer: C) "Since it is summer, they can swim in our pool."** It is important not to submerge head in water for 7 to 10 days while being treated for otitis externa. Complete the entire course of topical antibiotic otic drops and medication needs to absorb within ear canal wall for effectiveness. Refer to pediatric otolaryngologist if ear canal swells and unable to instill ear drops. Use a 50:50 solution of acetic acid (white vinegar) and rubbing alcohol to restore pH and prevent recurrence.

4. **Correct Answer: D) Bright red rash with sandpaper texture of skin.** Bright red rash with sandpaper-like rash is characteristic of scarlet fever. Other signs of scarlet fever are fever, abdominal pain, halitosis, and "strawberry tongue."

5. **Correct Answer: B) Have the child lie supine with head turned and pull pinna down and back, instill drops.** Due to the more horizontal position of the eustachian tube in children less than 3 years of age, pinna needs to be pulled down and back. The child should lie in a supine position with their head turned to the appropriate side; they should not sit on the caregiver's lap. Otic drops can be used for treatment of 2-year-old children.

6. **Correct Answer: C) Replace child's toothbrush after 24 hours of antibiotics.** Children are noninfectious after 24 hours of antibiotics. Waiting to replace the child's toothbrush for 10 days, allowing it to air dry, and soaking it in warm salt water will not prevent reinfection.

7. A nurse is assessing a child with obstructive sleep apnea. On assessment, the nurse would expect to find which of the following:

    A. Nasal congestion
    B. Mouth breathing
    C. Deep sleep
    D. Hypernasal speech

8. A nurse is providing discharge instructions to caregivers of a 10-year-old with recurrent epistaxis. What statement by the caregivers indicates the need for further teaching?

    A. "We will discourage nose picking."
    B. "They should lie down and rest during a nosebleed."
    C. "We should have them lean forward and pinch the soft part of the nose during a nosebleed."
    D. "We will put saline spray in the nose a couple of times each day to keep it moist."

9. A nurse is caring for a school-aged child recently diagnosed with SNHL. Her parents ask what they should tell the child's teacher about hearing loss. The nurse's best response is:

    A. "She does not need hearing aids."
    B. "She should sit in the front of the classroom."
    C. "She will need early intervention."
    D. "She has fluid in her ears."

10. A nurse is caring for a child with allergic rhinitis who on assessment has clear rhinorrhea and allergic shiners. Teaching caregivers about reducing exposure to allergens includes:

    A. Giving allergy shots
    B. Opening windows in the home
    C. Limiting smoking by family members to the garage
    D. Encasing child's pillows and mattress with dustproof covers

7. **Correct Answer: B) Mouth breathing.** Signs of obstructive sleep apnea include snoring, mouth breathing, restless sleep, hyponasal speech, difficulty swallowing, and enuresis. Nasal congestion is not a sign of obstructive sleep apnea.

8. **Correct Answer: B) "They should lie down and rest during a nosebleed."** When the nose is actively bleeding, the child should lean forward and either they or the caregiver should pinch the soft part of the nose for up to 15 minutes. Saline spray should be used a few times each day and nose picking should be discouraged.

9. **Correct Answer: B) "She should sit in the front of the classroom."** Preferential seating in the classroom is recommended for all school-aged children with hearing loss. Sensorineural loss' surgical treatment is a cochlear implant for extensive hearing loss which sends impulses to nerve (extremely sensitive to magnets). If the child is under 3 years of age, refer patient and family to early intervention.

10. **Correct Answer: D) Encasing child's pillows and mattress with dustproof covers.** Encasing child's pillows and mattress with dustproof covers will reduce allergen exposure. Allergy shots, opening windows, and smoking outside of the house does not reduce exposure to allergens.

CHAPTER 5

Neurologic Conditions

Gina Galosi

INTRODUCTION TO THE PEDIATRIC NEUROLOGIC SYSTEM FUNCTION

Central Nervous System Functions

- Sensory stimulus gathered from the environment: exteroceptors (external) and/or inter-receptors or proprioceptors (internal).
- The central nervous system (CNS) interprets, integrates, or retains the stimulus in memory.

Neurologic System—Pediatric Considerations

- Neural tube development in first weeks of gestational development; most susceptible time to infection, trauma, teratogens, and nutritional deficiencies from the pregnant individual.
- Development of nervous system and myelinization, proceeds in cephalocaudal, proximodistal progression.
- **Motor development:** Head and neck control develops first, then trunk, then extremities.
- Newborn reflexes (primitive) differentiate with maturity in normal infant/child.
- Head size larger in proportion to body, one-quarter of body height.
- Soft cranium, fontanels, and unfused sutures can result in change in shape of cranium in presence of intracranial pressure.
- Anterior and posterior fontanels provide information regarding intracranial pressure, fontanels close by 2 years of age.

Assessment Includes

- **Developmental history:** developmental age, milestones achieved and lost.
- Prenatal, perinatal (intrapartum), and family history must be investigated, including history of prenatal medications.
- Physical examination includes neurologic functioning for developmental age.
- Assessment of reflexes, cranial nerves, fontanels, and sutures if present (related to age and development).
- **Neurologic functions:** motor, sensory (vision and hearing), reflexes, and head circumference measurements.
- Assessments to include pain using pediatric pain scales.
- Glasgow Coma Scale (GCS) or Pediatric GCS Score (under 5 years old) and points as necessary.
- PERRLA (pupils equal, round, reactive to light and accommodation) exam.

Common Medical Treatments

- Physical/occupational/speech therapy
- Ventricular peritoneal shunt placement

- Ventilation, hyperventilation
- External ventricular drainage
- Ventricular tap
- Vagus nerve stimulator
- Ketogenic diet

PEDIATRIC SKILL 5.1: NEUROLOGIC ASSESSMENT

- Lumbar puncture, assist with
- Kernig's sign
- Brudzinski's sign
- Neurologic assessments
- Percussion of reflexes

AMBLYOPIA

Description

- Commonly referred to as lazy eye; reduced visual acuity in one eye, not related to defects and not immediately corrected with eye glasses
- Possibly resulting from strabismus
- Disuse of the affected eye may lead to loss of vision

Assessment

- Assess both eyes for bilateral symmetry of movement.
- Assess for visual acuity of each eye.
- Assess for central versus peripheral vision loss for the affected eye.

Diagnostics

- Eye exam, pupillary response, and red reflex; Snellen chart.
- Refer to ophthalmologist.

Nursing Interventions

- Cover the unaffected eye to strengthen the affected eye.
- Atropine eye drops to unaffected eye possible treatment inflicting blurriness, alternate to patch covering unaffected eye.

Special Considerations

The earlier the assessment of altered vision, the earlier the treatment can be implemented.

BRAIN TUMOR

Description

- Abnormal growth of tissue in brain; classification based on location and histology: infratentorial or posterior fossa; 60% (cerebellum or brain stem involvement), remaining supratentorial or non-posterior fossa (cerebrum)
- Low-grade gliomas, especially medulloblastoma (most common)

Assessment

- Assess neurologic symptoms based on location, size of tumor, and age of child.
  - Alteration in visual acuity and/or nystagmus, headaches, behavioral changes, loss of developmental milestones, irritability, or change in mood or affect.
  - May include decline in academic performance.
  - **Common neurologic symptoms:** Increased head circumference and bulging fontanelle, especially in infants with open sutures; vomiting; uncoordinated movement or gait; posturing; head tilt; altered vital signs (widening pulse pressure); seizures; cranial nerve palsies; vertigo; difficulty with dexterity of previously mastered skills.
- Assessment of neurologic function and possible obstruction of flow of cerebrospinal fluid (CSF) may show signs of increasing intracranial pressure (IICP) or hydrocephalus depending upon age and presence of fontanels.
- Headaches and pain upon spontaneous actions such as straining, sneezing, coughing, most often upon waking up in the morning.
- **Possible craniopharyngioma (pressure on the pituitary from tumor):** Diabetes insipidus, body temperature fluctuations in regulation, alteration in growth patterns as assessed on growth charts, and altered CSF pressure.

Diagnostics

Imaging studies, usually MRI (CT if MRI not available); tumor biopsy, blood serum tumor marker testing, may include analysis of CSF.

Nursing Interventions

- Preoperative Interventions
  - Preparation and education for child and family for CT or MRI scan
  - Surgical intervention as treatment
  - Radiation therapy (proton therapy) for tumor size reduction prior to surgical intervention for removal
  - Surrounding effects of chemotherapy (hair loss, facial edema)
  - Targeted immunotherapy if available and appropriate
- Postoperative Interventions
  - **Implement usual postoperative actions:** Vital sign assessment, pain management, incision care, neurologic assessment—neuro checks, level of consciousness (LOC).
  - Assess for signs and symptoms of IICP and administer steroids as ordered.
  - Prevent constipation to avoid straining and increasing IICP during elimination.
  - Implement seizure precautions as a safety measure.
  - **Postoperative positioning:** (Supratentorial) Nonoperative side to decrease pressure and prevent shifting of cranial contents into operative area. May elevate head of bed slightly to utilize gravity.
  - **Postoperative positioning:** (Infratentorial) Supine, flat on either side for stabilizing CSF levels.
  - Administer medications to treat diabetes insipidus for craniopharyngioma (discussed previously) as appropriate.

Special Considerations

- Children are hard to diagnose due to spongy, elastic cranial bones, and normal uncoordinated movement related to developmental level.
- Lumbar puncture contraindicated with IICP.

CEREBRAL PALSY

Description

- Neuromuscular disorder as a result of trauma or some sort of disruption to the area of the brain responsible for control of motor function; can cause cognitive disabilities.
- **Possible causes of cerebral palsy (CP):**
  - Birth trauma or anoxia/hypoxic event during pregnancy or surrounding the time of birth (before, during, after).
  - Infection surrounding time of birth (before, during, after).
  - Premature delivery may increase incidence.
- **Conditions associated with CP with varying degrees of severity:**
  - **Classifications:** Nonspastic, spastic, dyskinetic-athetoid, ataxic, or mixed.
    - Poor or abnormal muscle control and tone
    - Uncoordinated muscle movement
  - Intellectual disability may be present with varying degrees.
  - Possible speech, hearing, and/or visual conditions (comorbidities) may be present.
  - May have seizure disorder.
  - Poor dentition, dental anomalies.
  - Poor self-image and self-esteem.
- Nonprogressive disorder.
- In newborns, look for uncoordinated suck or difficulty with sucking while feeding.

Assessment (Mixed Forms Are Frequent)

- **Spastic (hypertonia) and nonspastic (ataxic and dyskinetic)**
  - **In spastic CP, assess for:**
    - Hypertonicity
    - Poor posture control
    - Scissoring of legs
    - Persistent reflexes of earlier developmental age
    - Speech difficulty due to altered muscle control
    - Poor coordination
    - Muscle contractures
  - **In athetotic CP (dyskinetic-athetotic), assess for:**
    - Involuntary, constant, wave-like movements (not during somnolence and increase with stress)
    - Abnormal facial and body movements
    - Decreased fine motor ability
    - Absence of contractures
  - **In ataxic CP, assess for:**
    - Ataxic movements, uncoordinated
    - Decreased equilibrium
    - Decreased muscle coordination
    - Unsteady, wide-based gait

Diagnostics

Based on history and physical examination and assessment of prenatal/perinatal history

Nursing Interventions

- Implement safety measures for uncoordinated movements and altered equilibrium (head gear, elbow pads, bed pads, bedside rails).
- Use short and direct instructions. Provide frequent rest periods and breaks. Provide time for child to complete activities.
- Increase caloric intake based on growth chart plotting as appropriate and based on feeding ability. Increase ease of feeding with easy-to-use appliances and food.
- Consider growth and development; adjust interventions to achieve highest possible developmental level.
- Provide support with actions to improve motor ability, verbal ability, and all forms of communication and educational activities. Employ all possible means for communication such as computers, whiteboards, preset recordings with words and phrases.
- Provide motivation and incentives for achieving small goals.
- Utilize passive and active range of motion (ROM), as appropriate, to decrease incidence of contractures.
- Consult therapies as appropriate, occupational, speech, nutritional, and physical.
- In case of contractures, surgical intervention may be necessary.
- Medications as ordered, such as muscle relaxants and pharmacologic therapy to decrease spasticity as appropriate.

Discharge Planning; Patient and Family Education

- Educate about safety measures, basic care, promotion of highest level of functioning.
- Educate on need for therapies, occupational, speech, physical, and nutritional.

HEADACHES

Description

- **Overview:** Pain in head described as sharp, throbbing, or dull; headaches with sensory implications such as overt sensitivity to light (flashing lights, auras, visual disturbances, may include loss of vision either during or before) and/or sound; often include gastrointestinal implications such as nausea and vomiting
- Considered temporary (hours to 2–3 days possible)
- May be caused by triggers such as food, hormones, lights, stress
- Identification of triggers and prevention

Assessment

- Investigate family history of headaches, migraines.
- Assess for location of headache (front, back, facial, periorbital—localized or generalized area).
- Assess for triggers: food, behaviors, incidents, time of month prior to occurrence of headaches.
- Timing of onset and duration.
- Use PQRST (provocation, quality, region, strength, and time course) for characteristics and gathering of information.
- Assess severity of pain scale; use pain scale specific to patient age and developmental level.
- Assess for factors affecting quality of life and ability to function (school, work, activity level, communication, ability to sleep).

- The clinical presentation of secondary headaches can be considered with the SNOOP(4)Y mnemonic: S—systemic symptoms, N—abnormal neurologic signs, O—acute onset, O—occipital signs, P—precipitated by Valsalva, positional, progressive, parents' lack of a family history, Y—years (patient age <6 years).

Diagnostics

May consider MRI, CT, and/or lumbar puncture if meningitis suspected or to rule out viral/bacterial infections

Nursing Interventions

- Activity and food diary for identification of triggers.
- Stress reduction, meditation, anxiety management strategies.
- Pharmacologic intervention as ordered based on identification of triggers.
- Possible hormonal implications and/or management, if necessary.
- Refer to neurologist for evaluation.

Special Considerations

- May refer to endocrinologist for hormonal link to headaches if appropriate.

HEAD INJURIES

Description

- Injury to the meninges, scalp, skull, or any part of brain/head
- Treatment dependent upon the extent of trauma, damage to the skull and soft tissues; stabilization of head and neck until extent and severity determined
- **Soft tissue injury could be attributed to two causes:**
  - Epidural hemorrhage is located in the space between dura mater and skull.
  - Subdural hemorrhage is located in the dura mater and arachnoid layer.
- **Skull fractures (trauma, accidents, falls, abuse):** interruption of skull integrity categorized by location and type:
  - Depression (caved in area)
  - Linear (simple fracture); most common
  - Basilar (skull base)
- **Concussion (trauma, accidents, falls, abuse):** soft tissues of brain swiftly shifted against skull interior sufficient enough to cause temporary neurologic brain injury or dysfunction with or without brief loss of consciousness and/or amnesia
  - May or may not include altered LOC.
  - Must completely heal or child at risk for continued brain injury (persistent postconcussive symptoms) and closed-head injury with possibility of sudden death.
- **Abusive head trauma (aka Shaken Baby Syndrome):** blood vessel injury within cranium accompanied by high rates of mortality and morbidity

Assessment

- Thorough history of recent head trauma (falls or accidents, possible abuse, or neglect).
- Vital sign assessment, pulse, and blood pressure (possible signs of increasing IICP) and shock.
- Assess signs and symptoms of IICP.

- Assess LOC; pain; decreasing score on GCS; Pediatric GCS; PERRLA if appropriate; unilateral and bilateral extremity movement; reflexes based on developmental level, age, and physical assessment; rhinorrhea; raccoon eyes; and Battle's sign (both related to Basilar fracture).
- Assess visual acuity and memory of incident if able and age appropriate.
- Assess behavior (physical coordination and emotional lability), possible aggression, irritability, withdrawal, opposite of normal, baseline behavior.
- Assess cognition and speech as appropriate, motor function, and for impaired memory, confusion, lethargy, sleep disturbances. Query change in school performance and daily behavior, sleep patterns.
- Assess for nausea and vomiting.
- Neuro checks and vital sign assessment frequently dependent upon severity of condition and injury report.
- Assess for presence of fluid drainage from ears and nose (possible CSF). If fluid present, collect for testing.

Diagnostics

- CT scan.
- Collect fluid—send to lab for CSF identification if present.

Nursing Interventions

- Promote bed rest limiting movement without restraining. Low Fowler's position, as needed.
- Implement seizure precautions as a safety measure until likelihood of seizure is ruled out.
- Decrease stimulation (sensory stimulation). Dim lights, quiet atmosphere, low volumes of speaking. Restrict or limit activities involving electronics such as laptops, phones, texting, reading, and television activity (decreases eye strain and sensory stimulation).
- Assess LOC every 2 hours, awaken child if necessary.
- If suspected intracranial hemorrhage, preparation and education about consult for possible surgical evaluation/intervention for either clot removal or ligation of bleeding vessel as appropriate.
- **Maintain strict intake and output (I&O)**
  - Nothing by mouth (NPO) or clear liquids dependent upon severity of injury, LOC, and presence of nausea and/or vomiting.
  - Initiate fluid restriction as appropriate based on presence of IICP.

Discharge Planning; Patient and Family Education

- Patient and family education as appropriate based on injury, history, age, and developmental level focusing on future injury prevention.
- Patient and family education as appropriate for signs and symptoms of IICP or behavioral changes requiring notification of healthcare clinician.

HYDROCEPHALUS

Description

- Increase of CSF within the four ventricles (area of production) of the brain and/or subarachnoid space (area of reabsorption) due to overproduction, malabsorption, or obstruction. Increased amounts of CSF cause expansion and increased intracranial pressure from ventricular enlargement.
- **Causative factors:** Majority obstructive (noncommunicating hydrocephalus) in nature such as structural abnormality; may be malabsorption of the arachnoid space/nonobstructive (communicative hydrocephalus).

- **Congenital (most common):** Structural malformations such as Arnold–Chiari malformation
- **Acquired:** May be caused by meningitis, prematurity of birth, trauma, and tumors

Assessment

- Depends on age of child; occurs prior to fusion of cranial sutures and closure of fontanels.
- Measurement of head circumference, across forehead above eyebrows (compare to birth measurement and increase of diameter).
- Assess for signs and symptoms of IICP (see Pediatric Pearls).
- Assess cranium, specifically widening sutures, tense, bulging fontanels (anterior), possible distended scalp veins, apnea, bradycardia, and irritability.
- Assess vocalizations of child noting high-pitched cry.
- Assess LOC, irritability, lethargy, possible confusion.
- Assess for "sunset sign" (sclera is visible above the iris) and papilledema.
- Asses for loss of developmental milestones.
- Assess for seizures, if possible.
- Assess for Parinaud syndrome, abnormal eye movements, and pupil dysfunction.

Diagnostics

Cranial ultrasound up to 12 months of age (separated sutures), MRI, CT of brain for emergent situation when MRI not available. Increased radiation exposure with CT.

Nursing Interventions

Focus on decreasing CSF fluid

- **Preshunt insertion:** Education of procedure, expectations of procedure
- **Postshunt insertion interventions**
  - Head circumference measurements above the eyebrows.
  - Postsurgical pain management as needed.
  - Maintain supine, flat position to decrease headache and shifting of CSF fluid (first 24 hours).
  - Avoid positioning on the side of shunt insertion.
- Provide head and neck support if positioned upright after the first 24 hours.
- Parent/caregiver education postoperative care.
- Parent/caregiver education of previously listed signs and symptoms of increased intracranial pressure, infection, possible blockage/malfunction of shunt.

Special Considerations

- Children with hydrocephalus require follow-up for monitoring of complications and/or progression of condition. Follow-up includes shunt imaging.
- Shunt overdrainage (uncommon) may result in headaches and subdural hematoma.

Discharge Planning; Patient and Family Education

Educate family, caregivers, and child (when age appropriate) on signs and symptoms of IICP and shunt infection and malfunction. May need replacement with growth.

INCREASED INTRACRANIAL PRESSURE

See Pediatric Pearls at the end of the chapter.

Description

- CSF pressure >20 mmHg
- Considered a medical emergency

Assessment

- Occurs after fusing of cranial sutures and closing of fontanels.
- **Assess for the following:**
  - LOC, lethargy, difficulty concentrating or following simple commands
  - Motor response and ability, ataxia, uncoordinated movements
  - Nausea and vomiting
  - Headache
  - Papilledema (swollen optic disc)
  - Blurred vision, papilledema, altered pupillary response (assess PERRLA)
  - **Vital signs:** Increased blood pressure in the presence of decreased pulse rate and respirations (Must continue vigilant assessment to avoid respiratory and cardiac arrest.)
  - Cushing reflex (hypertension, bradycardia, and irregular breathing)
- Assess for personality changes by interviewing caregivers.
- Assess for seizure activity.

Diagnostics

CT, lumbar puncture for CSF analysis, once possibility of herniation is ruled out. Possible external ventricular drain for monitoring and decreasing CSF. Surgical intervention, craniectomy for pressure reduction if other means to reduce pressure unsuccessful.

Nursing Interventions

- Position patient to facilitate lessening of intracranial fluid, low to semi-Fowler's position.
- Assess LOC, lethargy, confusion, (sedation may be used to treat agitation).
- Administer medications ordered for osmotic diuresis such as Mannitol, hypertonic saline, and/or corticosteroids (second line).
- I&O, consider limiting fluids as ordered.
- Assess fluid and electrolytes for imbalances.
- Perform hyperventilation with bag-valve-mask device as ordered (not for prolonged use).

Special Considerations

Consider age and presence of fontanels.

Discharge Planning; Patient and Family Teaching

- Teach child and caregivers regarding knowledge of conditions and activities which can increase IICP (fever, pain, seizures, crying, coughing, trauma, physical abuse, straining, strenuous exercise).
- Avoid activities which can increase IICP (constipation and straining, strenuous exercise, trauma, crying, coughing).

LEAD POISONING/PLUMBISM

Description

- Lead poisoning caused by consumption of paint containing lead and paint dust. Some instances caused by drinking water contaminated from lead pipes. Commonly found in older homes prior to the 1970s or when construction/rehabilitation occurs in older homes and with younger children (usually under the age of 5 due to hand-to-mouth developmentally appropriate behavior). Can also be from home remedies as well as unsealed pottery, ceramics, and cookware containing lead.

LEAD POISONING/PLUMBISM

- Lead ingestion may cause neurologic concerns at any blood level but usually at blood lead level (BLL) >5 mcg/dL.
- Screening and education are of highest importance for prevention of lead poisoning.
- Will result in chronic condition if not identified and treated in a timely manner. Can be acute or chronic depending upon exposure amount and length of time.
- Excretion takes place in urine and bile.
- Lead attaches to red blood cells, with deposits accumulating in bone and other tissues.
- Anemia, and damage in other organs such as kidneys and brain resulting in neurologic impairment such as sensory (vision and hearing) and behavioral changes (impulsivity, distractibility, hyperactivity, developmental delays, cognitive impairment); dependent upon length of time and amount of exposure/ingestion of lead.
- Paralysis, blindness, seizures, coma, and death are possible.

Assessment

- Investigate home environment and possibility of contact with lead paint, water from lead pipes, age of home environment, day care, family dwellings, or where child spends time.
- Assess for rehabilitation projects in the home, herbal remedies, and unsealed ceramic or pottery use.
- Assess for bluish discoloration of gingival border (Burtonian blue lines).
- Assess neurologic function, LOC, developmentally appropriate reflexes and milestones based on age and caregiver report of ability.
- Assess for signs and symptoms of neurologic impairment such as behavioral changes, irritability, learning or cognitive impairment, regression in motor ability, possible seizure activity, or coma with elevated levels.
- Assess for gastrointestinal symptoms such as decreased appetite, nausea, vomiting, constipation, and possible abdominal pain.
- Assess laboratory values for kidney function, complete blood count for anemia, and lead levels once suspected.
- Plot height and weight on growth charts assessing for lower percentiles of growth in the case of prolonged lead ingestion chronic exposure.
- Assess for pica or ingestion of nonfood items; approximately 90% of children also have pica.
- Assess for symptoms of anemia such as pallor, fatigue, low hemoglobin, pale mucous membranes, and possible tachycardia.

Diagnostics

- **Laboratory values:** lead levels, kidney and liver function
- Abdominal x-ray if suspected ingestion of lead-containing paint chips

Nursing Interventions

- Educate regarding sources for possible lead ingestion.
- Inclusion of routine screening for possible lead exposure starting at 6 months of age and/or day care.
- I&O
  - Increase of fluids for promotion of kidney function and lead excretion.
  - Assess urinary output amount for kidney function evaluation.
  - Provide specimens for urine testing to provide objective data to evaluate kidney function.
- Educate family and caregivers to decrease and prevent continued ingestion to lower existing lead levels.
- **Chelation treatment for lead poisoning based on blood levels:**

- Greater than 45 can be administered orally or intravenous (IV)
- Greater than 70 requires admission to hospital for treatment
■ Bowel decontamination may be considered for ingestion of lead paint chips or if abdominal x-ray shows radiopaque contents.
■ Education about home testing kits for lead. May also run water for at least 1 minute prior to consuming if water is considered the source of lead.

Special Considerations

■ Educate about lead poisoning contaminants and sources.
■ Activated charcoal does not bind to lead and not used for lead poisoning treatment.

MENINGITIS

Description

■ Inflammation of the meninges, transmitted by droplets:
- **Viral (aseptic) meningitis:** No bacterium identified; no antibiotics unless initiated prior to identification of underling cause (most common enteroviruses)
- **Bacterial (septic) meningitis:** Antibiotics as ordered and based on identification of causal agent

■ *Haemophilus influenzae* type B vaccine as a preventative measure to decrease incidence in children

Assessment

■ As soon as meningitis is suspected, implement isolation precautions and conduct continuing assessment utilizing isolation precautions.
■ Assess for signs and symptoms of IICP such as developmentally appropriate (see Pediatric Pearls).
■ Assess for seizure activity via query of caregivers.
■ Note purpura, petechiae, or purpuric rash (purple); may indicate meningococcal infection (bacterial). This is a medical emergency.
■ **Assess for postural signs that irritate meninges:**
- **Kernig's sign:** Resistance to leg extension from flexed position; positive for pain upon knees flexed and legs raised
- **Brudzinski's sign:** Positive upon passive/deliberate neck flexion, knees and hips flex
- **Opisthotonic position:** Hyperextension of the head, neck, and spine to relieve discomfort; may be a late sign of condition

■ Assess results of CSF specimen sent for evaluation.

Diagnostics

■ Blood culture and lumbar puncture with Gram stain to obtain CSF for evaluation (cloudy, high number of white blood cells [WBCs; mostly neutrophils] and protein counts, low level of glucose level for bacterial meningitis)
■ CT or MRI for IICP or abscess

Nursing Interventions

■ Implement and maintain isolation precautions for a minimum of 24 hours post-antibiotic administration and until determine viral or bacterial.
■ Implement seizure precautions for child safety.
■ Assist with lumbar puncture.

- Monitor vital signs and pain level, I&O, fluid status and neurologic checks every 2 hours, as necessary.
- Decrease stimulation (sensory stimulation). Dim lights, quiet atmosphere, low volumes of speaking. Restrict or limit activities involving electronics such as laptops, phones, texting, reading, and television activity (decreases eye strain and sensory stimulation).
- Position child supine (flat) in bed, limiting movements.
- Avoid coughing and straining.
- Administer antipyretics to reduce fevers and antibiotics (after obtaining cultures) as ordered.

Special Considerations

Immunizations for prevention

NEURAL TUBE DEFECTS (SPINA BIFIDA)

Description

- Group of abnormalities resulting from incomplete development of the neural tube during embryonic period. The neural tube becomes the CNS.
- Degree of the defect differs in severity and is associated with several factors.
- Prenatal care and testing will suggest possibility of neural tube defects (NTD). High amounts of alpha-fetoprotein in amniotic fluid from CSF leakage.
- Types of NTD (classified by involvement of section of CNS):
  - **Anencephaly:** Incompatible with life, usually intrauterine fetal demise or within hours of birth, comfort care measures implemented as appropriate based on gestational age
  - **Encephalocele:** Herniation
  - Spina bifida types (Figure 5.1)
    - **Occulta:** Not able to be seen with the eye. May see a tuft of hair or dimple on sacral area, uneven gluteal folds. Not associated with neurologic deficit.
    - **Meningocele:** Sac of meninges protruding, filled with CSF; no nerve or spinal cord involvement. Not usually associated with neurologic deficit but necessitates surgical intervention for repair of protruding sac.

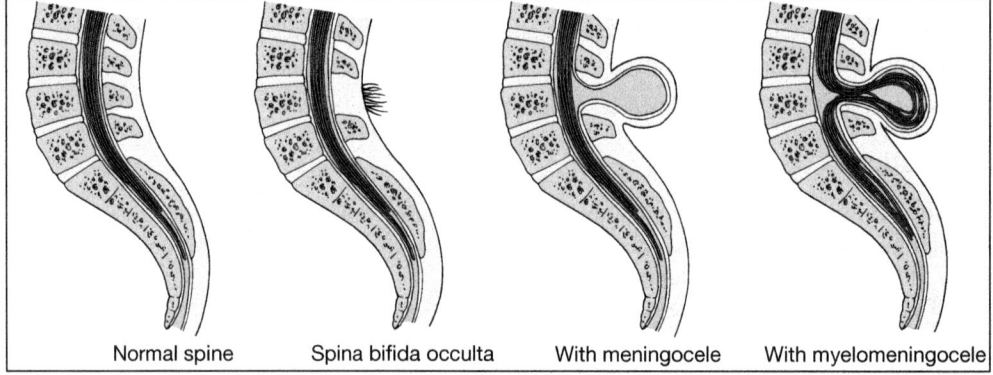

FIGURE 5.1: Normal spine and types of spina bifida

Source: Reprinted from Jnah, A. J., & Trembath, A. N. (2019). *Fetal and neonatal physiology for the advanced practice nurse* (1st ed.). Springer Publishing Company.

NEURAL TUBE DEFECTS (SPINA BIFIDA)

- **Myelomeningocele:** Sac of meninges filled with CSF, nerve, and part of spinal cord involved. Neurologic deficit dependent upon the site of protruding sac and amount of cord involvement. Necessitates surgical intervention for repair of defect.

Assessment

- For spina bifida:
  - **Occulta:** Dimple, tuft of hair; may necessitate an ultrasound of the area
  - **Meningocele and myelomeningocele:**
    - Assess sac for intactness, drainage, leakage.
    - Measure head circumference above the eyebrows for comparison (baseline data to assess for hydrocephalus prior to surgical intervention).
    - Assess for signs and symptoms of infection at sac site, CSF, and/or meninges (redness, exudate, odor, febrile status).
    - Assess for presence and level of motor and sensory deficit distal to the area of the defect.
    - Assess for functional ability for elimination (bowel and bladder function).

- **Preoperative Interventions**
  - Educate family and caregivers on surgical procedure, timing of surgical intervention (24 to 48 hours from delivery).
  - Implement strict aseptic technique to reduce infection.
  - Implement measures to prevent drying of sac (saline-soaked sterile dressing), utilize Silo (sterile plastic bag for protective environment).
  - Maintain prone and side positioning (head to side) to maintain sac integrity, prevent rupture. Avoid increasing pressure in sac and within brain with frequent positioning designed to avoid hydrocephalus and sac rupture.
  - Implement infection control measures. Position child on diaper with meticulous vigilance to decrease infection of sac from urine or stool.

- **Postoperative Assessment**
  - Assess for IICP, measure head circumference, and compare to preoperative measurement for early identification of hydrocephalus.
  - Assess for paralysis and sensation below defect such as spontaneous motor function and sensation of lower extremities in response to touch or pain.
  - **Assess I&O:** Assess for neurogenic bowel and bladder; distended bladder, leakage of urine and/or stool.
  - Consider growth and development and developmental milestones as appropriate.

- **Postoperative Interventions**
  - Postoperative care as required: vital signs, I&O, age-appropriate pain scale and administer ordered pain management therapy.
  - Integument and wound care as necessary maintaining aseptic technique and infection control measures for surgical site.
  - Assess integument for pressure injuries, especially when paralysis present. Implement sheepskin as a protective measure.
  - Assess for infection of surgical site (redness, edema, ecchymosis, drainage, and approximation).
  - Implement education about orthopedic appliances if ordered and as needed.
  - Implement measures to prevent constipation and distended bladder. Teach caregivers aseptic (clean) intermittent catheterization.

- Be aware of high incidence of latex allergies in pediatric population with numerous surgeries (use latex-free no-elastic pants, nipples, pacifiers, or any products with latex).

Diagnostics

Physical assessment and prenatal testing

Special Considerations

- Children with allergies; latex allergies common with pediatric population with multiple surgeries.
- Childbearing people should take 0.8 mg folic acid daily for prevention.

Discharge Planning; Patient and Family Education

Depends upon severity and level of neurologic deficit

SEIZURE DISORDER (COMMONLY REFERRED TO AS EPILEPSY)

Description

- Alteration in normal nerve cell function characterized by abnormal electrical activity in the brain leading to involuntary movement, sensory impairment, behavior disturbances, and possible loss of consciousness.
- Epilepsy refers to a condition of recurrent seizures; status epilepticus refers to a prolonged seizure lasting ≥30 minutes, or a child having several seizures without any consciousness periods (postseizure/postictal phase) in between each seizure.
- **Types of seizures:** Epileptic/infantile, absence (petit mal), clonic, tonic, clonic-tonic (grand mal), myoclonic, atonic, focal (with or without loss of consciousness), status epilepticus.

Assessment

- Gather information including a detailed assessment of changes in development, history of seizures, predisposing factors (fever or injury), and presence of auras, ascertain sensory information prior to seizure.
- Obtain information regarding the timing of seizure, activity before seizure, anatomy involved (muscle groups and extremities involved, bilateral versus unilateral involvement of the body).
- Assess behavior immediately following seizure (postseizure/postictal response) for awareness alert, oriented to person, place, time, and situation, lethargic, confused, uncoordinated motor response.
- Assess neurologic status for deficits.

Diagnostics

Blood laboratory studies to rule out metabolic conditions and provide baseline for anticonvulsant medications; EEG, clinical presentation, may consider MRI.

Nursing Interventions

- Referral to neurologist.
- Prepare environment to keep child safe in the event of seizure activity (pad crib, bed, area, to minimize physical trauma).
- Remain with child and family member, do not leave; use other means to request assistance without leaving.
- Do not try to control or interrupt seizure activity. Remove hazardous objects when possible.
- Do not confine or restrain individual during seizure activity.
- Maintain patient airway.
  - Do not put anything in child's mouth.

- After seizure, administer oxygen when necessary (hypoxia, cyanosis), and after respirations are spontaneous.
- May reposition child to lateral position for airway patency to minimize aspiration of salivary secretions and facilitate open airway, reduce airway blockage from tongue.
■ Documentation of neurologic activity.
  - Timing of start to end of seizure activity.
  - Movement as compared to staring or blinking.
  - Note unilateral or bilateral movement.
■ **Administer ordered medications**.
  - Phenytoin (Dilantin), carbamazepine (Tegretol), valproic acid (Depakote).
  - Diazepam (Valium), rectal suppository, or intranasal midazolam (Versed) if seizure greater than 5 minutes; IV diazepam should only be diluted with 0.9% sodium chloride to prevent precipitation.
■ Obtain serum levels of anticonvulsant medications assessing for therapeutic levels as compared to toxic or sub-therapeutic levels.
■ Prescribed dietary changes may be beneficial such as ketogenic, high fat, low carbohydrate diet.
■ Prepare for brain surgery, if necessary, for intractable seizures.
■ Additional therapy with antiepileptic medications: vagus nerve stimulator (VNS).
  - Indications made by age of patient: ≥4 years if pharmacologic therapy is unsuccessful.
  - Education necessary for child and caregivers regarding appliance and care of appliance.
  - Electrodes placed under skin to stimulate vagus nerve.

Special Considerations
See Pediatric Pearls: Febrile Seizures

Discharge Planning; Patient and Family Education
■ Educate caretakers about disorder, safety measures, activity restrictions, protective environment and timing of seizure activity, anticonvulsant medications, therapeutic levels, and side effects.
■ Teach about VNS.
■ Educate regarding ketogenic diet.
■ Stress importance of notification of schools and other caregivers of condition and wearing of notification bracelet or necklace.
■ Call 911 if first seizure, seizures last for >5 minutes and/or if the child stops breathing.

SENSORY IMPAIRMENT: HEARING IMPAIRMENT

Refer to Chapter 4.

SENSORY IMPAIRMENT: VISUAL IMPAIRMENT

Description
Sense of vision or sight. Provides spatial ability and sensory information; vision provides curiosity of surroundings and motivation for exploration; acuity between 20/70 and 20/200 in better eye (legal blindness <20/200).

Assessment of Vision

- In general, in a position face to face with child:
    - Assess for symmetry (bilateral).
    - Corner of eyes should be equal with pinna of ear.
    - Assess for strabismus and nystagmus.
    - Assess visual acuity using developmentally appropriate tools such as:
        - Sloan letters chart (for children who know the alphabet and letters)
        - Snellen chart
        - Picture chart; useful for preschoolers
        - For infants, use ability to track objects as developmentally appropriate

Assessment of Vision Impaired

- Assess growth and development including achievement of developmental milestones (assess for possible delays).
- Assess parental or caregiver interaction for initiation of eye contact, holding eye contact.
- **Assess for behavioral signs such as:**
    - Movement, purposeful movement, and hesitancy (e.g., accidents, bumping into furniture)
    - Dependency on other children or objects in environment
    - Fear, fear of falling, question if age appropriate of child's ability
    - Ability to focus on objects, reaching for objects, (too near or too far for grasp), ability to track people and/or objects
    - Squinting or blinking (school-aged children) and assess for distance to materials such as books or electronics

Nursing Interventions

- Announce self and others when entering room and when interacting with child.
- Verbalize intended actions clearly prior to initiation of actions.
- Explain all sounds to the child.
- Keep normal-to-bright lighting in child's environment.
- Prevent injury and provide information verbally about safety measures and room information such as furniture placement.
- For children with partial vision, educate child and family about potential aids available (sitting in front of classroom, large print materials, color blocking, and color-coding).

Discharge Planning; Patient and Family Education

Refer to "Nursing Interventions."

PEDIATRIC PEARLS

FEBRILE SEIZURES

- Occurs with fevers rapidly increasing at or above 39 °C (100.2 °F) in children less than 5 years of age with no CNS infection, metabolic disturbance, or history of afebrile seizure (usually benign)
  - **Simple febrile seizure** (65%–90% of febrile seizures) if all of the following criteria are met:
    - Generalized tonic-clonic activity with no focal component (staring, repetitive movements such as lip-smacking, blinking, grunting) and duration ≥15 minutes
    - Occurs no more than once in 24 hours with no previous neurologic problems
  - **Complex febrile seizure**: >15 minutes; has a focal component; or recurs within 24 hours
- Blood, urine, and lumbar testing (CSF to rule out meningitis) to identify source of infection
- Treatment focused on antipyretics

PEDIATRIC PEARLS

SIGNS AND SYMPTOMS OF INCREASED INTRACRANIAL PRESSURE

- Assess for signs and symptoms of IICP such as developmentally appropriate:
  - Vomiting, nausea if old enough to verbalize symptom, or diarrhea.
  - Infants and toddlers under 3 years of age (with patent fontanels) may have high-pitched or weak cry, assess fontanels for bulging (late finding). May possibly exhibit poor suck/swallow and feeding poor muscle tone, irritability, fever, temperature instability.
  - Older children and adolescents may complain of neck pain or nuchal rigidity, headache, possible sensitivity to light, and diplopia.
- **Early signs**
  - Headache; vomiting (possible projectile); altered pupil reaction times; diplopia (vision difficulties); vital sign changes (increased pulse and blood pressure, widening pulse pressure); "sunset sign"; altered LOC; seizure activity; for infants, fontanel, sutures, cranial vein assessment, and high-pitched or weak cry
- **Late signs**
  - Altered LOC, lower levels; altered motor, sensory, and reflex responses; bradycardia; irregular and/or Cheyne-Stokes respirations; fixed or dilated pupils; decerebrate or decorticate positioning

BIBLIOGRAPHY

DynaMed. (2018, November 30). *Febrile seizures*. EBSCO Information Services. Retrieved March 1, 2021, from https://www.dynamed.com/condition/febrile-seizure

DynaMed. (2018, November 30). *Elevated intracranial pressure (ICP) in children*. EBSCO Information Services. Retrieved March 4, 2021, from https://www.dynamed.com/condition/elevated-intracranial-pressure-icp-in-children

DynaMed. (2018, December 4). *Hydrocephalus in children*. EBSCO Information Services. Retrieved March 4, 2021, from https://www.dynamed.com/condition/hydrocephalus-in-children

Hockenberry, M. J., Wilson, D., & Rodgers, C. (2019). *Wong's nursing care of infants and children* (11th ed.). Mosby.

Ricci, S. S., Kyle, T., & Carman, S. (2021). *Maternity and pediatric nursing* (4th ed.). Wolters Kluwer.

Silbert-Flagg, J., & Sloand, E. D. (Eds.). (2017). *Pediatric nurse practitioner certification: Review guide, primary care* (6th ed.). Jones & Bartlett.

KNOWLEDGE CHECK

1. A nurse is caring for a 10-month-old child who is suspected of having hydrocephalus. What would the nurse most likely see in the child?

   A. Increased head circumference above the eyebrows
   B. Loss of verbal ability and low-pitched cry
   C. Increased temperature, shivers, and sweating
   D. Stabilization of head and neck until shunt placement

2. A nurse is assessing a 4-year-old child's neurologic system. Which finding would the nurse document as normal?

   A. Widening cranial sutures
   B. Patent anterior fontanel
   C. Showing interest in other children and fantasy play
   D. Toes flaring when sole stroked from bottom of foot to top

3. A nurse is caring for an infant diagnosed with a seizure disorder. Which statement by the parents indicates the need for further teaching?

   A. "My child will never play sports."
   B. "I will learn how to administer the medications to keep a stable blood level."
   C. "It may be possible for my child to be able to drive even with a seizure disorder."
   D. "The family can adjust to learn how to care for the child."

4. A nurse is teaching a family about providing care for a child with a ventriculoperitoneal shunt. The priority information for the nurse to include is:

   A. The child should be given anti-nausea medicine for gastrointestinal upset.
   B. If the child is difficult to rouse from sleep, the child must be allowed to rest.
   C. If vomiting and confusion occur, bring the child in for shunt evaluation.
   D. Once the shunt is placed, replacement is rarely necessary.

5. A child is brought to the emergency department, a brief history and chief complaint is obtained, and a nurse suspects a diagnosis of meningitis. What should the nurse do first?

   A. Implement isolation precautions until identification of causative factors.
   B. Perform a full neurologic examination for assessment and treatment purposes.
   C. Assess for signs and symptoms of increased intracranial pressure.
   D. Complete a history and physical including assess for allergies.

6. While assessing a child, the nurse notices the patient grimace in pain when the knees are flexed and legs raised. The nurse recognizes this as:

   A. A normal neurologic finding
   B. Impending seizure activity
   C. Kernig's sign
   D. Brudzinski's sign

7. A child is being examined because of increased incidence of headaches. What assessment question is a priority to determine cause?

   A. "What activities are you performing when headaches occur?"
   B. "How long do the headaches last?"
   C. "What activities make the headache better?"
   D. "What activities make the headache worse?"

KNOWLEDGE CHECK

1. **Correct Answer: A) Increased head circumference above the eyebrows.** In the infant, the most obvious indication is often a rapid increase in head circumference. A high-pitched cry is expected, not low; fever is not an expected assessment, nor is stabilization of the head and neck prior to shunt placement. Ten-month-old children are still beginning to display verbal ability with vocalizations.

2. **Correct Answer: C) Shows interest in other children and fantasy play.** Showing interest in other children and in fantasy play can indicate normal development for 4-year-old children. At this age, children should have fused sutures and no fontanels. A positive Babinski reflex should disappear once the child learns to walk.

3. **Correct Answer: A) "My child will never play sports."** There are several sports in which children diagnosed with seizure disorders can participate. Contact sports are to be avoided but other sports such as golf, running, etc. can be explored. The parents will learn about the medication regimen, and the family will adjust to providing care for the child. Driving is a possibility for this patient, but it is not an immediate concern.

4. **Correct Answer: C) If vomiting and confusion occur, bring the child in for shunt evaluation.** The nurse's priority is to address the patient's vomiting and confusion, as these symptoms may indicate IICP due to shunt infection or malfunction. Antiemetics are to be given if the child experiences nausea; they are not to be administered because the child has a shunt. Further assessment is necessary if the child does not easily rouse. Shunts may need replacement possibly due to infection, malfunction, or growth.

5. **Correct Answer: A) Implement isolation precautions until identification of causative factors.** Immediate isolation is warranted until the viral or bacterial cause is determined to prevent the spread of bacterial meningitis. Isolation is required before further neurologic assessment. Assessment of allergies will be necessary before antibiotics are given, but this is not the first priority. Assessment of IICP is not suspected in the question stem at this time but will be a priority assessment, but the first priority is to isolate the patient.

6. **Correct Answer: C) Kernig's sign.** Kernig's sign is tested by flexing legs at the hip and knee, then extending the knee. A positive report of pain along the vertebral column and/or inability to extend knee is a positive sign and indicates irritation of meninges. Brudzinski's sign is tested by the child lying supine with the neck flexed. A positive sign occurs if resistance or pain is met. The child may also passively flex hip and knees in reaction, indicating meningeal irritation. This assessment does not signify impending seizure activity and it is not a normal neurologic finding.

7. **Correct Answer: A) "What activities are you performing when headaches occur?"** It is important to ask which activities are associated with headache onset because it will help determine possible triggers for the headaches. Asking the patient about the duration of the headaches, and what makes the headaches better or worse direct the inquiry to after the headache has already occurred and do not address causative factors.

8. While examining a 10-month-old infant during a routine visit, the nurse notices the infant does not track objects. As part of the plan of care, the nurse should implement which priority intervention?

   A. Take steps to visualize the retina.
   B. Obtain an order for optic nerve imaging.
   C. Refer to an ophthalmologist for further evaluation.
   D. Interview the parent for a complete perinatal history.

9. A nurse is caring for a child diagnosed with a myelomeningocele preoperatively. What intervention is of highest priority?

   A. Maintaining the integrity of the protruding sac
   B. Vital signs and assessment of LOC
   C. Strict measurement of I&O
   D. Shift assessment of the head circumference

10. A lumbar puncture is ordered for a pediatric patient. The nurse understands that a lumbar puncture is performed to:

    A. Examine the cerebrospinal fluid for evaluation capabilities.
    B. Identify extent of neurologic involvement.
    C. Determine prognosis and length of treatment.
    D. Replace neurologic imaging for diagnosis.

KNOWLEDGE CHECK

8. **Correct Answer: C) Refer to an ophthalmologist for further evaluation.** A 10-month-old infant should be tracking objects visually (usually by 3 months of age). It is important for the nurse to refer the child for further investigation and obtain treatment as early as possible. The nurse's priority in the plan of care will not include visualization of the retina or optic nerve imaging since this is a routine visit and assessing developmental milestones. A complete perinatal history will not provide the priority information for further assessment of the lack of ability to visually track an object.

9. **Correct Answer: A) Maintaining the integrity of the protruding sac.** Rupture of the sac provides a portal of entry for infection that can lead directly to meningitis because of an opening into the brain and spinal cord of the myelomeningocele, complicating the impending surgery. Vital signs, LOC, I&O, and head circumference are important, but the integrity of the sac is the highest importance until the surgical repair.

10. **Correct Answer: A) Examine the cerebrospinal fluid for evaluation capabilities.** The lumbar puncture is the vehicle for obtaining the CSF specimen for examination and testing purposes. The CSF does not determine the extent of neurologic involvement, does not determine the prognosis or length of treatment, nor does it replace imaging.

CHAPTER 6

Respiratory Conditions

Barbara Butynskyi

INTRODUCTION

Respiratory disorders are the most common causes of illness and hospitalization in children and account for the majority of acute illnesses in children. In the pediatric patient, anatomical differences from the adult airway place the infant and child at greater risk and account for both the frequency and severity of respiratory illness.

INTRODUCTION TO PEDIATRIC MUSCULOSKELETAL SYSTEM

Because infants and children are not just little adults, anatomical differences can affect progression and severity of the illness.

- Infants and children have smaller, narrower airways, so inflammation, edema, and secretions can impede oxygenation.
- The tongue of an infant or child is large and can by itself occlude the airway patency.
  - Positioning is vital to support an open airway.
- Young infants until approximately 6 weeks of age are obligatory nose breathers, making nasal congestion and secretions a bigger threat for them.
- The neck muscles of an infant are not as developed, so airway support must be managed with optimal positioning.
- Children have enlarged tonsillar and adenoid tissue, which can lead to airway obstruction.
  - Airway lumen is smaller in infants and children than in adults, and when edema, mucus, or bronchospasm is present, the capacity for air passage is greatly diminished.
- Reduction in the diameter of a child's airway will result in a greater increase in resistance to airflow, causing increased work or breathing.
- Child's airway is highly compliant, making it quite susceptible to collapse during airway obstruction.
- Location of the trachea at the third thoracic vertebra in children (as opposed to the sixth in adults) has implications when suctioning children and assessing for risk for aspiration.
- Children have a significantly higher metabolic rate than adults and this affects normal oxygen transport.
- Exposure to environmental smoke can increase the incidence of respiratory illnesses such as asthma, bronchitis, and pneumonia.

PEDIATRIC PEARLS

- Nursing care is always directed at the priority of maintaining patent airway and providing adequate oxygenation.

RESPIRATORY ASSESSMENT PARAMETERS

Initial Assessment

- Assess for history/birth record for acquired, congenital, genetic disorders or circumstances that might affect the child's respiratory system.
  - Assess for exposure to secondhand smoke, close living quarters, vaccine history, daycare/school attendance, and urban or rural environment.
- Assess for respiratory symptoms, including onset, severity, precipitating factors, and illness exposures.
- Assess for signs and symptoms that may include:
  - Shortness of breath, cyanosis, assumed position of comfort to ease respiratory effort, chest pain, chest congestion, nasal congestion, and cough
  - Fever, irritability, difficulty feeding, and allergies

Physical Assessment

Inspection

- Infants and young children breathe regularly irregular, so a full minute is required to count the rate (Table 6.1). Note depth, quality, and work of breathing.
- Note inspiratory/expiratory ratio; inspiratory phase should be about 2x the expiratory phase. Prolonged inspiration could indicate foreign body obstruction; prolonged expiratory phase could indicate lower obstruction of airway such as asthma.
- Assess for signs and symptoms that may include:
  - Shortness of breath, cyanosis, assumed position of comfort to ease respiratory effort, chest pain, chest congestion, nasal congestion, and cough
  - Fever, irritability, difficulty feeding, and allergies
- **Observe for skin color:** Pallor, cyanosis, acrocyanosis (normal in newborns in first 4 hours of life), clubbing.
- **Rate and depth of respirations:** Tachypnea, bradypnea, or apnea.
- **Cough and other airway noises:** Quality of air movement (atelectasis), stridor, wheeze, rales, rhonchi.
- Note respiratory effort, expiratory grunting, nasal flaring, and retracting are hallmarks of infant respiratory distress.
  - Retractions (Figure 6.1)
  - **Supra sternal, and supra-clavicular:** Observed in upper airway inflammation and obstruction such as croup, epiglottitis, foreign body occlusion
  - **Sub-costal and sub-sternal, intercostal:** Observed in lower airway inflammation and obstruction such as asthma, pneumonia, newborn respiratory distress syndrome (NRDS)
  - See-saw respirations (paradoxical breathing) is a very ineffective pattern to support gas exchange. Chest falls on inspiration, rises on expiration

TABLE 6.1: Normal Respiratory Rates for Infants and Children

Age	Respiratory Rate (breaths/min)
Infant	30–60
Toddler	24–40
Preschooler	22–34
School-aged child	18–30
Adolescent	12–16

Source: Adapted from University of Iowa Stead Family Children's Hospital. (n.d.). *Vital signs: Normal respiratory rate (PICU chart)*. https://uichildrens.org/health-library/vital-signs-normal-respiratory-rate-picu-chart

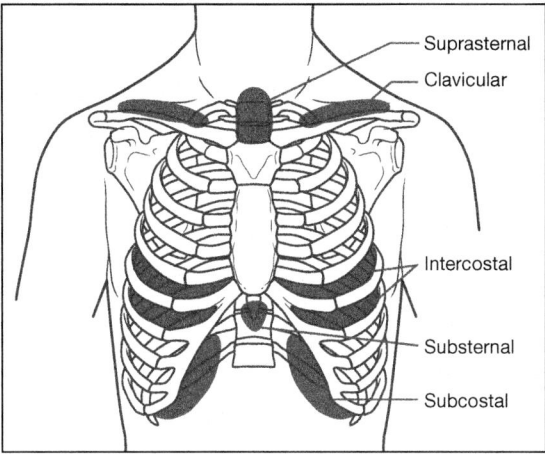

FIGURE 6.1: Anatomic locations of retractions
Source: Adapted from Chiocca, E. M. (2019). *Advanced pediatric assessment* (3rd ed.). Springer Publishing Company.

Auscultation

- Note location and intensity of adventitious breath sounds:
  - **Wheezing:** High-pitched whistling sound usually heard on expiration.
    - Results from lower airway obstruction. If wheezing clears with coughing it is usually the result of accumulation of secretions.
  - **Stridor**: Inflammation and narrowing of the upper airway.
  - **Rales**: Intermittent high-pitched sounds noted on inspiration or expiration.
    - Caused by fluid in the small airways or alveoli. Can also be heard with atelectasis as small airways open
  - **Rhonchi:** Low-pitched continuous breathing sounds that resembles snoring or gurgling. Rhonchi are best heard in the expiration phase.

PEDIATRIC PEARLS

- Infants and young children have very thin chest walls. When there is upper airway congestion, the noise may be transmitted throughout the lung fields. If heard, try to reevaluate after the child coughs or nasal suction has been performed.

Percussion

- A dull or flat sound would be percussed over partially consolidated lung tissue, as occurs with pneumonia.
- Fremitus (vibration felt over the chest wall), found on palpation as vibrations noticed during speech. Fremitus is abnormal when it is increased or decreased.
  - Because sound is transmitted more strongly through non-air-filled lung, increased fremitus suggests a loss or decrease in ventilation in the underlying lung.
- Tympany might be percussed with pneumothorax, and hyperresonance might be apparent with asthma.

Diagnostics for Respiratory Dysfunction

- **Pulse oximetry:** Oxygen saturation might be decreased significantly or be maintained. If O_2 saturation is maintained during periods of work of breathing, the child still may require

supplemental O₂ because respiratory fatigue is likely and the child may quickly desaturate with O₂ readings falling rapidly.
- **Chest radiograph:** Might reveal hyperinflation and patchy areas of atelectasis or infiltration.
- **Blood gases:** Might show carbon dioxide retention and hypoxemia.
- **Nasal-pharyngeal washings:** Positive identification of respiratory syncytial virus (RSV) can be made via enzyme-linked immunosorbent assay (ELISA) or immunofluorescent antibody (IFA) testing.
- Nasal and pharyngeal cultures can be done to detect virus and bacterial pathogens.
- **Sweat chloride test:** Considered suspicious if the level of chloride in collected sweat is above 50 mEq/L and diagnostic if the level is above 60 mEq/L.
- **Pulmonary function tests:** Might reveal a decrease in forced vital capacity and forced expiratory volume, with increase in residual volume.

Nursing Interventions: Oxygen Delivery Systems

- The administration of oxygen to children requires the selection of an oxygen delivery system that suits the child's age, size, needs, clinical condition, and therapeutic goals.
- Oxygen delivery systems are categorized as low-flow systems or high-flow systems.
    - With low-flow systems, 100% oxygen mixes with room air during inspiration, and room air is entrained, making the percentage of delivered oxygen variable.
    - High-flow devices provide such a high flow of premixed gas that the child is not required to inhale room air.
- Supplemental oxygen therapy is often recommended for children when peripheral oxygen saturation is consistently below 94%.
- Selection of delivery devices (Table 6.2).
- Oxygen can dry the respiratory system; many oxygen delivery systems allow for humidification. Especially in infants and younger children, humidity is recommended for oxygen delivery.

ASTHMA

Description

- Chronic inflammatory airway disease resulting from a hyper-responsiveness of the airway to irritants (triggers) characterized by swelling and excess mucous production, resulting in

TABLE 6.2: Oxygen Delivery Devices

Delivery Device	Description
1. Low-flow nasal cannula	• Used for pediatric patients who need oxygen concentrations 22%–60% • Allows child to eat, talk, and cough without interrupting oxygen delivery
2. High-flow nasal cannula	• Used when a higher FiO_2 with some end-expiratory pressure is required and ventilation is adequate
3. Simple face mask	• Low-flow device for children who need approximately 0.35–0.6 FiO_2
4. Partial rebreathing mask with reservoir, a nonrebreathing mask with reservoir, Venturi mask)	• Used for pediatric patients who need precise delivery of FiO_2 concentrations, not affected by airflow, particularly between 24% and 40%
5. Face tent and oxygen hood	• Deliver supplemental oxygen to children to treat hypoxia, respiratory distress, and respiratory failure with high humidity

narrowed airways. Initially there is a release of inflammatory mediators from the bronchial mast cells, followed by activation of additional inflammatory cell activity.
- Alterations in the autonomic neural control of airway tone create a hyper-responsiveness in the smooth muscle of the airway.
- Accounts for a majority of childhood disease and absence from school. Most children experience their first attack by 5 years of age.
- **Three components of altered airway functioning:** Bronchial spasm, inflammation/swelling, and mucous production.
- **Common triggers for an asthma attack include** (Note: non-exhaustive list):
  - **Allergens:** Dust, mold, animal dander, food, food preservatives
  - Viral infections
  - **Irritants:** Pollution, cigarette smoke, perfume, laundry detergent
  - **Environmental:** Rapid change in environmental temperatures, exercise, psychological stressors

Assessment

- Assess for exposure to triggers.
- Assess for wheezing, dyspnea, cough.
  - Could only be a cough in cough variant asthma
- Observe for use of accessory muscles, anxiety.
- Auscultate for decreased air movement or wheezes/other added breath sounds.

Diagnostics

- Classification (Table 6.3)

Nursing Interventions

- Stepwise approach towards treatment (Figure 6.2)
- **Medications:**

TABLE 6.3: Classification of Asthma Severity

				For adults and children aged >5 years who can use a spirometer or peak flow meter	
Classification	Step	Days With Symptoms	Nights With Symptoms	FEV1 or PEF* Percentage Predicted Normal	PEF Variability (%)
Severe persistent	4	Continual	Frequent	≤60	>30
Moderate persistent	3	Daily	>1/week	>60–<80	>30
Mild persistent	2	>2/week but <1 time/day	>2/month	≥80	20–30
Mild intermittent	1	≤2/week	<2/month	≥80	<20

Note: *Percentage predicted values for FEV1 and percentage of personal best for PEF.
FEV1, forced expiratory volume in 1 second; PEF, peak expiratory flow.
Source: Adapted from the Centers for Disease Control and Prevention.

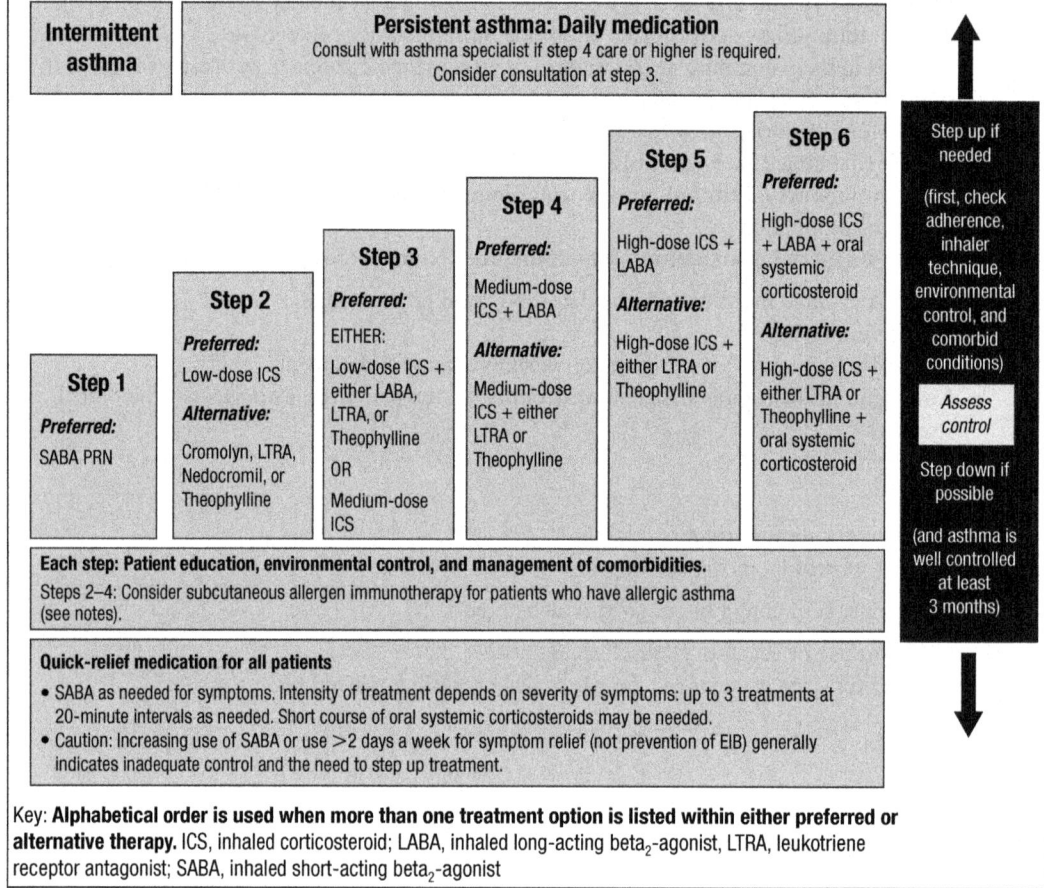

FIGURE 6.2: Stepwise approach for managing asthma in children 5 to 11 years of age

Source: Courtesy of National Asthma Education and Prevention Program, Third Expert Panel on the Diagnosis and Management of Asthma. National Heart, Lung, and Blood Institute (US); 2007 Aug.

- Bronchodilator (Albuterol)
- **Steroids:** Prednisone, Prednisolone (oral), Fluticonase, Budesonide, Beclomethasone, Mometasone
  - (Inhaled) corticosteroids oral/intramuscular (IM)/intravenous (IV; acute phase) and inhaled (maintenance) provide local and long-term anti-inflammatory action. Not for management of acute asthma attack.
    - Mouth should be rinsed thoroughly after inhalation to prevent the incidence of fungal infections.
- **Leukotriene receptor antagonist:** Monteleukast, zafirlukast. Used for treatment of nasal congestion and runny nose associated with allergies, common cold, and sinusitis
  - Nebulizers
  - Metered-dose inhalers (MDIs)
  - Dry powder inhalers
  - Diskus
- **Spacers (with a tight-fitting mask):** Should be used in the pediatric population to assure that medication is adequately administered. A crying child will still breathe in the medication (Figure 6.3).

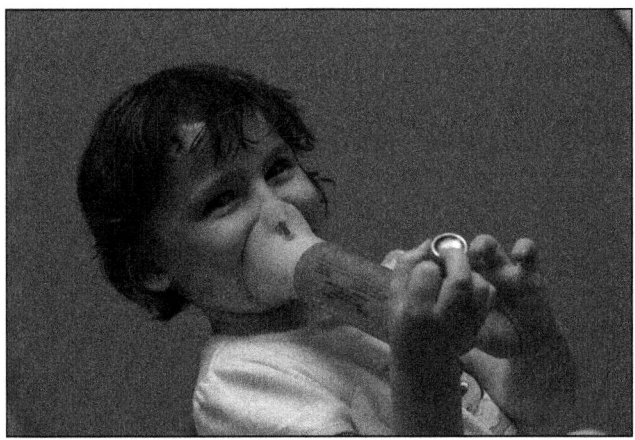

FIGURE 6.3: Pediatric asthma sufferers can use a spacer to inhale medicine
Source: Courtesy of Tradimus, licensed under CC BY-SA 3.0.

Special Considerations

- Steroids will reduce the immune response, so healthcare clinician should be notified if vaccinations are to be given during treatment with corticosteroids.
- Long-term steroids can increase the likelihood for peptic ulcer development and altered growth.
- Steroids can also elevate the blood sugar, and long-term use can affect bone growth and density.

PEDIATRIC SKILL 6.1: USE OF PEAK FLOW METER

- Readings from a peak flow meter can help recognize early changes that may be signs of worsening asthma.
- During an asthma attack, the smooth muscles that surround the airways tighten and cause the airways to narrow.
- The peak flow meter (Figure 6.4) alerts the patient/family to the tightening of the airways often hours or even days before asthma symptoms appear. By using the meter with the Asthma Action Plan at home, the patient/family will know when to take rescue (quick acting) asthma inhaler or other asthma medicine.

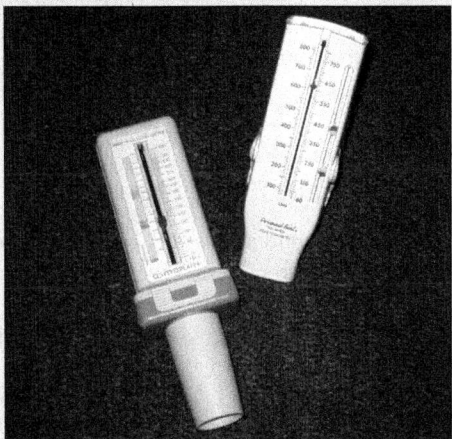

FIGURE 6.4: Peak flow meters
Source: Courtesy of Hosse.

(continued)

- Directions for use:
  1. Have the patient stand up or sit up straight.
  2. Make sure the indicator is at the bottom of the meter (zero).
  3. Take a deep breath in, filling the lungs completely.
  4. Place the mouthpiece in your mouth; lightly bite with your teeth and close your lips on it. Be sure your tongue is away from the mouthpiece.
  5. Blast the air out as hard and as fast as possible in a single blow.
  6. Remove the meter from your mouth.
  7. Record the number that appears on the meter and then repeat steps one through seven two more times.
  8. Record the highest of the three readings in an asthma diary. This reading is your peak expiratory flow (PEF).
- Interpretation of peak flow meter results:
  - **Green:** This zone is from 80% to 100% of the child's personal best peak flow reading. This is the zone the child should be in every day. This is a signal that air moves well through their airways. It means that the child can do their normal activities and go to sleep without trouble. When the peak flow readings are in this zone, the child should:
    - Stay away from asthma triggers.
    - Use controller medicines every day.
    - Use the reliever medicines 15 to 20 minutes before exercise if the child's asthma is triggered by exercise, as directed by the child's clinician.
  - **Yellow:** This zone is from 50% to 80% of the child's personal best peak flow reading. This is a clue that the airways are starting to narrow. The child may begin to have mild symptoms. The child may be coughing, feeling tired, feeling short of breath, or feeling like their chest is tightening. These symptoms may keep the child from their normal activities or from sleeping well. To keep the child's peak flow numbers from getting worse and get the child's asthma back under control, you will need to:
    - Keep using the controller medicine as the child's clinician has ordered and stay away from asthma triggers.
    - Use the reliever medicine as ordered by the child's clinician.
    - Make sure the child is using their inhaler and spacer correctly.
  - **Red:** This zone is less than 50% of the child's personal best peak flow reading. Readings in this zone are a medical emergency. The child will need to get help right away. This means there is severe narrowing of the airways. The child may be coughing, very short of breath, and wheezing, and may also have problems walking and talking. The child should use their reliever medicine and you should call the child's clinician, go to the hospital emergency department, or call 911.

Discharge Planning; Parent and Family Education

- **Patient and Family Education:** Instruct child and family on disease process, trigger exposure, signs, symptoms, and medication regimen. A well-developed Asthma Action Plan should be initiated (see Exhibit 6.1.).
- The family should be familiar with recognition of green, yellow, and red zones, and the appropriate actions for each zone.
- Advise the caregivers to keep this posted in a prominent place in the home (e.g., the refrigerator) for quick reference.
- Education and management are focused on identifying and avoiding triggers.
- Status asthmaticus is an acute, prolonged, severe asthma attack, which is unresponsive to usual treatments.
  - Priorities of care include maintaining the airway and adequate oxygenation and ventilation of the child.

Asthma Action Plan

For: _____ **Doctor:** _____ **Date:** _____
Doctor's Phone Number _____ **Hospital/Emergency Department Phone Number** _____

GREEN ZONE — Doing Well
- No cough, wheeze, chest tightness, or shortness of breath during the day or night
- Can do usual activities

And, if a peak flow meter is used,
Peak flow: more than _____
(80 percent or more of my best peak flow)

My best peak flow is: _____

Take these long-term control medicines each day (include an anti-inflammatory).

Medicine	How much to take	When to take it

Before exercise | ☐ _____ | ☐ 2 or ☐ 4 puffs _____ | 5 minutes before exercise

YELLOW ZONE — Asthma Is Getting Worse
- Cough, wheeze, chest tightness, or shortness of breath, or
- Waking at night due to asthma, or
- Can do some, but not all, usual activities

-Or-

Peak flow: _____ to _____
(50 to 79 percent of my best peak flow)

First Add: quick-relief medicine—and keep taking your GREEN ZONE medicine.
_____ (short-acting beta₂-agonist) ☐ 2 or ☐ 4 puffs, every 20 minutes for up to 1 hour
☐ Nebulizer, once

Second If your symptoms (and peak flow, if used) return to GREEN ZONE after 1 hour of above treatment:
☐ Continue monitoring to be sure you stay in the green zone.

-Or-

If your symptoms (and peak flow, if used) do not return to GREEN ZONE after 1 hour of above treatment:
☐ Take: _____ (short-acting beta₂-agonist) ☐ 2 or ☐ 4 puffs or ☐ Nebulizer
☐ Add: _____ (oral steroid) _____ mg per day For _____ (3–10) days
☐ Call the doctor ☐ before/ ☐ within _____ hours after taking the oral steroid.

RED ZONE — Medical Alert!
- Very short of breath, or
- Quick-relief medicines have not helped, or
- Cannot do usual activities, or
- Symptoms are same or get worse after 24 hours in Yellow Zone

-Or-

Peak flow: less than _____
(50 percent of my best peak flow)

Take this medicine:
☐ _____ (short-acting beta₂-agonist) ☐ 4 or ☐ 6 puffs or ☐ Nebulizer
☐ _____ (oral steroid) _____ mg

Then call your doctor NOW. Go to the hospital or call an ambulance if:
- You are still in the red zone after 15 minutes AND
- You have not reached your doctor.

DANGER SIGNS
- Trouble walking and talking due to shortness of breath
- Lips or fingernails are blue

- Take ☐ 4 or ☐ 6 puffs of your quick-relief medicine AND
- Go to the hospital or call for an ambulance _____ (phone) NOW!

See the reverse side for things you can do to avoid your asthma triggers.

EXHIBIT 6.1: ASTHMA ACTION PLAN

Source: Adapted from National Heart Lung and Blood Institute, a Division of the National Institute of Health; a United States Government agency.

BRONCHOPULMONARY DYSPLASIA

Description

- Chronic pulmonary disease in infancy, characterized by need for oxygen therapy beyond the first 28 days of life.
- Can affect neonates born before 30 weeks of gestation, especially those of very low birth weight and those with respiratory disorders such as meconium aspiration and respiratory distress syndrome.
- Exact cause is unknown but thought to be the result of early lung injury related to mechanical ventilation with high oxygen concentration and pressures. Positive airway pressures and high oxygen concentrations injure alveolar sacs small airway epithelium leading to fibrosis.
  - Airway smooth muscle hypertrophy leads to bronchospasm and interstitial edema.
- May have right-sided heart failure, hepatomegaly, periorbital edema, possibly pulmonary edema.
- Clubbing may be seen with severe disease.
- Pulmonary function test may reveal increased airway resistance and decreased lung compliance.

Assessment

- Assess for cyanosis, tachypnea, grunting, flaring, and retractions when breathing room air.
- Assess for increased anterior-posterior diameter of the chest.
- Assess for right-sided heart failure signs: periorbital edema, hepatomegaly, and/or jugular distention.
- Assess for left-sided heart failure signs: productive cough and pulmonary edema.

- Height and weight are generally in the lower 50th percentile.
  - May present as failure to thrive (FTT) from poor nutrition and prolonged hospitalization.

Diagnostics

- Pulmonary function testing may reveal increased airway resistance, decreased lung compliance (stiffness of lungs), and increased functional residual capacity.
- Chest x-ray reveals the characteristic streakiness, with areas of atelectasis and hyperinflation.
- EKG and echocardiogram results may show right sided heart failure.

Nursing Interventions

- Support safe oxygen weaning; wean as oxygen saturation allows and observe for increased evidence of respiratory distress.
  - Promote optimal oxygenation.
- Administer medications, usually bronchodilators, anti-inflammatory medications, and antibiotics (if indicated).
  - Diuretics are prescribed for symptoms of heart failure.
- Promote adequate nutrition; nasogastric tube (NG) feedings if oral feedings cause increased respiratory distress and increased work of breathing.

PEDIATRIC PEARLS

- There is a high rate of mortality associated with bronchopulmonary dysplasia (BPD) in the first year of life.
- The ability to wean mechanical ventilation and high oxygen concentrations as allowable will decrease the incidence of BPD.

Special Considerations

Surfactant administration in the preterm neonate has significantly reduced the time and pressures used in mechanical ventilation.

Discharge Planning; Patient and Family Education

- Support family coping and provide education on infant CPR instruction.
- Review of medication schedule and determine family's ability to obtain home medications.
- Have caregivers administer medications prior to discharge to ascertain correct dosing and understanding regarding the various medications.

BRONCHIOLITIS

Description

- Inflammation of the lower respiratory tract, associated with swelling of tissue, and increased mucous production. This constricts the lumen of the airway and can lead to air trapping and hyperinflation of the lungs.
- This can lead to atelectasis and alveolar collapse leading to impaired gas exchange.
- May have a hereditary aspect with possible type-2 collagen gene defects.
- Exact cause is unknown, self-limiting process.
- RSV accounts for a vast majority of cases of bronchiolitis.
  - Peak season for RSV is winter and early spring.
  - Severity of disease is usually greater in infants, with toddlers experiencing more upper airway symptoms.

CROUP SYNDROMES

- Common sources of infection include daycare centers and places where groups of children can be found.

Assessment

- Assess for rhinorrhea, harsh cough, wheezing, diffuse rhonchi or crackles, and intermittent fever.
- Onset of illness with a clear runny nose (sometimes profuse), pharyngitis, low-grade fever, poor feeding secondary to lethargy, and/or increased work of breathing.
- Assess for tachycardia, tachypnea, and the presence of fine crackles/rhonchi or wheezes upon auscultation.

Diagnostics

- Nasal swab to identify the RSV virus
- Chest x-ray if pneumonia is suspected
  - Findings usually demonstrate hyperinflation of the lungs.

Nursing Interventions

- Cluster nursing care; allow for rest and activities that diminish energy expenditure.
- Treatment is supportive; oxygen as needed, adequate hydration; monitor intake and output (I&O), normal saline solution (NSS) and suction to mobilize secretions, especially prior to oral feeding.
- Maintain head of bed elevated, keep nares patent.
- Tylenol as needed for fever or discomfort.
- IV hydration is recommended to maintain adequate hydration as well as to keep secretions loose and mobile.
- Institute contact and droplet precautions.

PEDIATRIC PEARLS

- For infants, when respiratory rates exceed 60/minute, oral feedings should be held to reduce the threat of aspiration.
- Fever could indicate super-infection (pneumonia) requiring antibiotic therapy.

Special Considerations

This virus is highly contagious especially in infancy, immune-compromised patients, and the preterm infant; implement precautions, children with RSV bronchiolitis may share a common room.

Discharge Planning; Patient and Family Education

- Preterm infants, and those born with chronic lung or congenital heart defects, may meet the requirements for receiving the medication paivizumab (Synagis) to prevent RSV infection.
- Prevention with good hand washing, avoid crowded areas during RSV season.
- Cough may persist for several weeks after an acute infection.
- Instruct caregivers about signs and symptoms of worsening respiratory distress.

CROUP SYNDROMES

Description

- Croup refers to an infection (usually viral) of the upper airway, which obstructs breathing and causes a characteristic barking cough.

CROUP SYNDROMES

- **Laryngotracheobronchitis (LTB):** Inflammation and narrowing of the laryngeal and tracheal areas of the airway.
  - Most common form of croup for children less than 6 years of age
- **Spasmodic croup:** Similar to LTB but tends to occur at night.
  - Seen most commonly in 3 months to 3 years of age
  - Usually occurs in children under 5 years old
- Self-limiting and generally lasts 3 to 5 days.

Assessment

- Assess for harsh barky cough and audible stridor.
- Assess for history of having an upper respiratory infection (URI) prior to the onset of symptoms.
- Assess for gradual onset of URI symptoms.
- Increased distress with stridor, or stridor at rest should be treated more emergently.

Diagnostics

- History and physical findings.
- Radiographs of chest may be performed; noted steeple sign indicates the glottic and subglottic narrowing of the airway typically seen in children with croup.

Nursing Interventions

- Cool mist humidity
- Steroids to reduce inflammation
- Racemic epinephrine (alpha-adrenergic)
  - Child should be observed for a period of 4 hours following the administration of racemic epinephrine. Children with croup who are treated with nebulized racemic epinephrine may develop reemergence of symptoms, but they are not worse than baseline (rebound effect was previously called). Current research suggests they do not have rebound phenomenon.
  - The reemergence of symptoms after treatment with nebulized racemic epinephrine is less pronounced in children who had concurrent treatment with oral or parenteral glucocorticoids. Hence children who have had moderate-to-severe croup receiving nebulized adrenaline should be given oral or parenteral glucocorticoids.

PEDIATRIC PEARLS

- When in doubt about severity, give racemic epinephrine and observe for 3 to 4 hours for recurrence of stridor. The biggest pitfall is not observing long enough and discharging the child only to see them back in the hospital or clinic several hours later with recurrent stridor.
- Be sure to discuss what to expect and close follow-up with parents if the child is to be discharged home.

Special Considerations

Cool mist humidification (not a warm vaporizer), such as that from a home freezer may assist with the suppression of laryngeal edema and narrowing of the airways.

Discharge Planning; Patient and Family Education

- Educate parent to provide cool (preferably) or warm, moist air to assist with breathing easier.
  - If your child has symptoms of croup, take him into the bathroom, close the bathroom door, and turn on a hot shower. Do not put your child under the shower. Sit with your child in the

warm, moist air for 15 to 20 minutes. If it is cool outside, take your clothed child outside into the cool, moist air for 5 minutes.
- Use a cool mist humidifier in the child's room. This may also make it easier for the child to breathe and help decrease cough.
- Educate parent to keep the child calm as possible, allow the child to rest as much as possible.
- Offer the child small amounts of room temperature liquids every hour.
- Do not let others smoke around the child. Smoke can make the child's breathing and coughing worse.

EPIGLOTTITIS

Description

- Acute and severe inflammation and swelling of the epiglottis (Figure 6.5) due to *Haemophilus influenza* type b (Hib) bacteria, which is the same bacteria that causes pneumonia and meningitis.
- It is a sudden onset with fever, lethargy, and dyspnea.
- Transmission of the bacteria is the same as with the common cold; droplets of saliva or mucus are spread into the air when a carrier of the bacteria coughs or sneezes.
- Emergent situation! DO NOT ATTEMPT TO VISUALIZE THE THROAT as this may precipitate airway closure.
- Seen most commonly in children 3 to 5 years of age.
- Child is more toxic appearing than in other croup syndrome.
  - With epiglottitis, children look worse than they sound (stridor may be present). whereas in croup, children sound worse than they look.
- Decreased incidence with introduction of Hib vaccine in infancy.

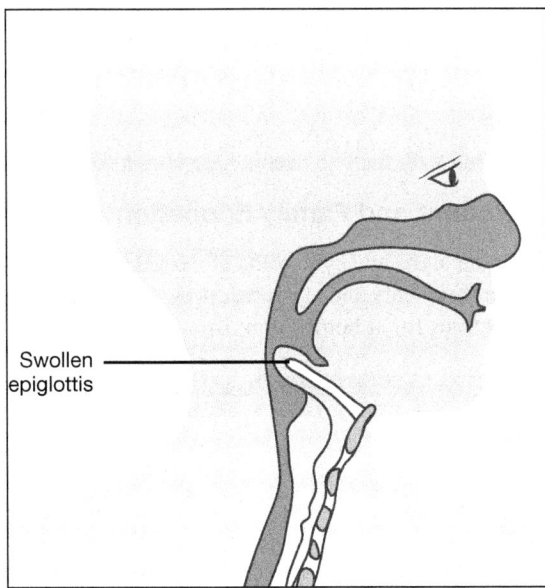

FIGURE 6.5: Swollen epiglottis in acute epiglottitis

Source: Adapted from Slota, M. (2018). *AACN core curriculum for pediatric high acuity, progressive, and critical care nursing* (3rd ed.). Springer Publishing Company.

Assessment

- Assess for anxious expression and severe shortness of breath/increased work of breathing.
- Child presents in tripod positioning, drooling, hyperextension of the neck, and making little to no sound; does not have a croup cough.
- Assess for stridor, this is a high-pitched sound when inhaling caused by the swelling.
- Other symptoms include fever, sore throat, and drooling, as well as difficulty breathing and swallowing.
  - Epiglottitis is a medical emergency, and if the child is having trouble breathing and swallowing, they should seek emergency medical attention.

Diagnostics

Radiography film; lateral neck x-ray may show a classic "thumb-sign" indicative of swollen epiglottis.

Nursing Interventions

- Cool air, supplemented with oxygen, cardio-respiratory monitor, do not leave child alone.
- Avoid interventions that cause the child to become upset and cry, which can further narrow the upper airway.
- Administer aerosolized bronchodilator.
- All efforts should be aimed at keeping the child quiet and comfortable.
- Place an emergency airway at the bedside (tracheostomy tray); may be required if airway closure occurs.
- Allow the child to assume a comfortable position, usually child is content on his parent's lap with either blow-by oxygen or if able to tolerate a mask without additional stress or crying, a mask delivery system; administer 100% O_2 in the least invasive manner.

PEDIATRIC PEARLS

- Do not place the child in a supine position.
- Allow child to assume a position of comfort—usually the tripod position.
- Do not attempt to visualize epiglottis.

Special Considerations

Children who are not immunized with the Hib vaccine are at risk for contracting acute epiglottitis.

Discharge Planning; Patient and Family Education

- Instruct the caregiver about signs and symptoms of worsening respiratory condition.
- Allow parents to express their fears and concerns; provide reassurance as appropriate.
- Provide medication directions for at home administration.

CYSTIC FIBROSIS

Description

- Chronic, multisystem disorder of the exocrine glands, characterized by abnormally thick pulmonary secretions.
- Cystic fibrosis (CF) also affects the exocrine glands of the pancreas, the gastrointestinal (GI) tract, salivary glands, and reproductive tract.
- It is an autosomal recessive disorder that leads to increased mucous viscosity and the mucous has abnormal electrolyte concentrations, especially sodium.

- The cilia move slower, and secretions accumulate in the respiratory tract resulting in obstruction, air trapping, and increased risk for bacteria and infection with retained secretions.
  - Common bacterial infections include *Pseudomonas aeruginosa*, *Burkholderia cepacia*, *Haemophilius influenza*, *Staphylococcus aureus*, and *Klebsiella pneumoniae*.
    - Recurrent infection leads to bronchiectasis and fibrosis.
- The pancreas, small intestines, bile duct, salivary glands, and reproductive system are also affected by thick mucus and blockage.

Assessment

- Assess for family history of CF.
- Assess for respiratory signs and symptoms, wheezing, dyspnea, cough, cyanosis atelectasis, and obstructive emphysema. Long-term barrel chest and clubbing of the fingers.
- Assess for gastrointestinal signs and symptoms, meconium ileus at birth; rectal prolapse; steatorrhea (loose, bulky, frothy, fatty stools); weight loss and wasting; failure to thrive (FTT); distended abdomen; vitamin A, D, E, and K deficiencies; and bowel obstruction (distal intestinal obstruction syndrome).
- Assess for reproductive signs and symptoms; females can have delayed puberty, and decreased fertility (increased viscosity of cervical mucous); males vas deferens blockage can cause infertility and sterility.
- Assess for electrolyte disturbances, hyponatremia, excessive amounts of sodium in excreted sweat results in loss of sodium, especially during periods of exercise, playing in hot temperatures, and febrile illness.

Diagnostics

- **Sweat chloride test:** The gold standard diagnostic test and considered suspicious if the level of chloride in collected sweat is above 50 mEq/L and diagnostic if the level is above 60 mEq/L.
- **Pulse oximetry:** Oxygen saturation might be decreased, particularly during a pulmonary exacerbation.
- **Chest radiography:** Might reveal hyperinflation, bronchial wall thickening, atelectasis, or infiltration.
- **Pulmonary function tests:** Might reveal a decrease in forced vital capacity and forced expiratory volume, with increase in residual volume.

Nursing Interventions

- Promote adequate oxygenation and breathing patterns.
- Monitor nutritional status; malabsorptive disorder, monitor height, and weight frequently.
  - Encourage double portion meals in-between respiratory treatments when energy levels are the highest.
  - Assess nutritional lab values, calorie counts, I&O monitoring.
  - Promote a diet high in protein and calories, moderate fat, with free use of salt and supplementation with fat soluble vitamins A, D, E, and K.
  - Encourage increased salt intake in hot weather or febrile illnesses when sweating can increase salt (sodium chloride) losses.
  - Administer prescribed meds; pancreatic enzymes with each meal and snack.
- Administer bronchodilators, especially prior to chest physiotherapy, antibiotics as indicated.
- Encourage fluid intake; as a rule, children with CF should have 6 to 12 ounces of fluid 15 minutes before exercise and every 15 to 20 minutes during exercise. Fluids should always be available, and planned fluid breaks are very important.

Special Considerations

Burkholderia cepacia is a bacteria found in soil and water that can be particularly harmful to patients who are immunocompromised. It has also been linked to faster decline in lung function for patients with CF. All efforts to minimize infection exposure, especially cepacia, should be taken to minimize the spread of contamination and worsening of lung function for these patients.

Discharge Planning; Patient and Family Education

- Provide child and family teaching and support; refer child and family to support group.
- Allow child and family to verbalize their concerns; reassure as appropriate.
- Develop a daily treatment plan that contains good pulmonary hygiene practices, good nutritional choices, and infection prevention measures.

RESPIRATORY DISTRESS/RESPIRATORY DISTRESS SYNDROME

Description

- Any pediatric illness or alteration in anatomical function can place infants and children at risk for respiratory distress.
- The premature infant is at risk for respiratory distress syndrome due to lung immaturity and surfactant deficiency.
  - Surfactant is a phospholipid protein developed in the fetal lung at about 35 weeks gestation. It adheres to alveolar wall and decreases surface tension, allowing inflation, deflation, and gas exchange to occur.
  - As the disease progresses, fluid and fibrin leak from the pulmonary capillaries, causing hyaline membrane formation in the bronchioles. This is seen as a "ground-glass" appearance on a chest x-ray. Long-term lung disease can result from the high pressures required in mechanical ventilation to maintain gas exchange.

Assessment

- Assess for symptoms of respiratory distress seen immediately after birth, or within hours of delivery.
- Assess for grunting on expiration, shallow breathing, nasal flaring, and retractions.
  - Hypoxia is detected by pulse oximetry.
- Assess for tachycardia, tachypnea, and the presence of fine crackles upon auscultation.

Diagnostics

Diagnosis is made based on clinical presentation, arterial blood gas results, and chest x-ray findings. There is a bell-shaped appearance to the lungs, with the possible ground-glass appearance associated with hyaline membrane formation.

Nursing Interventions

- Care is primarily supportive.
- Interventions are focused on maintaining optimal oxygenation and lung volumes.

Special Considerations

- Respiratory distress syndrome and/or prematurity place the infant at increased risk for respiratory illness in the first year of life.
- Maintain adequate infection prevention practices.

Discharge Planning; Patient and Family Education

- Emphasize importance of follow-up care and appointments.
- Ensure the family understands the medication regime; medications may include diuretics, bronchodilators, and oxygen therapy.
- Avoid exposing the child to any smoking in the home.
- Educate on signs of respiratory distress, have family complete the CPR course.
- Educate family on when they should contact their clinician; fever, diminished food or fluid intake, losing or not maintaining weight, any questions or concerns.

BIBLIOGRAPHY

Hinkle, J. L., & Cheever, K. H. (2018). *Brunner and Suddarth's textbook of medical-surgical nursing* (14th ed.). Wolters Kluwer.
Ricci, S. S., Kyle, T., & Carman, S. (2017). *Maternity and pediatric nursing* (3rd ed.). Wolters Kluwer.
Ricci, S. S., Kyle, T., & Carman, S. (2017). *Maternity and pediatric nursing* (4th ed.). Wolters Kluwer.
The Point (Wolters Kluwer): https://thepoint.lww.com/gateway

KNOWLEDGE CHECK

1. Which of the following statements, made by the primary caregiver of a child with asthma, indicates need for further teaching?

   A. "We need to identify things that trigger the attacks."
   B. "He should use the bronchodilator inhaler before the steroid inhaler."
   C. "We will make sure that the child avoids exercise to minimize attacks."
   D. "We should increase oral fluid intake to keep the mucous thin."

2. The administration of the Hib vaccine to infants has had the greatest impact on which respiratory condition in infants and children?

   A. LTB
   B. Epiglottitis
   C. Pneumonia
   D. RSV bronchiolitis

3. When developing a plan of care for the child diagnosed with CF, what priority should the nurse keep in mind?

   A. CF is an autosomal dominant heredity disorder
   B. Obstruction of the endocrine glands throughout the body occurs
   C. Elevated levels of potassium are found in the sweat of a child with CF
   D. Children with CF have abnormally thick pulmonary secretions

4. A patient requires low-flow supplemental oxygen therapy. Which delivery device should the nurse most likely expect to use?

   A. Simple face mask
   B. Nonrebreather mask
   C. Venturi mask
   D. Oxyhood

5. The nurse is percussing the chest of a child with a suspected respiratory disorder. What sound might the nurse note that would indicate pneumonia?

   A. Decreased fremitus
   B. Dull sound
   C. Tympany
   D. Hyperresonance

6. A patient diagnosed with asthma is in the yellow zone of the Asthma Action Plan. Which of the following symptoms should the nurse expect the patient to report to the nurse?

   A. No cough, wheeze, chest tightness, or shortness of breath
   B. Able to do some, but not all usual activities
   C. Peak flow is more than 80% or more of best peak flow reading
   D. Quick-relief medications have not helped

7. A child arrives in the emergency department in significant respiratory distress, sitting upright leaning forward, drooling, with a panicked facial expression. What is the priority nursing intervention?

   A. Provide cool, humidified air
   B. Initiate a racemic epinephrine aerosol treatment
   C. Notify the healthcare clinician and obtain intubation equipment on standby
   D. Have the patient lie flat and suction the airway

KNOWLEDGE CHECK

1. **Correct Answer: C) "We will make sure that the child avoids exercise to minimize attacks."** Additional teaching is needed to explain that although exercise can trigger an attack, children should be encouraged to exercise as tolerated. The use of the bronchodilator inhaler before exercise may be beneficial as well as avoiding any known triggers. It is correct for the caregiver to indicate the need to identify asthma triggers, to affirm the use of the bronchodilator inhaler before the steroid inhaler, and to note the intention to increase oral fluid intake to keep mucous thin.

2. **Correct Answer: B) Epiglottitis.** Epiglottitis is a bacterial infection of the epiglottis primarily caused by Hib. The ability to vaccinate infants against this bacterium has reduced the incidence of the disease.

3. **Correct Answer: D) Children with CF have abnormally thick pulmonary secretions.** CF is an autosomal recessive disorder, which involves obstruction in the exocrine glands. Abnormal secretion of salt is found in sweat of children with CF, but the pulmonary secretions are abnormally thick and require vigorous chest physiotherapy to loosen them for the lung wall.

4. **Correct Answer: A) Simple face mask.** Low-flow oxygen delivery systems consist of nasal cannula, nasal catheters, transtracheal catheters, and the simple face mask. The standard nasal cannula delivers an FiO_2 of 24% to 44% at supply flows ranging from 1 to 8 liters per minute (LPM). A simple face mask can deliver 35% to 60% oxygen with an appropriate flow rate of 6 to 10 LPM.

5. **Correct Answer: B) Dull sound.** Dull or flat sound would be percussed over partially consolidated lung tissue, as occurs with pneumonia. Decreased fremitus is found on palpation and may be found with barrel chest, as may occur with CF. Tympany might be percussed with pneumothorax, and hyperresonance, resonance increased above normal, and often of lower pitch, on percussion as a result of overinflation of the lung might be apparent with asthma.

6. **Correct Answer: B) Able to do some, but not all usual activities.** No cough, wheeze, chest tightness, or shortness of breath, as well as peak flow at more than 80% or more of best peak flow reading, places the patient in the green zone. Ineffective quick-relief medications places the patient in the red zone.

7. **Correct Answer: C) Notify the healthcare clinician and obtain intubation equipment on standby.** This child may be experiencing acute epiglottitis and intubation equipment should be available. Racemic epinephrine would be used to treat croup. The child should remain upright with no attempt to visualize the throat. Providing cool, humidified oxygen would be indicated, not air.

8. A newborn is admitted to the special care nursery with respiratory distress syndrome. What action by the healthcare team will minimize the development of BPD?

   A. Placing the infant on a radiant warmer to maintain thermoregulation
   B. Initiating early gastric feedings to promote optimal nutrition and healing
   C. Initiating bag-valve-mask (BVM) with 100% oxygen
   D. Assisting with the administration of surfactant and weaning ventilator pressures as the infant improves

9. The nurse reads a lateral neck x-ray report for a patient indicating a "steeple sign" noted in the upper airway. What intervention does the nurse anticipate?

   A. Albuterol nebulizer treatment
   B. Antibiotic therapy
   C. Corticosteroids
   D. Vigorous nasopharyngeal suction

10. What observation of the chest during breathing would most likely indicate that the gas exchange is impaired?

    A. Eupnea respiratory pattern
    B. Pectus carinatum
    C. See-saw respirations
    D. Pectus excavatum

KNOWLEDGE CHECK

8. **Correct Answer: D) Assisting with the administration of surfactant and weaning ventilator pressures as the infant improves.** BPD results from damage to the lung from high oxygen and pressure. Administering surfactant will reduce surface tension of the alveoli and allow for less pressure to maintain gas exchange. Placing the infant on a radiant warmer, initiating early gastric feedings or utilizing a short-term BVM device for respirations will not contribute to the development of the disease process of BPD. BPD is caused by damage to the delicate tissue of the lungs. This damage most often occurs in infants who have required extended treatment with supplemental oxygen or breathing assistance with a machine (mechanical ventilation), such as infants who are born prematurely and have acute respiratory distress syndrome.

9. **Correct Answer: C) Corticosteroids.** The steeple sign is a radiologic sign found on a frontal neck radiograph where subglottic tracheal narrowing produces the shape of a church steeple within the trachea itself. The presence of the steeple sign supports a diagnosis of croup, where there is airway inflammation. A type of steroid (glucocorticoid) may be given to reduce this inflammation in the airway. Benefits will typically be felt within a few hours. A single dose of dexamethasone is usually recommended because of its long-lasting effects. Albuterol breathing treatments do not help the subglottic swelling caused by croup. Antibiotics do not treat viruses, which cause most cases of croup. Croup or epiglottitis (which has a bacterial cause) are considered absolute contraindications to nasopharyngeal suctioning.

10. **Correct Answer: C) See-saw respirations.** See-saw respirations (paradoxical breathing) is a very ineffective pattern to support gas exchange. In see-saw respirations, the chest falls on inspiration, and rises on expiration. Eupnea respiratory pattern is an expected respiratory pattern associated with adequate oxygenation. Pectus excavatum refers to a chest wall deformity, commonly known as funnel chest or concave chest, where the breastbone is pushed inward resulting in a sunken chest appearance but is not expected to result in impaired gas exchange. Pectus carinatum is another chest wall deformity, commonly referred to as pigeon chest or raised chest, and results in a condition where the breastbone and ribs protrude. Similar to pectus excavatum, this condition would most likely not impair any gas exchange.

CHAPTER 7

Cardiovascular Conditions

Kevin J. Nusspickel

INTRODUCTION

The cardiac system is responsible for perfusion and bringing oxygenated blood to the peripheral tissues. The pediatric nurse should be aware of and knowledgeable about assessment parameters, diagnostics, treatment modalities, and nursing interventions for those diseases and disorders of the circulatory system.

INTRODUCTION TO THE PEDIATRIC CARDIOVASCULAR SYSTEM

- **Obtaining a Relevant History:**
  - **Feeding pattern:**
    - Duration, frequency, associated distress, choking, or diaphoresis, volume consumed, stopping to rest or breathe during meals, and caloric supplementation required to sustain growth.
    - Children with compromised cardiac function may only tolerate small feeding volumes and often appear distressed while eating.
  - **Impaired growth:**
    - Children with congenital heart disease (CHD) are in a state of increased energy expenditure.
    - Failure-to-thrive patients need 125 to 150 kcal/kg/day of caloric intake with fortified feeds.
    - Monitoring trends using a percentile growth chart is the best representation of overall health.
  - **Dyspnea or tachypnea:**
    - At rest or on exertion (eating, crying, and playing)
  - **Cyanosis:**
    - Cyanosis is typically evident when the saturation on pulse oximetry (SpO_2) falls below 85%, indicating that ≥5 g/dL of the hemoglobin is desaturated or not bound with oxygen.
    - Questions about a patient's baseline SpO_2 reading can reveal clinically significant deviations.
    - Note that the degree of visible cyanosis depends on total hemoglobin and level of saturation.

- Cyanosis may appear milder in a child with a cyanotic heart defect due to compensatory *polycythemia* or increased red blood cell (RBC) count. Conversely, cyanosis in an anemic child may be more challenging to detect, even during states of profound hypoxemia.
- Skin tone and oxygen saturations remain unaffected in certain cardiac lesions (i.e., acyanotic).

- **Squatting:**
  - Position assumed in cyanotic heart defects when repairs are delayed or remain undiagnosed

- **Recurrent respiratory infections:**
  - More susceptible due to increased risk of congestive heart failure (CHF)

- **Focused Physical Examination:**
  - Assess for physical characteristics of chromosomal defects (e.g., Down syndrome, DiGeorge).
  - Examine the chest and precordium for visible pulsations or heaves, suggesting volume overload.
  - Inspect nails for signs of *clubbing*—a flattened angle of the nail base exceeding 180° attributable to a prolonged state of decreased oxygen saturation. A normal finding is approximately 160° (Figure 7.1).
  - Note the presence of edema, which is more common in the periorbital and sacral areas of infants.
  - Palpate the abdomen for areas of tenderness, distension, ascites, or hepatosplenomegaly.
  - **Neurovascular assessment:**
    - **Skin:** Note pallor, cyanosis, flushing, jaundice, or mottling.
    - **Temperature:** Influenced by the environment but may indicate decreased perfusion.
    - **Capillary refill:** Evaluated by applying moderate pressure to a distal extremity and noting the time required for the blanched area to reperfuse. Normal findings are <2 to 3 seconds. A prolonged capillary refill time may denote reduced cardiac output (CO).
    - **Pulses:** Note rate, regularity, and strength (0–4 scale) in both upper and lower extremities. Assess the brachial pulse in neonates or infants and the carotid pulse in older children.

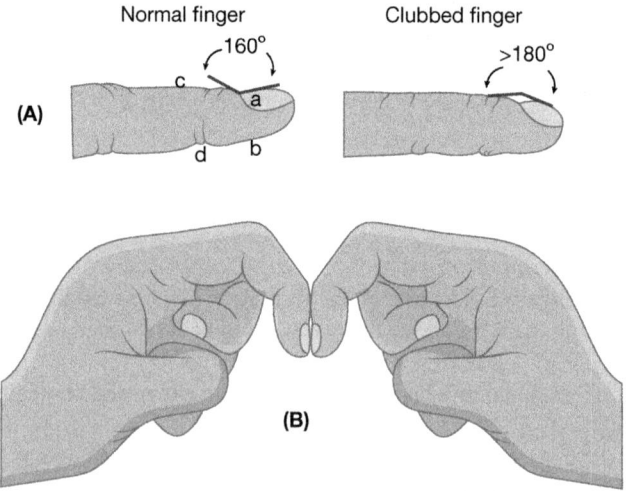

FIGURE 7.1: Nail clubbing

Source: Reprinted from Gawlik, K. S., Melnyk, B. M., and Teall A. M. (2021). *Evidence-based physical examination: Best practices for health and well-being assessment* (1st ed.). Springer Publishing Company.

- Analyze resting heart rate (HR) in the context of patient age and clinical condition.
  - Sinus tachycardia is a common, nonspecific response to a variety of clinical conditions such as fever, anemia, anxiety, and crying.
    - *Tachycardia* associated with signs of circulatory compromise such as hypotension, altered mental status, or signs of shock requires prompt evaluation and medical intervention.
- **Auscultate for the presence of normal heart sounds:**
  - S_1: Closure of the atrioventricular valves (tricuspid and mitral) during systole
  - S_2: Closure of the semilunar valves (pulmonic and aortic) during diastole
- Listen for *murmurs*. Consider patient age, clinical presentation, history, and overall health.
  - Note timing (systole and/or diastole), location of highest intensity, and sound quality with patient positioning.
  - Innocent murmurs may occur in high-output states (e.g., fever, anemia), usually during systole, and become louder with adjustments in patient position.
- **Pulse oximetry:**
  - Measures the percent of total hemoglobin that is fully saturated with oxygen but does not indicate oxygen delivered to tissues nor effectiveness of ventilation (CO_2 elimination).
  - When the device is unable to detect a consistent pulse under conditions of diminished distal perfusion, it generates a suboptimal waveform which is deemed an unreliable reading.
- **Blood pressure (BP):**
  - Systolic BP readings in the lower limbs may be slightly higher when compared to the arms. This normal variation in BP is referred to as a *pressure gradient*.
  - In general, a pressure gradient ≥20 mmHg often warrants further clinical investigation.

PEDIATRIC PEARLS
Definition of hypotension by systolic BP and age:
- **Term neonates (0–28 days):** <60 mmHg
- **Infants (1–12 months):** <70 mmHg
- **Children (1–10 years):** <70 mmHg + (age in years × 2)
- **Children >10 years:** <90 mmHg

- **Normal Heart:**
  - **Right side:**
    - **SpO_2:** 70 to 75% (deoxygenated blood).
    - **Low-pressure system:** Right ventricle only needs to pump a short distance to the lungs.
    - Pulmonary vascular resistance (PVR) within the lungs reaches its nadir or lowest point between 8 weeks and 6 months of age.
  - **Left side:**
    - SpO_2: 95% to 100% (oxygenated blood).
    - **High-pressure system:** Left ventricle pumps a greater distance to achieve end-organ perfusion.
    - Systemic vascular resistance (SVR) within the body is considerably higher than the PVR.

PEDIATRIC PEARLS

The kidneys are one the most highly perfused organs per tissue mass—receiving roughly 20% to 25% of CO. Urine output is therefore considered an indirect measure of CO.

Low CO → reduced renal perfusion → low urine output (oliguria)

Expected urine output: 1 to 2 mL/kg/hour, measured by weighing a soiled diaper and subtracting that number from a dry diaper. Recall that 1 g on the scale is equal to 1 mL of urine. Note that normal urine output per hour is age-dependent:

- **Infants and young children:** 1.5 to 2 mL/kg/hour
- **Older children and adolescents:** 1 mL/kg/hour

- **Physiology Overview:**
  - Blood tends to travel the *path of least resistance*.
  - Cardiac defects may involve an anatomic connection between pulmonary and systemic circuits.
  - The defect can disrupt the balance between the once separated pulmonary and systemic circuits.
    - As a result, blood shunts preferentially from an area of *high resistance* to *low resistance*.
- **Congenital Heart Defects:**
  - Defects in the embryological development of the heart or its associated major blood vessels.
  - **Acyanotic subgroup:**
    - Oxygenated systemic blood flow on the left side of the heart shunts preferentially to the partially deoxygenated pulmonary blood flow on the right side of the heart.
    - Blood travels from left-to-right across the defect causing *increased* pulmonary blood flow.
    - Interventions such as supplemental oxygen (O_2) and inhaled nitric oxide (iNO) reduce PVR—increasing pulmonary blood flow, which can exacerbate the state of volume overload.
  - **Cyanotic subgroup:**
    - Partially deoxygenated pulmonary blood flow on the right side of the heart shunts preferentially to the oxygenated systemic blood flow on the left side of the heart.
    - Blood travels right-to-left across the defect causing *decreased* pulmonary blood flow.

ATRIAL SEPTAL DEFECT

Description

- Communication between the right and left atria (Figure 7.2)
  - May occur in isolation or, more commonly, in conjunction with other heart defects
  - Results in left-to-right shunting at the atrial level
    - Degree of shunting is determined by the size of the defect and ventricular compliance.
    - Shunting increases with age as ventricles become more compliant.
  - Classified as an *acyanotic* defect by way of increased pulmonary blood flow
    - Oxygen-rich blood from the left atrium flows through the defect in the septal wall.
    - Diverted blood flow causes a state of recirculation or an "extra trip" through the lungs.

ATRIAL SEPTAL DEFECT

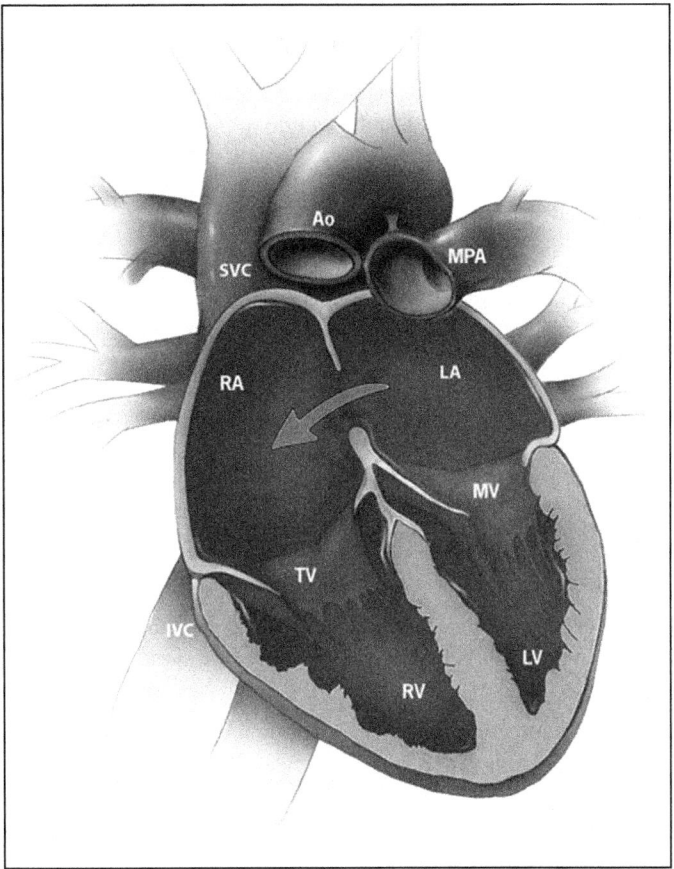

FIGURE 7.2: Atrial septal defect
Source: Reprinted from Gawlik, K. S., Melnyk, B. M., and Teall, A. M. (2021). *Evidence-based physical examination: Best practices for health and well-being assessment* (1st ed.). Springer Publishing Company.

Assessment

- Systolic ejection murmur at left sternal border (LSB) and widely split S_2 due to delayed pulmonic valve closure.
  - Often apparent at two to three years of age. Classic findings are rare in the term neonate.
- Assess for signs and symptoms of acute CHF.
  - Term neonates with isolated atrial septal defects (ASDs) are usually asymptomatic and rarely require intervention.
  - Clinical presentation for children includes fatigue, shortness of breath (SOB), exercise intolerance, and palpitations.
  - Children with profound CHF develop respiratory distress, poor growth, and hepatomegaly.

Diagnostics

Echocardiogram is the diagnostic tool of choice. Additional testing is usually not indicated.

Nursing Interventions

- Cluster care and limit crying to decrease oxygen demands.
- Bottle-feed with fortified (high calorie) formula or breastmilk to promote optimal growth.
  - Limit feeding attempts to ≤30 minutes. Prolonged attempts increase energy expenditure.
  - Reinforce education to ensure proper formula mixing.

- Monitor strict intake and output, weigh all diapers, and obtain daily weights.
  - Diuretics are the first-line treatment. Monitor for signs and symptoms of dehydration and associated electrolyte imbalances, which can lead to rhythm disturbances.
  - Obtain reliable weights by using the same weighing devices with each encounter.

Special Considerations

- Exercise clinical judgment when using supplemental O_2.
  - Respiratory distress is due to *volume overload* from blood preferentially shunting to lungs.
  - Oxygen is a pulmonary vasodilator that will only further decrease resistance within the lungs. The resultant drop in PVR causes additional left-to-right intracardiac shunting of blood.

Discharge Planning; Patient and Family Education

- ASD closure is not common until at least two years of age, with both device closure in the catheterization lab and surgical closure having exceptional outcomes.
  - Surgery requires the breastbone to be split by an instrument to obtain access to the heart. Once repaired, stainless steel wires are used to secure the sternal bone back together.
- *Sternal precautions* are techniques aimed to avoid using or putting stress on the muscles and bones attached to the sternum. Adherence to sternal precautions may prevent healing time delays.
  - Patients and families are advised to avoid pushing or pulling through the sternal area, prone positioning, or lifting under arms until cleared by the medical clinician.
  - Utilize the "scoop up" method to displace sternal pressure for the prescribed time period.

VENTRICULAR SEPTAL DEFECT

Description

- Communication between the right and left ventricles (Figure 7.3)
- May occur in isolation or in conjunction with other heart defects
- Most common; accounts for approximately 20% to 30% of congenital heart defects
- Results in left-to-right shunting at the ventricular level
  - Degree of shunting is determined by the size of the defect and PVR.
- Classified as an *acyanotic* defect by way of increased pulmonary blood flow
  - Oxygen-rich blood from the left ventricle flows through the defect in the septal wall.
  - Diverted blood flow causes a state of recirculation or an "extra trip" through the lungs.

Assessment

- Harsh holosystolic murmur at left sternal border.
  - Size of the defect is inversely related to the intensity of the murmur heard on auscultation.
  - For instance, a large ventricular septal defect (VSD) may produce a soft murmur owing to minimal blood turbulence.
- Assess for signs and symptoms of acute CHF.
  - Infants and children with a small restrictive VSD may remain asymptomatic.
  - Patients with a large nonrestrictive VSD may develop severe CHF characterized by feeding intolerance, respiratory distress, irritability, impaired perfusion, and failure to thrive.

COARCTATION OF THE AORTA

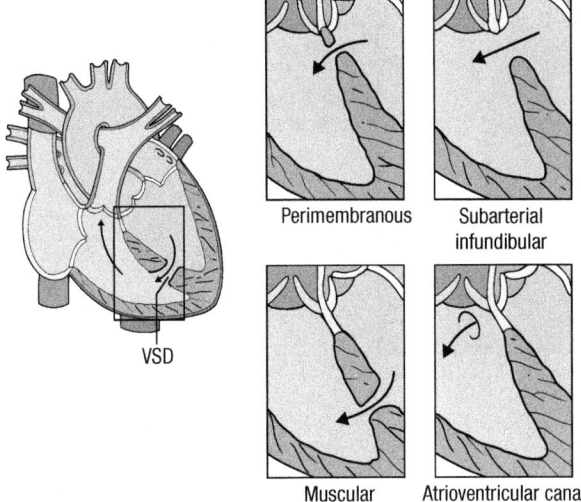

FIGURE 7.3: Ventricular septal defect

Source: Reprinted from Hoffman, J., Thompson-Bowie, N., and Jnah, A. J. (2019). The cardiovascular system. In A. J. Jnah and A. N. Trembath (Eds.), *Fetal and neonatal physiology for the advanced practice nurse* (1st ed.). Springer Publishing Company.

Diagnostics

- Echocardiogram is the diagnostic tool of choice. Additional testing is usually not indicated.
    - Cardiac catheterization may be used to quantify the amount of shunting.

Nursing Interventions

Refer to section under "Atrial Septal Defect."

Special Considerations

Refer to section under "Atrial Septal Defect."

Discharge Planning; Patient and Family Education

- Up to 45% of VSDs close spontaneously during the first year of life. For those lesions that become hemodynamically significant, open-heart surgical closure is the primary option.
    - Refer to sternal precautions section under "Atrial Septal Defect."

COARCTATION OF THE AORTA

Description

- Narrowing or "kink" in the descending aorta directly past the point of the left subclavian artery (Figure 7.4)
    - Note that the narrowing typically occurs before the patent ductus arteriosus (PDA).
    - The PDA is a normal fetal structure providing a vascular connection between the left pulmonary artery and descending aorta, which may close functionally within 24 hours.
- Classified as an *acyanotic* defect secondary to a systemic outflow obstruction
    - Deoxygenated blood from the right ventricle preferentially flows through the PDA to the lower body due to a paradoxical reduction in SVR directly past the narrowed aortic segment.
    - Deemed "ductal-dependent" when PDA provides sole blood flow to lower half of the body.

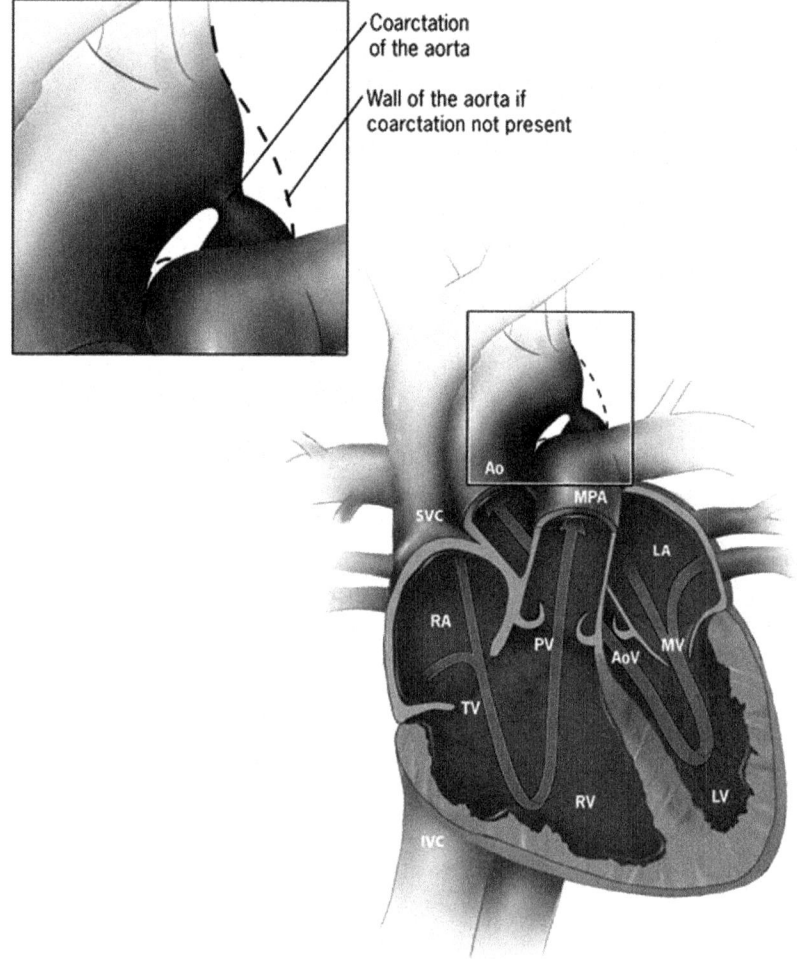

FIGURE 7.4: Coarctation of the aorta

Source: Reprinted from Gawlik, K. S., Melnyk, B. M., and Teall, A. M. (2021). *Evidence-based physical examination: Best practices for health and well-being assessment* (1st ed.). Springer Publishing Company.

Assessment

- **Neurovascular Assessment:**
  - Assess for bounding upper extremity pulses in the setting of weak lower extremity pulses.
  - Assess lower extremities for signs of impaired perfusion such as cyanosis, cold temperature, and delayed capillary refill time.
- **BP Discrepancy:**
  - The hallmarks of **coarctation of the aorta (CoA)** are absent **leg** pulses and a difference in **BP** between the arms and **legs** (high **BP** in the arms and **low** to normal **BP** in the **legs**).
  - A pressure gradient ≥ 20mmHg raises clinical suspicion for CoA.
- **Pre-and Post-Ductal Saturation Discrepancy:**
  - Assess SpO_2 reading on right hand (preductal) and toe (postductal) to infer ductal patency.

Diagnostics

Echocardiogram is the diagnostic tool of choice.

Nursing Interventions

- Perform four-extremity BP to determine degree and site of the narrowed aortic segment.
  - Obtain readings within a close time frame and ensure constant patient disposition (i.e., calm).

Special Considerations

- In cases of severe narrowing or "critical coarctation," adequate systemic CO can only be maintained by the right ventricle shunting blood across the existing PDA.
  - Neonates present in shock with hypotension, acidosis, and tachypnea as the ductus closes—emergently requiring prostaglandin (PGE_1) to open the PDA and restore systemic perfusion.

Discharge Planning; Patient and Family Education

- Repair may include surgical resection of the stenotic segment and end-to-end aortic anastomosis.
- Patients and families are instructed to monitor for signs and symptoms of CoA recurrence.

TETRALOGY OF FALLOT

Description

- Four (4) components: Overriding aorta, pulmonary stenosis, right ventricular (RV) hypertrophy, and VSD (Figure 7.5).
  - Broad continuum of clinical presentation—from mild cases ("pink Tet") to severe ("Tet spell")
    - Shunting is largely dependent upon the degree of *pulmonary stenosis*.

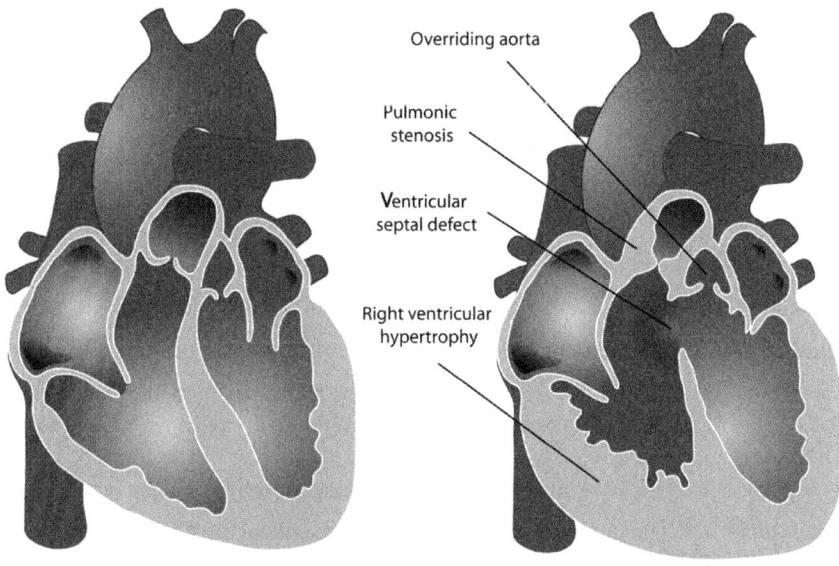

FIGURE 7.5: Tetralogy of Fallot

Source: Reprinted from Gawlik, K. S., Melnyk, B. M., and Teall, A. M. (2021). *Evidence-based physical examination: Best practices for health and well-being assessment* (1st ed.). Springer Publishing Company.

- Classified as a *cyanotic* defect typically characterized by decreased pulmonary blood flow.
- Hypercyanotic or "Tet" spells are theorized to result from infundibular muscle spasms. High PVR induces right-to-left shunting of deoxygenated blood via the VSD and enters systemic circulation.
  - Episodes of profound cyanosis are often triggered by a decrease in SVR (i.e., hypotension) or a sudden rise in resistance to pulmonary blood flow seen with crying or agitation.

Assessment

- Harsh systolic ejection murmur the over pulmonic area, indicating pulmonary stenosis.
- Monitor for exertional dyspnea, trend SpO_2, and observe signs of acute and/or chronic cyanosis.
  - Clubbing is a flattened angle of the nail base due to prolonged states of hypoxemia.
  - Chronic cyanosis stimulates erythropoiesis eliciting a rise in RBC count or polycythemia.
  - Squatting is evident in children with delayed surgical repair or who remain undiagnosed.

Diagnostics

Echocardiogram is the diagnostic tool of choice.

Nursing Interventions

- **Tet Spell Management:**
  - Oxygen, calming strategies (e.g., parental involvement, feeding), sedation (promotes venous dilation), and intravenous (IV) fluids (volume expansion to increase SVR)
  - *Knee-chest position* → compresses femoral artery → increases SVR → left-sided pressure now exceeds right → reverses shunt → blood directed to lungs → improved oxygenation

Special Considerations

Phenylephrine is given for refractory Tet spells to increase SVR and reverse shunt direction.

Discharge Planning; Patient and Family Education

Even after complete surgical repair, patients require lifelong cardiology surveillance due to increased risk for pulmonary valve regurgitation which can ultimately lead to RV dilation.

CONGESTIVE HEART FAILURE

Description

- Reduced ability of the heart to fill and/or eject blood to meet the body's metabolic demands.
  - Blood unable to be pumped forward eventually results in congestion within the circuits.
- The etiology and pathogenesis of CHF vary significantly between children and adults.
  - A common cause of CHF in neonates is congenital heart defects with a left-to-right shunt (i.e., ASD, VSD) where pulmonary blood flow progressively rises with the predicted drop in PVR.
  - In children, heart failure is most often due to CHD, cardiomyopathies, and sepsis.
- "Compensatory mechanisms" are initially beneficial in enhancing CO and end-organ perfusion but inevitably become maladaptive and promote progression of CHF over time.
  - SNS activation → vasoconstriction and tachycardia → end-organ perfusion and CO maintained initially → increased afterload and myocardial O_2 demand
  - Renin-angiotensin aldosterone system activation → salt and water retention → increased preload → enhanced CO (Frank-Starling mechanism) → increased myocardial O_2 demand

Assessment

- Clinical presentation for infants is characterized by feeding difficulties (e.g., decreased volume, prolonged feeding time, diaphoresis); impaired growth; tachypnea; and hepatomegaly.
- Clinical presentation for older children mainly manifests as fatigue, SOB, tachypnea, exercise intolerance, edema, and oliguria.
- Physical exam may yield delayed capillary refill, peripheral edema, tachycardia, tachypnea, crackles, gallop rhythm (S_3), and hepatomegaly.

Diagnostics

- Echocardiogram is used to assess ventricular systolic and diastolic function and other elements.
- Blood tests for brain natriuretic peptide (BNP), a cardiac hormone secreted in response stretch conditions, is a useful prognostic indicator of both disease progression and response to therapy.

Nursing Interventions

- Reduce preload, volume returning back to the heart, with diuretics (e.g., Lasix).
  - Monitor urine output, which is considered an indirect measure of CO.
- Fluid restriction. Closely monitor fluid status. Optimize judiciously only if clinically indicated.
  - Fluid bolus (5–10 mL/kg). Reassess for signs of fluid overload (e.g., crackles, hepatomegaly).
- Reduce afterload, resistance the heart pumps against, with antihypertensive medications.
- Optimize CO with inotropic agents such as Digoxin aimed to enhance heart contractility.

Special Considerations

- Electrolyte tests may reveal hyponatremia as owing to hemodilution from free water retention.
  - Dilution of serum electrolytes secondary to fluid retention may incite rhythm disturbances.

Discharge Planning; Patient and Family Education

- Provide education for taking an apical pulse when prescribed a cardiac glycoside. Digoxin has a narrow therapeutic index which increases the overall risk for drug toxicity.
  - Report signs and symptoms such as bradycardia, nausea/vomiting, and visual disturbances.
- Discuss signs and symptoms of clinical dehydration and when to contact the medical team.

SEPSIS (SEPTICEMIA)

Description

- Sepsis is a leading cause of morbidity, mortality, and healthcare utilization for children globally.
- Sepsis is life-threatening organ dysfunction caused by a dysregulated host response to infection.
  - Septic shock is circulatory and cellular dysfunction associated with a greater mortality risk.
- Septic shock is the most common form of distributive shock. Infectious organisms release byproducts termed endotoxins resulting in vasodilation and increased capillary permeability.

- Since children are heavily reliant upon elevation of HR to optimize CO, tachycardia is a significant finding in pediatric sepsis. When increasing HR is no longer able to sustain CO, systemic vasoconstriction occurs in response to the declining stroke volume and contractility.
  - *Hypotension* is therefore considered a relatively late and ominous sign in sepsis, signifying the failure of crucial compensatory mechanisms intended to bolster CO and enhance SVR.
- Risk factors include but are not limited to chronic conditions such as CHD, immunosuppression, asplenia, organ/bone marrow transplant, neonates, prematurity, and indwelling central venous catheter (CVC).

Assessment

- In the *early* stages, signs of septic shock are often subtle and difficult to detect since peripheral perfusion often appears to be adequate during this "warm shock" phase.
- Clinical presentation with "warm shock" may include warm and flushed skin, flash capillary refill, bounding pulses, tachycardia, tachypnea, altered mental status, hypotension with a wide pulse pressure, oliguria, fever or hypothermia, and a distinctive petechial or purpuric rash.
- Progression to "cold shock" is comparable except now with pale or mottled skin, cold extremities, delayed capillary refill, thready pulses, and hypotension with a narrow pulse pressure.

Diagnostics

Clinical signs of sepsis, source identification (e.g., blood cultures and antigen testing) and control. Biomarker marker evaluation (e.g., white blood cell [WBC], erythrocyte sedimentation rate (ESR), C-reactive protein, and lactate levels).

Nursing Interventions

- **Recommendations for sequential elements of early goal-directed therapy for sepsis include:**
  - Prompt recognition of decreased mental status and perfusion with early O_2 administration, securing IV/intra-osseous (IO) access, fluid bolus, and broad-spectrum antibiotics within the first hour.
  - Best practice recommends obtaining blood cultures before initiating antimicrobial therapy under circumstances where this does not substantially delay administration.
  - Administering up to 40 to 60 mL/kg fluid boluses in increments is recommended over the first hour, titrating to clinical markers of CO and discontinued if signs of fluid overload develop.
  - Vasoactive infusions (e.g., epinephrine, norepinephrine) are recommended after fluid resuscitation if evidence of abnormal perfusion persists.
- Therapeutic endpoints include brisk capillary refill, normal central and peripheral pulses, warm extremities, normotensive for age, urine output >1 mL/kg/hour, and improved mental status.

Special Considerations

Neonates presenting with decreased femoral pulses may be erroneously suspected and worked up clinically for CoA when they are, in fact, in a critical state of septic shock.

Discharge Planning; Patient and Family Education

Infection control with meticulous hand hygiene and aseptic technique with indwelling CVCs.

INFECTIVE ENDOCARDITIS

Description

- Infection of the endothelial surface of the heart.
  - Heart valves are most commonly affected but can develop on or within any heart structure.
- Risk factors include prosthetic valves, previous endocarditis infection, complex cyanotic CHD, injection drug use, indwelling CVC, recent surgical repair or palliation, and residual heart lesions.
- Damage to endocardium → thrombus forms → circulating pathogens adhere to clot (vegetation).
- Mitral valve is most commonly affected. Tricuspid valve is often damaged due to intravenous (IV) drug use.
- Infective endocarditis (IE) is primarily classified by the manner in which it presents; acute versus subacute.
  - Acute IE describes a toxic-appearing child with high fever and hemodynamic instability.
  - Subacute IE includes nonspecific low-grade fever, anorexia, myalgia, arthralgia, and fatigue.

Assessment

- Clinical presentation includes fever plus a new or changing heart murmur from valve damage.
- Parts of the vegetation may detach, forming septic emboli that circulate and lodge in the body.
  - Splinter hemorrhages are deposits of the septic emboli under nailbeds.
  - Janeway lesions are red, painless lesions on the palms and soles from septic emboli deposits.
  - Osler nodes are raised painful lesions on finger and toe pads from immune complex deposits.
  - Roth spots are retinal hemorrhages from immune complex deposits visible on an eye exam.

Diagnostics

Peripheral blood cultures. Echocardiogram for pathologic evidence of intracardiac vegetation.

Nursing Interventions

Obtain three peripheral blood cultures from different areas; first culture before antibiotic therapy.

Special Considerations

Cultures yielding a bacterial pathogen may require four to eight weeks of IV antibiotic therapy. Antibiotic therapy is challenged with penetrating the robust fibrin mesh which encloses the vegetation.

Discharge Planning; Patient and Family Education

Antibiotic therapy before invasive dental work prevents IE in designated high-risk patients.

KAWASAKI DISEASE

Description

- Self-limiting systemic vasculitis in children typically between the ages of six months and five years.
  - Etiology remains unknown. Theorized that infectious and genetic components play a role.
- Inflammation of the medium-sized vessels can lead to necrosis and coronary artery aneurysms.

Assessment

- A persistent (≥5 days) sudden onset of high fever often unresponsive to antipyretics plus at least four of the specific criteria is required for clinical diagnosis.
  - Bilateral conjunctivitis without discharge, nonspecific polymorphous rash; cervical lymphadenopathy; mucous membrane changes (injected pharynx, cracked lips, strawberry tongue); and distal extremity changes (erythema and edema of hands and feet) are classic signs and symptoms. Hands and feet may desquamate or peel during the convalescent phase.

Diagnostics

Nonspecific supporting lab tests. Echocardiogram to assess for evidence coronary abnormalities.

Nursing Interventions

- Monitor urine output and encourage adequate intake to prevent dehydration secondary to fever.
- Treatment regimen may include **IV immunoglobulin** and **high-dose aspirin**.

Special Considerations

Aspirin is inadvisable for children due to link with Reye syndrome, except in Kawasaki disease.

Discharge Planning; Patient and Family Education

Prompt recognition and early treatment of suspected cases promote reassuring clinical outcomes.

ACUTE RHEUMATIC FEVER

Description

- Acquired condition occurring two to four weeks after a group A beta-hemolytic *Streptococcal* infection.
  - May develop when a strep throat infection remains untreated or partially treated.
- Theories support the concept of molecular mimicry, whereby antibodies produced against the streptococci toxin mistakenly launch an attack and destroy similar appearing healthy tissue.

Assessment

Clinical presentation may include fever, migratory polyarthritis, pancarditis with valve involvement (new systolic murmur), subcutaneous nodules, erythema marginatum (painless nonpruritic rash), and Sydenham's chorea (non-rhythmic involuntary movements).

Diagnostics

- No single confirmatory test exists. Jones criteria were developed to guide diagnosis of acute rheumatic fever (ARF).
  - Initial diagnosis of ARF requires documentation of a recent streptococcal infection with either a positive throat culture or antistreptolysin-O titer (ASO) blood test.

Nursing Interventions

- Provide analgesia, positioning, warm baths, and gentle range-of-motion exercises for joint pain.
- Monitor closely for signs of carditis such as chest pain, SOB, fatigue, friction rub, and gallop.
  - Endocarditis with resultant heart valve damage may increase risk for recurrent infections.

Discharge Planning; Patient and Family Education

- Offer primary prevention education on early detection and completion of the entire antibiotic course.
- Discuss compliance with long-term prophylactic antibiotic regimen to prevent recurrence.

BIBLIOGRAPHY

Colombo, J. N., & McCulloch, M. A. (2018). Acyanotic congenital heart disease: Left-to-right shunt lesions. *NeoReviews*, *19*(7), e375–e383. https://doi.org/10.1542/neo.19-7-e375

Flocco, S. F., Lillo, A., Dellafiore, F., & Goossens, E. (2019). *Congenital heart disease: The nursing care handbook*. Springer Nature. https://doi.org/10.1007/978-3-319-78423-6

Garcia, R. U., & Peddy, S. B. (2018). Heart disease in children. *Primary Care: Clinics in Office Practice*, *45*(1), 143–154. https://doi.org/10.1016/j.pop.2017.10.005

Hueckel, R. M. (2019). Pediatric patients with congenital heart disease. *The Journal for Nurse Practitioners*, *15*(1), 118–124. https://doi.org/10.1016/j.nurpra.2018.10.017

Kline-Tilford, A., & Haut, C. (2016). *Pediatric acute care nurse practitioner: Lippincott certification review*. Wolters Kluwer.

Lantin-Hermoso, M. R., Berger, S., Bhatt, A. B., Richerson, J. E., Morrow, R., Freed, M. D., & Beekman, R. H. (2017). The care of children with congenital heart disease in their primary medical home. *Pediatrics*, *140*(5), e20172607. https://doi.org/10.1542/peds.2017-2607

Masarone, D., Valente, F., Rubino, M., Vastarella, R., Gravino, R., Rea, A., Russo, M. G., Pacileo, G., & Limongelli, G. (2017). Pediatric heart failure: A practical guide to diagnosis and management. *Pediatrics and Neonatology*, *58*(4), 303–312. https://doi.org/10.1016/j.pedneo.2017.01.001

Prusakowski, M. K., & Chen, A. P. (2017). Pediatric sepsis. *Emergency Medicine Clinics of North America*, *35*(1), 123–138. https://doi.org/10.1016/j.emc.2016.08.008

Puri, K., Allen, H. D., & Qureshi, A. M. (2017). Congenital heart disease. *Pediatrics in Review*, *38*(10), 471–486. https://doi.org/10.1542/pir.2017-0032

Ungerleider, R., Meliones, J. N., McMillan, K. N., Cooper, D. S., & Jacobs, J. P. (2019). *Critical heart disease in infants and children* (3rd ed.). Elsevier.

Weiss, S. L., Peters, M. J., Alhazzani, W., Agus, M. S., Flori, H. R., Inwald, D. P., Nadel, S., Schlapbach, L. J., Tasker, R. C., Argent, A. C., Brierley, J., Carcillo, J., Carrol, E. D., Carroll, C. L., Cheifetz, I. M., Choong, K., Cies, J. J., Cruz, A. T., De Luca, D., … Tissieres, P. (2020). Surviving sepsis campaign international guidelines for the management of septic shock and sepsis-associated organ dysfunction in children. *Intensive Care Medicine*, *46*(1), 10–67. https://doi.org/10.1007/s00134-019-05878-6

KNOWLEDGE CHECK

1. When developing a health prevention plan to address a primary prevention strategy for rheumatic fever, the nurse should include:

   A. Early treatment with IV immunoglobulin and high-dose aspirin
   B. Empiric antibiotic therapy prior to gastrostomy tube placement
   C. Long-term oral anticoagulation therapy after mechanical valve implant
   D. Antibiotic therapy to treat a confirmed streptococcal throat infection

2. The nurse is rendering care to an infant at risk for CHF secondary to a congenital heart defect that increases pulmonary blood flow. Which of the following cardiac conditions would most likely result in pulmonary overcirculation?

   A. VSD
   B. Tetralogy of Fallot (TOF)
   C. CoA
   D. Pulmonary arterial hypertension (PAH)

3. The nurse is admitting a toddler with an unrepaired ASD. Which of the following would the nurse most likely expect to find within the patient's past medical history?

   A. Baseline O_2 saturations of 85%
   B. Assumes squatting position
   C. Weight-for-age at 98th percentile
   D. Tachypnea with congested cough

4. A nurse is caring for a 4-year-old male recently diagnosed with Kawasaki disease. What classic finding does the nurse expect to find on physical examination?

   A. Intermittent low-grade fever which responds to antipyretics
   B. Diffuse, erythematous, blanching, sandpaper-like rash
   C. Cracked lips, strawberry tongue, with edematous hands and feet
   D. Unilateral conjunctivitis with purulent drainage

5. An infant is admitted with acute CHF secondary to a large VSD. The nursing plan of care should include:

   A. Supplemental O_2 for respiratory distress
   B. Cluster care to decrease oxygen demands
   C. Twice maintenance IV fluids for oliguria
   D. Bottle feed slowly over one hour to conserve energy

6. An 8-week-old infant presents to the emergency department with respiratory distress and decreased oral intake. Vital signs are as follows: heart rate (HR): 175 bpm, respiratory rate (RR): 70/min, SpO_2: 96%, blood pressure (BP): 81/44 mmHg. On physical exam, the nurse notes a grade I/VI systolic murmur, crackles, and hepatomegaly. The diagnosis of a large VSD is confirmed with echocardiography. Which intervention does the nurse anticipate will most likely be ordered?

   A. Furosemide (Lasix)
   B. Albuterol
   C. Ceftriaxone (Rocephin)
   D. NSS bolus (20 mL/kg)

KNOWLEDGE CHECK

1. **Correct Answer: D) Antibiotic therapy to treat a confirmed streptococcal throat infection.** Rheumatic fever is an acquired condition that occurs weeks after a streptococcal infection. The condition may emerge when a strep throat infection remains untreated or partially treated. Antibodies formed against the streptococci toxin mistakenly launch an attack and destroy similar appearing healthy tissue. Primary prevention should emphasize the importance of early detection and completion of prescribed antibiotics. IV immunoglobulin and high-dose aspirin best describe the treatment plan for Kawasaki disease. Antibiotic therapy prior to invasive dental, not gastrointestinal, work aims to prevent IE in patients who meet criteria for high-risk conditions. Long-term oral anticoagulation is prescribed for patients with a mechanical valve or an implanted cardiac assist device such as a left ventricular assist device (LVAD).

2. **Correct Answer: A) VSD.** Recall that resistance is normally higher on the left side of the heart. Blood tends to travel the path of least resistance. Cardiac defects disrupt the balance between the pulmonary and systemic circuits, allowing blood to shunt preferentially from an area of high resistance to low resistance. In acyanotic defects such as a VSD, ASD, or PDA, the resultant left-to-right shunt causes an *increase* in pulmonary blood flow. In both TOF and PAH, the increased resistance on the right side of the heart causes a *decrease* in pulmonary blood flow. CoA is an acyanotic defect that may decrease circulation to lower extremities but does not explicitly enhance pulmonary blood flow.

3. **Correct Answer: D) Tachypnea with congested cough.** An ASD is classified as an acyanotic defect with increased pulmonary blood flow. Clinical presentation may include fatigue, SOB, tachypnea, and exercise intolerance. The left-to-right shunting may contribute to recurrent respiratory infections and a predisposition to heart failure. Children with profound CHF develop respiratory distress, poor growth, and hepatomegaly. The weight-for-age percentile for a child with an unrepaired ASD is projected to be substantially lower given the state of increased energy expenditure. High-calorie formula or breast milk to promote sustained weight gain is often recommended. Baseline O_2 saturations in acyanotic defects are expected to be normal. In cyanotic defects such as TOF, transient elevations in PVR may induce right-to-left shunting of deoxygenated blood which enters systemic circulation causing profound hypoxemia. Squatting may manifest in children with delayed TOF surgical repair or who remain undiagnosed.

4. **Correct Answer: C) Cracked lips, strawberry tongue, with edematous hands and feet.** Kawasaki disease is a self-limiting systemic vasculitis in children typically between the ages of six months and five years. A persistent (≥5 days) sudden onset of high fever often unresponsive to antipyretics plus at least four of the specific criteria are required for clinical diagnosis. Bilateral conjunctivitis without discharge; nonspecific polymorphous rash; cervical lymphadenopathy; mucous membrane changes (injected pharynx, cracked lips, strawberry tongue); and distal extremity changes (erythema and edema of hands and feet) are classic signs and symptoms. Hands and feet may desquamate or peel during the convalescent phase. The diffuse, red, blanching, sandpaper-like rash describes a classic finding seen in scarlet fever.

5. **Correct Answer: B) Cluster care to decrease oxygen demands.** Concerted efforts should be made to consolidate nursing care when possible to reduce O_2 demands. Similarly, bottle feeding attempts should not exceed 30 minutes as this increases energy expenditure. Respiratory distress in acyanotic defects may be due to volume overload from blood preferentially shunting to the lungs. Providing supplemental O_2, a pulmonary vasodilator further drops resistance within the lungs and exacerbates intracardiac shunting.

6. **Correct Answer: A) Furosemide (Lasix).** CHF in neonates is often due to acyanotic heart defects with a left-to-right shunt (i.e., ASD, VSD) whereby pulmonary blood flow progressively increases with the expected decline in PVR. Recall that PVR within the lungs reaches its lowest point between eight weeks and six months of age, expediting the onset and severity of CHF symptoms. The faint murmur suggests minimal blood turbulence in the setting of a

7. An infant diagnosed with Tetralogy of Fallot is awaiting a date for surgical repair. The inconsolable infant suddenly appears profoundly cyanotic. To improve oxygenation, the nurse should place the infant in which strategic position?

   A. Semi-Fowler
   B. Knee-chest
   C. Reverse Trendelenburg
   D. Left lateral recumbent

8. A 2-day-old baby with Turner syndrome arrives at the emergency department with decreased urine output in the setting of respiratory distress. Parents report that the newborn has not produced a wet diaper today. Upon assessment, the nurse notes bounding brachial pulses coupled with weak, thready femoral pulses. Lower extremities are dusky and cool with a 4 second capillary refill time. The nurse anticipates management to include:

   A. SpO_2, knee-chest maneuver, and phenylephrine infusion
   B. ECG, labs (troponin, CK-MB), and tPA infusion
   C. SpO_2, four-extremity BP, and PGE_1 infusion
   D. Echocardiogram, labs (BNP), and Lasix infusion

9. A child diagnosed with hypoplastic left heart syndrome (HLHS) is scheduled to undergo a staged surgical palliation. Baseline oxygen saturations typically range from 75% to 80% in room air. Given the state of chronic hypoxemia, the nurse expects to find which of the following upon physical examination and routine laboratory studies?

   A. Splinter hemorrhages
   B. Anemia
   C. Osler nodes
   D. Nail clubbing

10. An infant recently underwent surgical repair of a congenital heart defect without incident. On postoperative day (POD) #3, the patient transitioned to the step-down unit to start the discharge planning process. The patient seems inconsolable despite receiving as needed (PRN) analgesics for presumed post-operative pain through a PICC line. Vital signs are as follows: T: 39 °C (102.2 °F), HR: 188 bpm, RR: 68/min, SpO_2: 94% in room air, BP: 81/22 mmHg. The nurse notes bounding pulses, warm and flushed skin, with a flash capillary refill. Calculated urine output for the shift is 0.5 mL/kg/hr. The appropriate initial interventions include which of the following in sequential order?

    A. Provide O_2, establish intravenous (IV)/intra-osseous (IO) access, start vasoactive drugs, rapid fluid administration, antibiotics
    B. Provide O_2, establish central venous access, obtain cultures, rapid albumin administration
    C. Provide O_2, establish central venous access, rapid blood administration, start vasoactive drugs
    D. Provide O_2, establish intravenous (IV)/intra-osseous (IO) access, obtain cultures, rapid fluid administration, antibiotics

large VSD. In a state of volume overload as evidenced by crackles and hepatomegaly, both reduction in preload with diuretics and implementation of a fluid restriction are paramount. For patients considered to be high risk for CHF, fluid would be optimized judiciously with a 5 to 10 mL/kg bolus coupled with frequent reassessments for signs of volume overload. Prompt administration of empiric broad-spectrum antibiotics such Ceftriaxone (Rocephin) would be most appropriate for suspected sepsis. Using a short-acting beta agonist such as Albuterol in the absence of wheezing is generally not recommended for CHF.

7. **Correct Answer: B) Knee-chest.** A hypercyanotic or "Tet" spell is theorized to be caused by infundibular muscle spasms, resulting in right-to-left shunting of deoxygenated blood through the VSD. Episodes can be provoked by a decrease in SVR (i.e., hypotension) or an increase in resistance to pulmonary blood flow such as crying or agitation. The knee-chest position compresses the femoral artery causing a transient increase in SVR, thereby reversing the shunt of blood back toward the lungs to improve oxygenation. The remaining answer choices are not clinically indicated for medical management.

8. **Correct Answer: C) SpO_2, four-extremity BP, and PGE_1 infusion.** The vignette best describes the clinical presentation for CoA. This acyanotic cardiac defect involves a narrowing in the descending aorta directly past the point of the left subclavian artery. Bounding upper extremity pulses in the setting of weak lower extremity pulses are classic findings. Lower extremities may reveal signs of impaired perfusion such as cyanosis, cold temperature, and delayed capillary refill time. The systemic outflow obstruction can impede renal perfusion which would account for decreased urine output. Comparing SpO_2 readings on the right hand (pre-ductal) and toe (post-ductal) can infer ductal patency. Four-extremity BPs serve as an invaluable tool for assessing the degree and approximate site of the narrowed aortic segment. A systolic pressure gradient $\geq 20mmHg$ raises clinical suspicion for CoA. The correlation between the age of the neonate and symptom onset is clinically significant. The timing infers that the cardiac defect may be "ductal-dependent" in nature as the predicted closure of the PDA seems to restrict blood flow to lower half of the body. A PGE_1 infusion is used to maintain ductal patency to restore systemic perfusion. The choice including SpO_2, knee-chest maneuver, and phenylephrine infusion best describes some of the interventions for Tet spells. The selection comprising of ECG, labs (troponin, CK-MB), and tissue plasminogen activator (tPA) infusion aligns most closely with the management for an acute myocardial infarction. The option containing echocardiogram, labs (BNP), and Lasix infusion clearly outlines the management of acute CHF.

9. **Correct Answer: D) Nail clubbing.** Clubbing is a flattened angle of the nail base as a result of a prolonged state of decreased oxygen saturation. Polycythemia, rather than anemia, may occur in response to chronic states of hypoxemia often associated with cyanotic cardiac defects such as TOF, transposition of the great arteries (TGA), pulmonary atresia, HLHS, and others. Splinter hemorrhages (deposition of emboli under nailbeds) and Osler nodes (painful antigen-antibody complex deposits in the pads of digits) are classic signs associated with IE.

10. **Correct Answer: D) Provide O_2, establish IV/IO access, obtain cultures, rapid fluid administration, antibiotics.** Tachycardia associated with signs of circulatory compromise such as hypotension, altered mental status, or signs of shock requires prompt evaluation and medical intervention. The vignette best describes the clinical presentation for a patient in the "warm shock" phase of septic shock as evidenced by an abnormal neurovascular exam and wide pulse pressure in the setting of a fever and central line. Recall that conditions of low CO may cause reduced renal perfusion which, in turn, results in low urine output. The urine output is suboptimal since the expected urine output for an infant is 1.5 to 2 mL/kg/hour. According to the 2020 Surviving Sepsis Campaign, the sequential components of early goal-directed therapy include prompt recognition of decreased mental status and perfusion with early administration of O_2, establishment of IV/IO access, fluid administration, and empiric broad-spectrum antibiotics

within the first hour of recognition. Best practice recommends obtaining blood cultures before starting antimicrobial therapy under circumstances where this does not substantially delay administration. Administering up to 40 to 60 mL/kg in bolus fluid in increments is recommended over the first hour; titrating to clinical markers of CO and discontinued if signs of fluid overload develop. Vasoactive infusions (e.g., epinephrine, norepinephrine) are recommended after fluid resuscitation if evidence of impaired perfusion persists.

CHAPTER 8

Hematologic and Oncologic Conditions

Terri Giordano

INTRODUCTION TO PEDIATRIC HEMATOLOGY AND ONCOLOGY

- Hematopoiesis is the process by which the cellular elements of blood are formed.
- The major hematopoietic organs of the body are the red bone marrow (myeloid tissue) and the lymphatic system which consists of lymph (fluid), lymphatic vessels and lymphoid structures (lymph nodes, spleen, thymus, and tonsils).
- Blood is composed of fluid portion called plasma and cellular portion.
  - Plasma is 90% water and 10% solutes.
  - Principal solutes are albumin, electrolytes, and proteins.
- The major function of red blood cells (RBCs) is to transport hemoglobin, which carries oxygen to all cells of the body; normal RBCs' life span is 120 days; hematocrit is the volume of RBCs in blood.
- Anemia is lack of RBC or hemoglobin in the blood.
- Polycythemia is an increase in the number of RBCs in the blood causing the blood to be thicker, slowing blood flow.
- Pediatric cancer is rare.
- Incidence of pediatric cancer varies according to age, sex, and race/ethnicity.

LEUKEMIAS: ACUTE LYMPHOBLASTIC LEUKEMIA AND ACUTE MYELOGENOUS LEUKEMIA

Description

- Leukemias are a broad term given to a group of malignant diseases of the bone marrow, blood, and lymphatic system, especially an overproduction of immature white blood cells.
- **Two types:** Acute lymphoblastic leukemia (ALL) and acute myelogenous leukemia (AML).
  - *ALL*
    - Occurs more often in boys than girls and in White individuals more than African American individuals, with peak onset between 2 and 5 years of age
    - Most common type of leukemia and most common childhood cancer
    - **Features:** Low-grade fever, fatigue, malaise, irritability, anorexia, bone or joint pain, listlessness, pallor, purpuric petechial skin lesions, hepatosplenomegaly, lymphadenopathy
  - *AML*
    - Accounts for 15% to 20% of all cases of childhood leukemia; incidence similar for males and females

♦ Fever, night sweats, shortness of breath, fatigue, easy bruising, petechiae, bone or joint pain

Assessment

- Assess for any signs of infection, fatigue, headache, bleeding.
- If petechiae or bruising present, assess for any recent falls or trauma.
- In AML, assess for leukemia cutis (painless blue/purple lumps that may appear on neck, underarm, abdomen, or groin; blue/green around eye known as chloromas).

Diagnostics

- Obtain complete blood count (CBC) with differential (presence of blast cells) and complete metabolic panel.
- Obtain bone marrow biopsy.
- If diagnosis of ALL/AML confirmed, obtain lumbar puncture to determine if any central nervous system (CNS) involvement.

Nursing Interventions

- Administer chemotherapy medications as ordered.
- Assist with intrathecal chemotherapy administration and/or radiation therapy if necessary for CNS prophylaxis.
- May need bone marrow transplant.

Special Considerations

More common in children with certain chromosomal abnormalities such as Down syndrome, Bloom syndrome, ataxia-telangiectasia, and Fanconi anemia.

Discharge Planning; Patient and Family Education

- Educate caregivers on importance of monitoring child's temperature closely.
- Educate caregivers on prophylaxis against pneumocystis pneumonia with antibiotics is routinely given to children during treatment.
- Educate caregivers on frequent blood transfusions are necessary during treatment to increase hemoglobin levels.
- Refer to Pediatric Pearls for more information.

PEDIATRIC PEARLS

BLOOD PRODUCT ADMINISTRATION

- Explain the procedure to the patient and caregivers; verify prescribers order for transfusion; obtain blood product from blood bank.
- Take vital signs before administration of blood, 15 minutes after initiation of transfusion, hourly while blood is infusing and at completion of transfusion.
- With another RN, check blood product label against original order and patient identifiers, verifying patient's name and medical record number, type of blood component, patient's ABO group and Rh factor, donor's ABO group and Rh factor, blood product unit number, expiration date of blood product, special requirements (e.g., cytomegalovirus negative).
- Don appropriate protective apparel, open tubing infusion set and appropriate blood filter, prime tubing and place in intravenous (IV) controlled infusion pump, set the rate of infusion and begin infusion, infuse unit of blood or specific amount within 4 hours.
- If any transfusion reaction is suspected, stop transfusion, take vital signs, maintain a patent IV with normal saline, notify clinician and do not restart transfusion until child's condition has been medically evaluated.
  - **Signs of transfusion reaction:** Fever, chills, urticaria, tachycardia or bradycardia, hypotension, headache, restlessness, dyspnea, abdominal pain, oliguria

APLASTIC ANEMIA

Description

- Condition in which the production of the formed elements of the blood is depressed
- Can be primary (congenital) or secondary (acquired); referred to as Fanconi anemia, best-known type

Assessment

- Assess for any signs of infection.
- Assess for any bruising, petechiae, bleeding.

Diagnostics

- Obtain CBC with differential and complete metabolic panel.
- Obtain bone marrow biopsy to confirm diagnosis (decreased or abnormal cells).

Nursing Interventions

- Administer immunosuppressive therapy, blood transfusions as ordered.
- Monitor blood in urine/stool.
- May need hematopoietic stem cell transplantation (HSCT).

Discharge Planning; Patient and Family Education

- Provide emotional support to patient and family.
- Provide education on safety priorities for child to prevent injury/bleeding.

BETA THALASSEMIA

Description

- Autosomal recessive disorder resulting in abnormal hemoglobin production; inherited mutation in globin gene
- Abnormalities in chain synthesis; decreased/absent
- **Types:**
  - **Thalassemia minor:** Generally asymptomatic, silent carrier.
  - **Thalassemia trait:** Mild microcytic anemia.
  - **Thalassemia intermedia:** Homozygous or heterozygous abnormalities, splenomegaly, moderate to severe anemia; requires blood transfusions.
  - **Thalassemia major:** Also known as Cooley anemia; severe anemia, chronic hypoxia, not compatible with life without transfusion support and chelation therapy; focus on this type.

Assessment

- Assess for pallor, listlessness, unexplained fever, poor feeding, decreased exercise tolerance.
- Observe for jaundice and hepatosplenomegaly.
- Assess growth in height and weight.
- Assess for skeletal facial abnormalities (frontal bossing/prominent forehead) due to iron overload.
- Assess for hemosiderosis (iron overload) if patient receiving frequent transfusions.

Diagnostics

- Obtain CBC with differential.
- Obtain hemoglobin electrophoresis to confirm diagnosis and type and severity.

Nursing Interventions

- Monitor hemoglobin and hematocrit, blood iron levels.
- Administer blood products (packed red blood cells [PRBCs]) as ordered; chronic therapy, monitor for any reactions.
- Administer chelation therapy of deferoxamine IV or subcutaneously as ordered to remove excessive intracellular iron (thalassemia major subtype) as ordered.
- Refer to hematologist and/or pediatric surgery in severe splenomegaly.

Discharge Planning; Patient and Family Education

- Provide emotional support for patient and family, discuss the importance of having all family members tested for thalassemia trait.
- Educate on the importance of compliance with transfusion and chelation therapy.
- If splenectomy is required, review most children often require prophylactic antibiotics, discuss the importance of obtaining pneumococcal and meningococcal vaccines in addition to regularly scheduled vaccines.

BONE CANCER—EWING'S SARCOMA AND OSTEOSARCOMA

Description

- Malignant cells can proliferate in all tissues such as osteoid, blood vessels, and cartilage; affect bone growth.
  - **Types:** Ewing's sarcoma and osteosarcoma
  - *Ewing's sarcoma:*
    - Develops in the marrow spaces of the bone.
    - Tumors originate in shaft of long and trunk bones, most often femur, tibia, fibula, pelvis, ulna, humerus, vertebra, scapula, ribs, and skull.
    - Occurs in those under age 30 years, affecting White individuals more than those of other races.
    - Treated with multiagent chemotherapy.
  - *Osteosarcoma*
    - Solid tumor that grows in osteoid matrix of bone, especially metaphysis of long bones, most often femur.
    - Most common bone cancer in children; peaks at growth spurts.
    - Managed with chemotherapy (before and/or after surgery) and limb-sparing surgery or amputation.

Assessment

- Assess for any pain in bones, any painless swelling, or masses.
- Assess for presence of limp, decreased physical activity, or inability to hold heavy object.

Diagnostics

- If swelling or mass present, rule out trauma or infection.
- Obtain x-ray, CT scan, or MRI.
- Needle or surgical biopsy for definitive diagnosis.

Nursing Interventions

- Administer chemotherapy agents as ordered.
- Assess for presence of side effects of chemotherapy including nausea, vomiting, hair loss, peripheral neuropathy, and cardiotoxicity.
- May treat with local radiation; assess skin for irritation.
- **Osteosarcoma:** Provide preoperative teaching and care; provide postoperative care including wound care and monitor for infection; administer pain medications as ordered.

Discharge Planning; Patient and Family Education

Refer to Pediatric Pearls for more information.

PEDIATRIC PEARLS
SIDE EFFECTS OF RADIATION THERAPY

SITE	SIDE EFFECTS	DISCHARGE PLANNING
Skin	• Dry or moist desquamation followed by hyperpigmentation • Alopecia (hair loss)	• Discuss wearing loose fitting clothing, protect area from sunlight, wind, and cold • Review wearing a wig or head covering • Discuss washing daily, using soap sparingly • Avoid use of lotions and creams • Educate to not remove skin markings for radiation fields
Gastrointestinal	Nausea, vomiting, anorexia, diarrhea	• Review use of antiemetics before chemotherapy • Encourage foods and fluids as tolerated
Oral cavity	Mucositis, xerostomia (dry mouth), ageusia (loss of sense of taste), sore throat	• Encourage oral hygiene, dental care • Provide pain medication as needed
Bone marrow	Myelosuppression	Assess for fever, signs of infection

---

HEMOPHILIA

Description

- Refers to a group of bleeding disorders resulting from congenital deficiency, dysfunction, or absence of specific coagulation proteins or factors
- **Types:**
  - *Hemophilia A:* Classic hemophilia, factor VIII deficiency
  - *Hemophilia B:* Christmas disease, factor IX deficiency
- X-linked recessive disorder

Assessment

- Assess for prolonged bleeding, especially after circumcision.
- Assess for hemorrhage after minor trauma such as loss of deciduous teeth, slight fall, or bruise.

- Assess for presence of hematuria (blood in urine) and/or epistaxis (nosebleed).
- Assess for signs of internal bleeding, headache, slurred speech, loss of consciousness (cerebral bleeding), and black tarry stools (gastrointestinal [GI] bleeding).
- Assess for hemarthrosis (bleeding into joint cavities), especially in knees, ankles, and elbows; assess for numbness and tingling in joints.
- Assess for decreased ability to move or walk.

Diagnostics

Obtain CBC with differential, bleeding time, factor VIII and IX assays, prothrombin time (PT), partial thromboplastin time (PTT).

Nursing Interventions

- Administer clotting factors (factor replacement therapy) as ordered; prophylactic basis to prevent hemorrhage.
- Administer DDAVP (desmopressin) as ordered.
- Encourage active range of motion exercises to strengthen muscles around joints.

Discharge Planning; Patient and Family Education

- Provide emotional support to patient and family; educate on prevention of bleeding episodes, using protective equipment such as helmets, face mask, skin/wrist/elbow guards, knee pads.
- Educate on avoiding use of nonsteroidal anti-inflammatory drugs (NSAIDs) because they inhibit platelet function; encourage use of rest, ice, and elevation of joints and muscles.
- Encourage participation in noncontact sports such as swimming, golf, bowling, walking, jogging, fishing; contact sports such as hockey football, soccer, boxing, rugby are discouraged; encourage daily active range of motion exercises.
- Educate on oral hygiene using soft-bristled toothbrush, water irrigating device, or using sponge tipped disposable toothbrush; in adolescents, encourage use of electric shaver.
- Provide patients and caregivers with resources on support groups and genetic counseling.

HYPERBILIRUBINEMIA

Description

- Excessive level of bilirubin in the blood due to the breakdown of RBCs; characterized by jaundice/icterus (yellow discoloration of skin).
- Common finding in newborns.
- **Risk factors:** East Asian or Asian American ethnicity, prematurity, exclusive breastfeeding (breast milk jaundice), G6PD, maternal diabetes, sepsis.
- **Two forms:** Unconjugated (indirect) bilirubin—toxic; conjugated (direct) bilirubin—nontoxic.
- **Complications:** Encephalopathy (kernicterus) results in brain damage from high levels of bilirubin spreading to brain.

ASSESSMENT

- Assess for jaundice of skin and sclera, especially in the first 24 hours of birth.
- Assess for presence of cephalohematoma, hepatosplenomegaly.
- Monitor for sepsis, polycythemia, neurologic status.

Diagnostics

- Obtain total serum bilirubin.
- Obtain Coombs test to rule out blood incompatibilities.

Nursing Interventions

- Provide phototherapy as ordered exposing as much skin surface as possible; reposition infant frequently; apply properly sized opaque eye shield; remove eye shield during feedings; monitor and assess skin surfaces.
- Monitor temperature, intake and output (I&O), dehydration, daily weights.
- Feed infant frequently.
- May need exchange transfusion for high levels of bilirubin.

Discharge Planning; Patient and Family Education

- Provide caregivers with emotional support.
- Encourage breastfeeding; if home phototherapy is prescribed, reassure caregivers infants under phototherapy are warm and comfortable, teach application of eye shields and discuss removing eye shields during feedings, review serum bilirubin levels every 24 hours.

IDIOPATHIC OR IMMUNE THROMBOCYTOPENIA

Description

- Acquired hemorrhagic disorder characterized by thrombocytopenia, mucosal bleeding, petechiae, menorrhagia
- Most common thrombocytopenia of childhood, cause unknown

Assessment

- Assess for mucosal bleeding, presence of petechiae, purpura, or easy bruising.
- Assess for splenomegaly.

Diagnostics

Obtain CBC with platelet count and bleeding time.

Nursing Interventions

If prescribed, administer high dose prednisone, IV immune gamma globulin (IVIG), and anti-D antibody as ordered.

Discharge Planning; Patient and Family Education

- Provide emotional support to patient and caregivers; educate caregivers on limiting child's activities if platelet count is >50,000/mm^3.
- Educate on the importance of not participating in any contact sports, bike riding, skateboarding, gymnastics, climbing, or running.
- Discuss the importance of obtaining prompt medical attention if child sustains head or abdominal trauma.

IRON DEFICIENCY ANEMIA

Description

- Anemia due to an inadequate supply of iron, impaired iron absorption, increase in body's demand for iron or blood loss.
- Iron is required for production of hemoglobin; if iron stores are deficient, production of hemoglobin is reduced.

Assessment

- Assess for excess milk ingestion, pica (nonnutrious foods).
- Assess for irritability, fatigue, tachycardia, koilonychia (concave or spoon fingernails).

Diagnostics

Obtain CBC with differential, reticulocyte count, total iron-binding capacity (TIBC), serum iron concentration, and ferritin level.

Nursing Interventions

- Maintain nutritional intake.
- Administer oral iron supplementation as ordered, 1 hour before or 2 hours after meals; if liquid preparation, administer through a straw or syringe.

Special Considerations

- In cultures in which tea is a common beverage, administer iron with other liquid as the tannins in tea form an insoluble complex that limits absorption of nonheme iron.
- **American Academy of Pediatrics (AAP) guidelines:** Screen at 9 to 12 months.

Discharge Planning; Patient and Family Education

- Educate caregivers on limiting quantity of milk, using iron fortified infant formulas, and the importance of introducing solid foods.
- Teach oral administration of liquid preparation of iron using a syringe or straw, encourage brushing teeth after administration to decrease teeth discoloration.
- Educate patient and caregivers oral iron supplementation should be given 1 hour before or 2 hours after meals; may turn stools green or black.

LYMPHOMA

Description

- *Hodgkin lymphoma:* Malignancy originates in the lymphoid system and primarily involves the lymph nodes.
- *Non-Hodgkin lymphoma:* Malignancy in lymphoid system.

Assessment

- Assess for painless enlargement of lymph nodes.
- Assess for persistent, nonproductive cough, low-grade fever, anorexia, nausea, weight loss, night sweats, pruritus, pain.

Diagnostics

- Obtain CBC with differential, uric acid levels, liver function tests, erythrocyte sedimentation rate, C-reactive protein, alkaline phosphatase, and urinalysis.
- Obtain CT scan of neck, chest, abdomen, and pelvis.
- Obtain PET scan to identify metastatic disease.
- Obtain bone marrow aspiration and lumbar puncture.

Nursing Interventions

- Administer chemotherapy as ordered.
- Encourage regular diet as tolerated.
- Administer pain medication as ordered and evaluate effectiveness of pain relief.

Discharge Planning; Patient and Family Education

- Refer to Pediatric Pearls for more information.
- Encourage return to school and normal activities.

PEDIATRIC PEARLS

SIDE EFFECTS OF CHEMOTHERAPY

Skin	Alopecia (hair loss)
Gastrointestinal	Nausea, vomiting, anorexia, diarrhea, constipation
Oral cavity	Stomatitis (oral ulcers)
Hematologic	Anemia, thrombocytopenia, leukopenia
Cardiac	Hypertension, hypotension
Musculoskeletal	Neuropathy, paresthesia, joint pain
Metabolic	Fever, weight loss
Other	Hearing loss, anaphylaxis, headache, may affect fertility

---

NEUROBLASTOMA

Description

- Most common extracranial solid tumor of childhood.
- Tumors originate from embryonic neural crest cells.
- Primary site is within abdomen but can be found in head and neck region, chest, and pelvis.
- "Silent" tumor in more than 70% cases diagnosis made after metastasis occurs.

Assessment

- Assess for firm, nontender, irregular mass in abdomen that crosses the midline.
- Assess for urinary frequency or retention as tumor may compress kidney, ureter, or bladder.
- Assess for pallor, irritability, anorexia, weight loss, weakness, lymphadenopathy.
- Observe for proptosis and periorbital ecchymoses (raccoon eyes) indicating metastases.

Diagnostics

- Obtain CT of abdomen, pelvis, and chest.
- Obtain bone scan and meta-iodobenzylguanidine (MIBG) scan to evaluate presence of skeletal metastases.
- Obtain tissue biopsy and/or bone marrow biopsy.
- Check serum or urine catecholamine levels for tumor markers.

Nursing Interventions

- Pre- and postoperative care for operative procedures.
- Encourage food and fluids as tolerated; assess for dehydration.
- Administer chemotherapy agents as ordered; administer blood products as ordered.
- Assess for presence of side effects of chemotherapy including nausea, vomiting, hair loss, peripheral neuropathy, and cardiotoxicity.
- Assess for complications of radiation therapy.

Discharge Planning; Patient and Family Education

- Educate caregivers on frequent blood transfusions are necessary during treatment to increase hemoglobin levels.
- Refer to Pediatric Pearls in this chapter for more information.

RETINOBLASTOMA

Description

- Embryonal malignancy of the retina; most common intraocular tumor in children
- Can be unilateral or bilateral; hereditary or sporadic

Assessment

- Assess pupil for leukocoria or cat's eye reflex (i.e., a yellow-whitish glow in the pupil; Figure 8.1).
- Assess for strabismus, decreased vision, and pupil irregularity.

Diagnostics

Obtain orbital CT, MRI, or ultrasound.

Nursing Interventions

- Refer to ophthalmology.
- Refer to genetics if hereditary.
- Administer radiation and/or chemotherapy if ordered.
- **If enucleation (removal of the eye) is performed postoperative care:** Monitor I&O, assess for bleeding, pain, and infection.

Discharge Planning; Patient and Family Education

- Refer to Pediatric Pearls in this chapter for more information.
- Educate caregivers that radiation therapy can be used.
- Educate caregivers that chemotherapy can be used to decrease tumor size to allow treatment to allow treatment with local therapies such as plaque brachytherapy, photocoagulation, or cryotherapy.

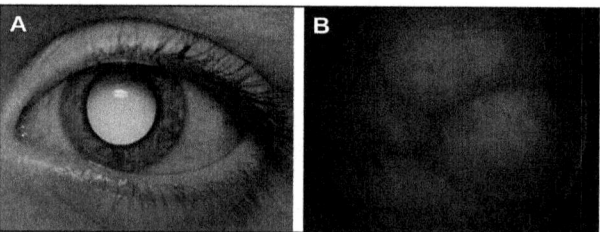

FIGURE 8.1: Retinoblastoma. Gross appearance of leukocoria (A) with an enucleated eye; (B) maximally dilated pupil shows large retinoblastoma filling the posterior chamber, vitreous seeds, and retinal detachment

Source: Reprinted from Rodriguez-Galindo, C., Orbach, D. B., and VanderVeen, D. (2015). Retinoblastoma. *Pediatric Clinics of North America, 62*(1), 201–223. https://doi.org/10.1016/j.pcl.2014.09.014. Reprinted from Jnah, A., and Trembath, A. (2018). *Fetal and neonatal physiology for the advanced practice nurse.* Springer Publishing Company.

- If enucleation was performed, educate caregivers on having infants and children wear eye patch to protect the socket; if child is fitted for a prosthesis, educate caregivers that prosthesis does not need to be removed unless cleaning is necessary; to remove prosthesis, gently pull down the lower lid and apply pressure to the upper lid.
- Educate caregivers to clean prosthesis, place in hot water and soak for several minutes; reinsertion is easier if prosthesis remains wet.
- For children with unilateral disease, educate caregivers on the importance of protecting the unaffected eye, avoid contact sports, and wear protective eyewear.
- Educate caregivers and patients on the late effects of cancer treatment that include peripheral neuropathy (tingling sensation in hands and feet, footdrop); cardiomyopathy; thyroid dysfunction; amenorrhea; delayed puberty; gonadal damage; growth retardation; hearing loss; dental caries; and second malignancies.

SICKLE CELL DISEASE

Description

- Group of hemoglobinopathies in which normal adult hemoglobin A (HgbA) is partially or completely replaced by abnormal sickle hemoglobin (HgbS); autosomal recessive condition.
- Obstruction in vessels caused by sickled RBCs, vascular inflammation, and increased RBC destruction.
- **Sickle cell anemia (SCA):** Most common genetic form.
- **Sickle cell trait:** Children have the same defect but only 35% to 45% of the total hemoglobin is HgbS; normally these children are asymptomatic.
- **Complications of sickling:** Thickening of blood causing obstruction of blood flow and hypoxic tissues; tissues and organs become ischemic and cause severe pain.

Assessment

- Assess hydration status to prevent sickling.
- Assess for infection, pain (vaso-occlusive crisis), hypoxemia.
- Assess for fever, pallor, fatigue, headache, signs and symptoms of anemia.
- Monitor for hepatosplenomegaly (sequestration), jaundice.

Diagnostics

- Universal screening of newborns for sickle cell disease is standard in the United States.
- Obtain CBC.
- Hgb electrophoresis may be ordered.

Nursing Interventions

- Monitor for dehydration; encourage fluid intake, can give children special cup or water bottle.
- Encourage frequent handwashing, infection prevention.
- Administer blood transfusion as ordered; monitor for transfusion reaction.
- Administer oral penicillin prophylaxis as ordered.
- **If splenectomy performed, postoperative care:** Monitor I&O, assess for bleeding, infection, pain; administer pain medication as ordered.
- May treat with HSCT.

Special Considerations

- **Monitor for acute chest syndrome:** Severe chest pain, fever 101.3°F or higher, cough, dyspnea, tachypnea, retractions, decreased oxygen saturation.

- **Monitor for stroke:** Severe unrelieved headache; severe vomiting; jerking or twitching of face, legs, or arms; seizures; strange behavior; inability to move arm or leg; stuttering or slurred speech; changes in vision.

Discharge Planning; Patient and Family Education

- Educate caregivers on the importance of obtaining childhood vaccinations.
- Emphasize importance of maintaining adequate hydration to prevent sickling; encourage drinking, review and provide written instructions on how many glasses or bottles per day are required; discuss foods such as soup, popsicles, yogurt, ice cream, and pudding can count as fluid; stress importance of adequate nutrition.
- Educate caregivers on signs of dehydration such as decreased number of wet diapers, dry mucous membranes, decreased tears, and sunken fontanel in infants.
- Educate patient and caregivers on the importance of infection prevention, taking oral penicillin prophylaxis as ordered, frequent handwashing, seeking medical attention if child has a fever, and routine immunizations.
- Educate patient and caregivers on minimizing tissue deoxygenation by taking frequent rest breaks during physical activities, avoiding contact sports if spleen is enlarged, avoiding environments with low oxygen concentrations such as high altitudes.
- Educate patient and caregivers on signs of sickle cell crisis, teach how to palpate spleen to monitor if spleen is enlarging; if patient prescribed hydroxyurea to improve oxygenation to tissues and reduce frequency of acute pain episodes, discuss the importance of taking medication as prescribed.
- Educate patient and caregivers on assessment for pain and taking pain medications as prescribed.
- Educate patient and caregivers on the importance of transcranial Doppler ultrasound annually as primary stroke prevention starting at age 2 years.

VON WILLEBRAND DISEASE

Description

- A hereditary bleeding disorder characterized by a deficiency of or defect in a protein called von Willebrand factor (VWF); classified as Type 1, Type 2, or Type 3.
- Type 1 Von Willebrand disease (VWD) is most common.
- Most common clinical feature is increased bleeding from mucous membranes; most common signs are epistaxis (nose bleeds), gingival bleeding, easy bruising, and menorrhagia (excessive menstrual bleeding).
- Autosomal dominant, affects males and females.

Assessment

- Assess for signs of bruising, bleeding from mucous membranes.
- If child requires surgery, refer to hematology to develop plan of care.

Diagnostics

- No single test can reliably diagnosis VWD.
- Obtain VWF antigen, VWF activity, VWF activity/antigen ratio, Factor VIII activity, and VWF multimers repeated at intervals a few weeks apart.

Nursing Interventions

Administer desmopressin (DDAVP) to stop bleeding.

Special Considerations

If child requires surgery, treatment with DDAVP and/or specialty concentrated clotting factor such as Humate-P may be indicated.

Discharge Planning; Patient and Family Education

- Provide emotional support to patient and caregivers, teach administration of DDAVP.
- Educate adolescent females with menorrhagia on using tampons and double sanitary pads.

WILMS TUMOR (NEPHROBLASTOMA)

Description

- The most common primary malignant renal tumor of childhood, also known as nephroblastoma.
- Can affect single kidney or be bilateral; most common initial clinical feature is incidental finding of asymmetric abdominal mass by parents while bathing or dressing of child.

Assessment

- Assess for abdominal mass.
- Assess for pallor, anorexia, lethargy, weight loss, fever, hypertension.

Diagnostics

- Obtain abdominal x-ray, ultrasound, CT or MRI of abdomen, CT of chest to evaluate for lung metastases, Doppler ultrasound of inferior vena cava.
- Obtain CBC with differential, complete metabolic panel, urinalysis.

Nursing Interventions

- Administer chemotherapy as ordered.
- Pre- and postoperative care for radical nephrectomy or partial nephrectomy.
- Encourage food and fluids as tolerated; assess for dehydration.
- Assess for presence of side effects of chemotherapy including nausea, vomiting, hair loss, peripheral neuropathy, and cardiotoxicity.
- Assess for complications of radiation therapy.

Special Considerations

Most important preoperative concern is not to palpate the tumor unless absolutely necessary because manipulation of mass may cause dissemination of cancer cells to adjacent and distant sites.

Discharge Planning; Patient and Family Education

- Educate patient and caregivers that chemotherapy and radiation therapy (if ordered) are usually begun immediately after surgery.
- Educate caregivers that frequent blood transfusions are necessary during treatment to increase hemoglobin levels.
- Refer to Pediatric Pearls for more information.

PEDIATRIC PEARLS

DISCHARGE PLANNING: PATIENT/FAMILY EDUCATION FOR CHILDREN RECEIVING CHEMOTHERAPY

Provide emotional support to patient and family
Educate that nausea and vomiting may occur; review antiemetics can be given 30 minutes to 1 hour prior to chemotherapy to prevent nausea and vomiting
• Discuss supportive nutritional measures such as increasing calories, cooking with butter, giving whole milk or PediaSure®, peanut butter, trail mix, dried fruit • Teach enteral feeding administration if required
Provide support in having head shaved or wearing a wig or head covering
Review while receiving chemotherapy, child should not receive any live, attenuated vaccines; inactivated vaccines can be given
Discuss interventions for stomatitis: soft diet, using soft sponge instead of toothbrush, rinsing mouth with chlorhexidine mouthwash, using sucralfate or solution of diphenhydramine and Maalox, avoid using lemon glycerin swabs and hydrogen peroxide
Review that children receiving steroids may develop mood changes, moon face, red cheeks, fluid retention, and weight gain; reassure that symptoms will resolve when medication is stopped
Provide resources for support groups and cancer survivorship programs
Provide education on late effects or later complications of treatment which can include musculoskeletal effects, delayed growth, dental caries, hearing loss, cardiac toxicity, thyroid dysfunction, pulmonary disease, delayed puberty, amenorrhea, reproductive problems, renal dysfunction, and the development of secondary malignant neoplasms such as leukemia and cancer of the digestive organs and breast

BIBLIOGRAPHY

Bowden, V. R., & Greenberg, C. S. (Eds.). (2016). *Pediatric nursing procedures*. Lippincott Williams & Wilkins.

Burns, C., Dunn, A., Brady, M., Starr, N., Blosser, C., & Garzon, D. (2017). *Pediatric primary care* (6th ed.). Elsevier Health Sciences.

Flint, P. W., Francis, H. W., Haughey, B. H., Lesperance, M. M., Lund, V. J., Robbins, K. T., & Thomas, J. R. (Eds.). (2021). *Cummings otolaryngology: Head and neck surgery* (7th ed.). Elsevier Inc.

Hockenberry, M. J., Wilson, D., & Rodgers, C.C. (2019). *Wong's nursing care of infants and children* (11th ed.). Elsevier Inc.

Kliegman, R. M., St. Geme, J. W., Blum, N. J., Shah, S. S., Tasker, R. C., & Wilson, K. M. (Eds.). (2020). *Nelson textbook of pediatrics* (21st ed.). Elsevier Inc.

Pizzo, P. A., & Poplack, D. G. (Eds.). (2016). *Principles and practice of pediatric oncology* (7th ed.). Wolters Kluwer.

Richardson, B. (2017). *Pediatric primary care* (3rd ed.). Jones & Bartlett Learning.

KNOWLEDGE CHECK

1. A nurse is caring for an infant with hyperbilirubinemia. What would the nurse most likely expect to assess for in the infant?

   A. Jaundice
   B. Purpura
   C. Black tarry stools
   D. Hematuria

2. When administering oral iron supplementation to a 6-year-old, the nurse should do all of the following except?

   A. Give 1 hour before meals
   B. Administer through a straw or syringe
   C. Give with breakfast
   D. Encourage brushing teeth after administration

3. A nurse is caring for a 3-year-old with hemophilia. What would the nurse most likely assess for in the child?

   A. Petechiae
   B. Excessive indigestion
   C. Dehydration
   D. Prolonged bleeding

4. A nurse is caring for a 16-year-old with sickle cell anemia. Which statement by the patient indicates the need for further teaching?

   A. "I should limit my drinking to 32 ounces every day."
   B. "I will need to be checked for stroke prevention yearly."
   C. "I should avoid going to Denver for a ski vacation."
   D. "I need to palpate my spleen to check that it is not enlarging."

5. A nurse is caring for a 4-year-old child recently diagnosed with acute ALL. Which physical examination finding is not expected to be seen in this child?

   A. Petechiae
   B. Urticaria
   C. Lymphadenopathy
   D. Hepatosplenomegaly

6. A nurse is caring for a 2-year-old child with neuroblastoma. Which statement by the parents indicates the need for further teaching?

   A. "We can continue to get the recommended inactivated vaccines."
   B. "To increase calories, we can give whole milk or PediaSure."
   C. "Using lemon glycerin swabs will help mouth pain."
   D. "More blood transfusions will be needed to get the hemoglobin level normal."

KNOWLEDGE CHECK

1. **Correct Answer: A) Jaundice.** Excessive bilirubin in the blood causes jaundice/icterus, that is, the yellow discoloration of skin. Purpura, black tarry stools, and hematuria will not be expected in an infant with hyperbilirubinemia.

2. **Correct Answer: C) Give with breakfast.** Oral iron is not absorbed if given with meals so it should be administered 1 hour before or 2 hours after meals. If oral iron supplementation is a liquid, administer it through a straw or syringe.

3. **Correct Answer: D) Prolonged bleeding.** The effect from hemophilia is prolonged bleeding anywhere from or in the body. Petechiae, excessive indigestion, and dehydration are uncommon findings in hemophilia.

4. **Correct Answer: A) "I should limit my drinking to 32 ounces every day."** Maintaining adequate hydration is important to prevent sickling. Splenomegaly is a complication of SCA. Minimizing tissue deoxygenation by taking frequent rest breaks during physical activities, avoiding contact sports if spleen is enlarged, and avoiding environments with low oxygen concentrations such as high altitudes are important considerations for patients with SCA. Annual primary stroke prevention is encouraged starting at 2 years of age.

5. **Correct Answer: B) Urticaria.** Urticaria is not associated with acute ALL. Petechiae, lymphadenopathy and hepatosplenomegaly are often seen in children with ALL.

6. **Correct Answer: C) Using lemon glycerin swabs will help with mouth pain.** Lemon glycerin swabs should be avoided due to their drying effect on oral mucosa. Making sure the child continues to receive inactivated vaccines, using whole milk or PediaSure to increase calories, and facilitating the impending need for blood transfusions are all correct discharge teaching.

7. When caring for a child with Wilms tumor, a priority for the nurse is to:

    A. Assess for a firm, nontender irregular mass
    B. Check for black tarry stools
    C. Administer antibiotics as ordered
    D. Not palpate the tumor unless absolutely necessary

8. A nurse is providing postoperative teaching to parents of a 12-month-old who underwent an enucleation for retinoblastoma. It is important to include all of the following in the patient teaching except:

    A. Protecting the unaffected eye
    B. Removing the prosthesis daily
    C. Cleaning the prosthesis in hot water
    D. Avoid contact activities

9. A nurse is caring for a 15-year-old beginning chemotherapy treatment for Hodgkin lymphoma. They ask the nurse if their hair is going to fall out. The best response from the nurse is:

    A. "Hair loss can be a side effect of many chemotherapy agents."
    B. "Your chemotherapy does not cause hair loss."
    C. "Do not worry, it will grow back."
    D. "Many people just wear a wig."

10. A nurse is caring for a 17-year-old undergoing radiation therapy for Ewing's sarcoma. It is important to include the following care instruction in the discharge teaching:

    A. Protect skin from sunlight, wind, and cold
    B. Wear tight fitting clothing
    C. Apply Vaseline to the skin daily
    D. Avoid showering

KNOWLEDGE CHECK

7. **Correct Answer: D) Not palpate the tumor unless absolutely necessary.** Preoperatively, it is important not to palpate the tumor unless absolutely necessary because manipulation of the mass may cause dissemination of cancer cells to adjacent and distant sites. Common findings upon assessment would include abdominal swelling or a mass in the kidney that can be felt upon physical examination. Some affected children have abdominal pain, fever, a low number of RBCs (anemia), blood in the urine (hematuria), or high blood pressure (hypertension). Additional signs of Wilms tumor can include loss of appetite, weight loss, nausea, vomiting, and tiredness (lethargy). Black, tarry stools would be associated with GI bleeding which is not observed with this tumor; antibiotics may be ordered for surgical resection but not a priority at this time.

8. **Correct Answer: B) Remove prosthesis daily.** Prosthesis does not need to be removed unless cleaning is necessary. Educate caregivers to clean prosthesis, place in hot water and soak for several minutes; reinsertion is easier if prosthesis remains wet. For children with unilateral disease, educate caregivers on the importance of protecting the unaffected eye, avoid contact sports, and wear protective eyewear.

9. **Correct Answer: A) "Hair loss can be a side effect of many chemotherapy agents."** Hair loss is a side effect of several chemotherapy agents. While not all children lose their hair during treatment, retaining hair is the exception. Dismissing the child's concern by saying it will grow back or saying that people wear a wig are not validating the child's feelings or answering the question asked by the child.

10. **Correct Answer: A) Protect the skin from sunlight, wind, and cold.** Radiation therapy often causes skin reactions of dry or moist desquamation. Protecting the skin from sunlight, wind, and cold is most important. Patient should be instructed to wear loose fitting clothing. Applying Vaseline to the skin and avoiding showering are not related to nursing care during radiation therapy.

CHAPTER 9

Gastrointestinal and Nutritional Conditions

Maureen Fitzgerald

INTRODUCTION TO PEDIATRIC GASTROINTESTINAL SYSTEM

- The gastrointestinal (GI) system functions in digestion, nutrient absorption, and waste elimination.
- Newborns have an immature gut and, therefore, are at risk for GI disturbances more frequently than other children; their GI system matures around two years of age.
- Most common result of GI conditions is dehydration (refer to Chapter 10).

ACETAMINOPHEN DOSING AND POISONING

Description

- An over-the-counter (OTC), nonopioid analgesic (pain reliever) for mild to moderate pain and used as an antipyretic (fever reducer) medication
  - Exact action unknown
  - **Dosage:** 10 to 15 mg/kg/dose every four to six hours, but no more than five times a day (24-hour period)
  - May be used for headaches, fevers, arthritis, musculoskeletal injuries/pain

Assessment

- **Assess pain using a developmentally appropriate pain scale:** Location, intensity, duration.
- If suspect poisoning/toxicity, assess for GI-related disturbances such as abdominal pain, nausea, vomiting, and diarrhea.

Diagnostics

Based on patient history and clinical features/presentation

Nursing Interventions

- Administer orally or rectally as ordered; may be ordered intravenously after surgery in hospital.
- Evaluate the effectiveness of acetaminophen on pain after administration.
- If suspect poisoning/toxicity, administer acetylcysteine/mucomyst as an antidote, as ordered.

Special Considerations

- Do not use aspirin in children due to risk for Reye's syndrome, a rare disorder that causes brain and liver damage.

- Acetaminophen does not have anti-platelet effects like aspirin, so it is safe for infants and children.

Discharge Planning; Patient and Family Education

- Educate caregivers on proper dosing of acetaminophen; toxicity or overdosing may cause hepatotoxicity.
- Instruct caregivers on reading medication bottle labels carefully and use the measuring device provided in order to give proper dose.

APPENDICITIS

Description

- Inflammation of the appendix caused by obstruction; may cause infection if perforates/ruptures
  - Treatment requires surgery.
  - Most commonly occurs in children 9 to 11 years of age.

Assessment

- **Assess pain level using a developmentally appropriate pediatric pain scale:** location, intensity, duration; patient complains of persistent pain without relief; difficulty walking.
- Assess for McBurney's point (located in right lower abdominal area with localized pain); patients complain of right lower quadrant pain—acute pain.
- Assess for nausea, vomiting, decreased appetite.

Diagnostics

- CT scan of abdomen
- Complete blood count (CBC), basic metabolic panel (BMP)

Nursing Interventions

- Preoperative care.
- Postoperative care may include intravenous (IV) antibiotics for 48 to 72 hours.

Special Considerations

If pain is relieved, may indicate rupture of appendix.

PEDIATRIC PEARLS

- At risk for appendix perforation/rupture and peritonitis if not treated quickly.

Discharge Planning; Patient and Family Education

Educate caregivers on the need for IV antibiotic therapy if appendix ruptured.

BILIARY ATRESIA

Description

- Condition in early infancy affecting the bile ducts (missing all or some) inside and/or outside the liver
  - Bile duct inflammation causes bile flow obstruction → cholestasis resulting in fat malabsorption → liver cirrhosis → may lead to death
  - **Features:** Jaundice without improvement, itching, irritability, difficulty gaining weight leading to failure to thrive

Assessment

- Assess for jaundice.
- Palpate for hepatomegaly; assess abdomen for firmness and distension; watch for splenomegaly.
- **Observe urine and stool appearance:** dark brown urine; stool will be clay colored/light beige/white (acholic) without bile in stools.
- Monitor lab values for increased liver enzymes, bilirubin.

Diagnostics

- Exploratory laparotomy/operative cholangiogram with liver biopsy
- Ultrasound and biliary scan

PEDIATRIC PEARLS

- Early identification is important for survival.

Nursing Interventions

- Pre- and postoperative care, including long-term antibiotics.
- Feed infants with formulas containing medium-chain triglycerides (MCT); add MCT oil to foods and/or liquids.
- Monitor for complications such as infection or ascites.

Special Considerations

A palliative treatment is the Kasai procedure to form alternate route for bile flow; most children will need a liver transplant.

Discharge Planning; Patient and Family Education

- Offer support to family.
- Educate family on the need for fat-soluble vitamins A, D, E, and K and increased calories; may need to feed infant via nasogastric tube.

CELIAC DISEASE

Description

- Condition where the body forms an autoimmune response to gluten injuring the villi of the small intestine
  - **Risk factors:** Family history for celiac disease, type 1 diabetes
  - **Features:** GI signs and symptoms: steatorrhea (fatty stools), chronic diarrhea/constipation, abdominal distension/bloating, nausea/vomiting, anorexia/weight loss leading to failure to thrive with vitamin deficiencies

Assessment

- **Assess GI status:** Painful, firm, distended abdomen, vomiting/diarrhea, thin extremities, nutritional deficiencies.
- Assess for anemia and osteoporosis.

Diagnostics

- **Genetic testing:** Antigen binding DQ2 (90% of patients) and/or DQ8 human leukocyte antigen (HLA)

- **Serum tests:** Tissue transglutaminase IgA (most indicative) and antiendomysium IgA tests
- Upper endoscopy with biopsy of small intestine

Nursing Interventions

- Refer to gastroenterologist, dietician/nutritionist.
- Discuss strict gluten-free diets.
- Monitor for nutritional deficiencies and normal growth and development.

Special Considerations

Only treatment is gluten-free diet.

Discharge Planning; Patient and Family Education

- Educate family on importance of maintaining the child on a gluten-free diet for lifetime, avoiding wheat, rye, and barley products since they contain the protein gluten.

CLEFT LIP AND PALATE

Description

- Birth defect where there is an opening in the roof of the mouth or a split lip; these facial structures did not fuse together in utero (Figure 9.1).
  - **Cleft lip:** Upper lip notch (partial)/opening/complete separation; opening may extend into the nose.
  - **Cleft palate:** Holes in the hard and soft palate.
  - Infants can have one or both defects; lip can be unilateral or bilateral.
  - Occurs often with other congenital malformations and syndromes.
  - Cause unknown; consider possible risk factors of maternal smoking, infections, and medications used during early pregnancy, such as antiseizure medications.

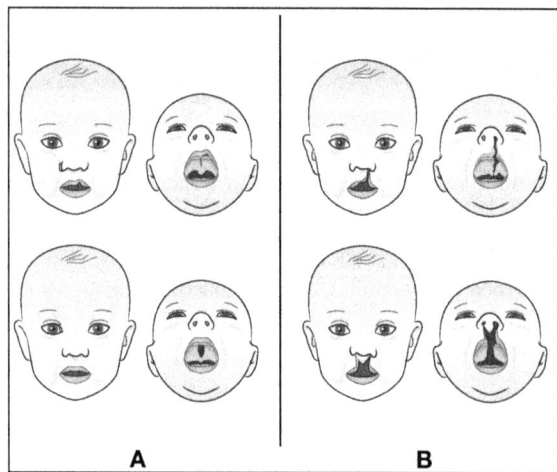

FIGURE 9.1: **(A)** Cleft lip may be minimal or extend past the upper border of the lip, or **(B)** It may be unilateral or bilateral and extend into the nares

Source: Reprinted from Chiocca, E. M. (2021). *Advanced pediatric assessment* (3rd ed.). Springer Publishing Company.

Assessment

- Inspect the oral cavity for orofacial defects.
- Assess for feeding difficulties (inadequate suck and swallow, unable to provide negative pressure for proper sucking; large amount of air intake; gagging/regurgitating/choking).
- Assess growth and development; be alert for weight loss, speech problems.

Diagnostics

- Prenatal ultrasound
- Clinical features/presentation on assessment

Nursing Interventions

- Monitor infant closely during feedings (risk for aspiration; respiratory distress).
- Educate families on appropriate feeding techniques with specialized nipples (e.g., Haberman feeder, cross-cut nipples [small frequent feedings, slower pace]); frequent burping may be necessary to help infant release excess air intake during feedings; may need a palatal obturator during feedings.
- Pre- and postoperative care; surgery is primary treatment to close structures:
  - Cleft lip usually repaired within first few months of life (rules of 10: 10 weeks, ≥10 lbs., hemoglobin >10 g, white blood cell [WBC] count <10,000 mm^3).
  - Cleft palate repaired around 9 to 12 months to avoid speech delays.
  - Protect the sutures on the lip and place the infant supine; may need arm restraints to avoid grabbing and rubbing at the repaired lip; avoid hard objects in the mouth after a cleft palate repair; keep the incision site clean by rinsing with water after feedings; feed via syringe or cup during the first postop day; decrease irritability and crying.
- Encourage breastfeeding.

Special Considerations

At risk for frequent upper respiratory infections such as otitis media, feeding issues, dental problems, and speech difficulties; interprofessional care team to manage these complications

Discharge Planning; Patient and Family Education

- Offer family emotional support and encourage parent–infant bonding; parents may grieve the loss of the "perfect" child.
- Refer to support group for cleft lip and/or cleft palate.
- Educate the family on pre- and postoperative care, the surgical treatments, and the positive outcome of minimal scarring.
- Long-term follow-up care with interprofessional team to monitor hearing, speech development, and dentition.

CONSTIPATION

Description

- Decrease in the number of bowel movements with an increase in the hardness and size of stool or trouble passing stool
  - Cause may be due to child holding stool in (functional constipation) after experiencing a painful bowel movement or from encopresis which is when impacted stool leaks from bowel into outer garment, unknowingly; can lead to loss of voluntary stooling or urge to have bowel movement.
  - **Other causes:** Intestinal malformations, GI conditions such as Hirschsprung disease, metabolic and neurologic issues, stress.

Assessment

- Assess abdomen for pain, bloating, distention; note bowel sounds and abdominal girth.
- Assess stool for consistency, blood, amount, duration, frequency; note if having bowel movements in school.
- Inspect anus for skin breakdown.
- Monitor for fever, nausea, vomiting.
- Determine diet and eating patterns, behavioral patterns.

Diagnostics

- Rectal examination as needed
- X-ray of abdomen to visualize stool in GI tract; may need a barium enema

Nursing Interventions

- Administer medications to soften stool and/or enemas as ordered.
- Ensure child is increasing fiber and fluids in diet.

Special Considerations

- Infants may have issues with certain formulas.
- Can offer prune juice to children >6 months of age.

Discharge Planning; Patient and Family Education

- **Educate child and family about**:
  - The development of constipation, signs, and symptoms of constipation in general and what to look for related to functional constipation and/or encopresis.
  - **Diet and eating patterns:** Increase fiber and fluids.
  - Bowel training with rewarding behaviors may be needed.
- Offer support to the family.

DIARRHEA

Description

- Increase in bowel movements and stool consistency is loose and watery; the injured intestinal mucosa is not able to absorb fluids.
  - **Types:** Acute or chronic (lasts more than two weeks)
  - **Causes:** Viruses most common; allergies, malabsorption, bacteria, parasites, medications such as antibiotics

Assessment

- Assess abdomen for pain, bloating, distention, bowel sounds.
- Assess stool for consistency, blood, amount, duration, frequency.
- Monitor for fever, nausea, vomiting.
- Assess for dehydration and metabolic acidosis.

Diagnostics

Stool studies including the presence of blood, if necessary; clinical features/presentation on assessment

Nursing Interventions

- Monitor hydration status via intake and output (I&O), daily weights.
- If child is dehydrated, begin oral rehydration therapy (ORT).

- Encourage normal diet.
- Treat any infectious process as ordered.

Special Considerations
Do not give child sugary drinks as this will make diarrhea worse.

Discharge Planning; Patient and Family Education
- Educate caregivers to contact clinician if child gets worse.
- Teach prevention strategies such as proper hand hygiene.

ESOPHAGEAL ATRESIA AND TRACHEOESOPHAGEAL FISTULA

Description
- Types of transesophageal malformations (TEM); congenital malformations that occur during fetal development where the esophagus is not a continuous structure to the stomach; the upper and lower sections of the esophagus are separate structures, and/or involves a connection between the esophagus and trachea
  - Different types of esophageal atresia (EA); most common is tracheoesophageal fistula (TEF).
  - Associated with other malformations in the kidney, heart.
  - The newborn's feeding does not enter the stomach because of the disconnect, may have trouble breathing, especially if there is a TEF; infants have excessive oral secretions.
  - Treatment is surgery (may be several stages) to connect the esophagus to the stomach and/or close the connection of the trachea to the esophagus.

Assessment
- Monitor newborn during feedings; be aware of key signs such as coughing, gagging, vomiting, choking, and cyanosis.
- Assess for respiratory distress.
- If newborn is having difficulty with feedings, try to insert a naso-gastric/oro-gastric tube; if it does not go very far, >9 to 12 cm, and meets resistance, then may suspect TEF.
- Assess newborn for other congenital anomalies/malformations.

Diagnostics
- Prenatal ultrasound (note polyhydramnios)
- Clinical features/presentation
- Chest and abdominal x-rays
- Esophageal endoscopy and/or tracheobronchoscopy

Nursing Interventions
- Feedings are stopped, and newborn is ordered nothing by mouth (NPO) and intravenous fluids (IVF).
- Provide continuous suction via catheter in the esophagus as ordered; be sure to raise the head of bed.
- Administer oxygen and support as needed.
- Perform pre- and postoperative care.
- Administer antibiotics as ordered.
- Postoperatively, feed child total parental nutrition (TPN) via G-tube until ready to start oral feedings; monitor for aspiration and swallowing difficulties.

Special Considerations

- **TEM associated with infants diagnosed with VACTERL defects**:
  - V = vertebral
  - A = anorectal
  - C = cardiac
  - TE = TEF/EA
  - R = renal
  - L = limb

PEDIATRIC PEARLS

- Stop feeding newborn immediately if showing signs and symptoms of possible TEF/EA.

Discharge Planning; Patient and Family Education

- Educate family on newborn's condition.
- Offer support pre- and postoperatively; infants may need repeated, staging surgeries depending on malformations and gastrostomy tube.
- Discuss palliative care if necessary, depending on the prognosis.

GASTROENTERITIS

Description

- Infection/inflammation of the stomach; can be acute and infectious
  - **Features:** Mostly diarrhea; may have abdominal pain, fever, nausea, vomiting
  - **At risk:** Antibiotics, day-care centers, immunocompromised infants/children, poor sanitation, sharing infected items, touching contaminated surfaces, travel, exposure to others who are sick
  - Usually resolves on own

PEDIATRIC PEARLS

- *Rotavirus* is a common infectious agent; prevention includes the *Rotavirus* vaccination.

Assessment

- Refer to the section on "Diarrhea."
- Assess for dehydration (daily weights, skin turgor); refer to Chapter 10.
- Assess for fever.

Diagnostics

- Clinical features/presentation on assessment
- May obtain stool sample, urine analysis (UA), CBC, electrolytes

Nursing Interventions

- Monitor for dehydration, I&O; obtain daily weights.
- Administer ORT as ordered; provide small amount of feedings often (refer to Chapter 10).
- Encourage breastfeeding.

Special Considerations

Do not give anti-diarrheal medications, especially children under two years of age. Contact healthcare clinician.

Discharge Planning; Patient and Family Education

- Educate families on prevention strategies—handwashing, breastfeeding, proper handling, and cooking of food.
- Inform parents/caregivers on the importance of cleaning practices in day-care centers.
- Educate families about promoting hydration using oral rehydration solutions (ORS); refer to Chapter 10.
- Discuss signs and symptoms of dehydration and worsening symptoms.
- Teach parents/caregivers to give child usual diet as tolerated; "bowel rest" is not recommended.

GASTROESOPHAGEAL REFLUX DISEASE

Description

- A disease where gastric acid and contents easily flow back up into the esophagus and may even enter the oropharynx; can cause discomfort and injury to the mucosa
  - Can occur in infants as gastroesophageal reflux (GER; normal) due to immature lower esophageal sphincter, without a disease process diagnosis, that resolves as child's GI system matures and has a solid diet around 12 to 18 months.
  - Infants may have been premature, have an allergy to formula.
  - Features most often include painless regurgitation of feeding with GER or may be irritable with gastroesophageal reflux disease (GERD); at risk for reflux-induced asthma, pneumonia, and esophagitis.

Assessment

- **Assess for GERD within one hour of feeding (note may not have any symptoms):** Vomiting, irritability, posturing.

PEDIATRIC PEARLS

- **Sandifer syndrome:** Look for abnormal neck posturing in infant by arching the back with feedings.

- Assess growth and development; at risk for failure to thrive with GERD.
- **Monitor for respiratory distress (at risk for aspiration):** choking, gagging, coughing, wheezing, cyanosis.
- Observe emesis and stool for blood; monitor labs for anemia.

Diagnostics

- History and clinical features.
- Esophageal pH probe may be ordered to determine acid versus non-acid reflux and the amount of reflux at the time.

Nursing Interventions

- Encourage breastfeeding.
- Consider thickening formula with rice cereal to decrease vomiting and be sure to enlarge nipple hole for less effort in suck–swallow technique.
- Administer reflux medications (famotidine, omeprazole) as ordered, often 30 minutes before feedings.

Special Considerations

Do not overfeed infant; try to offer smaller feedings more often; burp infant often when feeding.

Discharge Planning; Patient and Family Education

- Educate parents and caregivers to maintain infant in upright position (e.g., raise head of bed, hold in arms) during and after feedings for 30 minutes to 2 hours.
- Encourage avoidance of equipment that increases intra-abdominal pressure after feedings, such as infant swings.
- Encourage adherence to follow-up appointments to monitor growth.
- Offer emotional support to caregivers.
- Instruct to contact clinician if child experiences complications such as an apparent life-threatening event (ALTE).

PEDIATRIC PEARLS

- In severe cases of GERD, child may need surgery—a Nissen fundoplication, where the upper stomach (fundus) is sutured around the lower sphincter of the esophagus.

HEPATITIS (VIRAL CAUSE)

Description

- Liver inflammation, caused by five viral types:
    - **Hepatitis A (HAV;** most common in children)
        - **Features:** Found in contaminated water/poor sanitation, fecal–oral route, raw shellfish, travelers to developing countries, day-care centers
    - Hepatitis B (HBV)
        - **Features:** Blood and body fluid transmission, mother to fetus (vertical transmission), IV substance use, unprotected sex
    - Hepatitis C (HCV)
        - **Features:** Blood, IV substance use
    - Hepatitis D (HDV)
        - **Features:** Only HBV diagnosed persons can be infected
    - Hepatitis E (HEV)
        - **Features:** Found only in Asia, Africa, Mexico; oral–fecal transmission
- **Prevention:** Vaccines for HAV, HBV; good handwashing, drink noncontaminated water, use protection during intercourse, and avoid substance use
- Often asymptomatic; may have nausea, vomiting, diarrhea, anorexia, hepatomegaly, flu-like symptoms

Assessment

- Ask families about features/risks (listed previously).
- Assess for any mild signs and symptoms (listed previously).
- Assess skin and eyes for jaundice, cirrhosis (may have abdominal pain).
- Monitor for changes in urine (dark) and stool (light) color.

Diagnostics

- Liver enzymes
- Serologic antigen/antibody testing
- Ultrasound of liver
- Biopsy

Nursing Interventions

- Monitor for progression of hepatitis, cirrhosis.
- Monitor for dehydration.
- Emphasize importance of good nutrition.
- Administer vaccinations according to vaccine schedule, as prescribed by clinician.

Special Considerations

Newborns are often vaccinated with HBV before leaving hospital; give hepatitis B immunoglobulin (HBIG) if mom is Hepatitis B + within 12 of hours of birth.

Discharge Planning; Patient and Family Education

- Educate families on viral hepatitis, transmission, and prevention strategies, including sanitation and good handwashing.
- Monitor vaccination schedule.

HIRSCHSPRUNG DISEASE (CONGENITAL AGANGLIONIC MEGACOLON)

Description

- A congenital condition where the bowel is missing ganglion, or nerve cells, for motility of bowel contents through the intestine; loss of peristalsis causes obstruction (Figure 9.2).

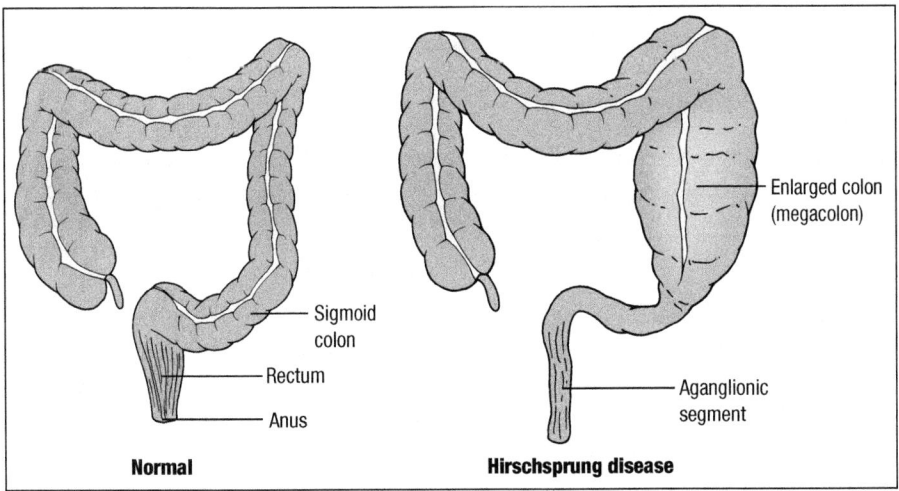

FIGURE 9.2: Normal intestine and manifestations of Hirschsprung disease. Hirschsprung disease results from failed migration of neural crest cells to the distal colon. As a result, submucosal and myenteric plexuses fail to develop, rendering the distal colon nonfunctional

Source: Reprinted from Jnah, A. J., & Trembath, A. N. (2019). *Fetal and neonatal physiology for the advanced practice nurse* (1st ed.). Springer Publishing Company.

- **Features:** Usually occurs within the first day of life; infant does not have a meconium bowel movement; may have small, "ribbon-like" stools (not diarrhea) as stool tries to push through obstruction.
- Treatment is surgery.

Assessment

- Assess newborn for bowel movement within 24 to 48 hours of life.
- Assess GI status: hypoactive bowel sounds, distended abdomen, may be able to palpate mass of stool.

PEDIATRIC PEARLS

- May have explosive stool after digital rectal exam; test for blood in stool if that happens.

Diagnostics

May need barium enema; rectal biopsy confirms diagnosis via pathology for aganglionic cells.

Nursing Interventions

- Perform pre- and postoperative care; may need ostomy, surgery may be done in stages.
- Monitor for infection, skin breakdown around ostomy site, failure to thrive.
- Monitor I&O.
- Provide referral to wound care/ostomy care nurse.

Special Considerations

Mostly seen in males; at risk are those with a family history, Trisomy 21/Down Syndrome and other anomalies

Discharge Planning; Patient and Family Education

- Educate the family on ostomy care if necessary.
- Instruct caregivers to contact clinician if child has signs and symptoms of infection (enterocolitis).
- Provide support and resources to families.

INFLAMMATORY BOWEL DISEASE—CROHN'S DISEASE AND ULCERATIVE COLITIS

Description

- A chronic condition in which the intestines become inflamed causing damage in the GI system (autoimmune issue); can have acute exacerbations; at-risk population are children with family histories for inflammatory bowel disease (IBD), usually diagnosed between 10 and 20 years of age
  - Diarrhea is main clinical feature/presentation; may have other symptoms not related to GI (extraintestinal; e.g., uveitis/iritis, arthritis, skin lesions)
  - Two types (Table 9.1 and Figure 9.3):
    - **Crohn's disease (CD):** Inflammation and injury occurs deep into the lining of the intestinal mucosa causing thickness and is seen anywhere in the intestinal tract; images show a "cobble-stone" appearance or skip pattern of normal and inflamed areas.
    - **Ulcerative colitis (UC):** Inflammation is seen only in the lining of the intestine, not thick within it; images show ulcers and inflammation found continuously along the mucosa.

INFLAMMATORY BOWEL DISEASE—CROHN'S DISEASE AND ULCERATIVE COLITIS

TABLE 9.1: Comparison of Types of Inflammatory Bowel Disease

	Crohn's Disease	Ulcerative Colitis
Features: Endoscopic view	• Transmural—all layers of bowel; can even affect any part of GI tract • Most common in distal ileum • Inflammation areas and thickening of bowel • "Cobble-stone" or "skip" pattern • Strictures, fistulas	• Mucosa and submucosa (only lining, not transmural) • Rectum and colon • Ulcerations • Inflammation—continuous • Abscesses
Assessment: Signs and symptoms (UC may be categorized as mild, moderate, and severe)	• Diarrhea • RLQ pain • Fissures and/or abscesses • Fever • Anorexia, malnutrition	• Bloody diarrhea • LLQ pain • Fever • Anorexia, weight loss • Anemia, can be severe • Hypovolemia • Hypoalbuminemia

CD, Crohn's disease; GI, gastrointestinal; RLQ, right lower quadrant; LLQ, left lower quadrant; UC, ulcerative colitis.

Assessment

- Assess growth and development (delayed puberty), weight loss, nutritional deficiencies.
- Monitor for infection especially with UC.
- Monitor for dysrhythmias.

Diagnostics

- **Labs:** Anemia, ↑ WBCs, ↓ protein and albumin (hypoalbuminemia)
- **Combination of tests:** Upper GI and small bowel series/endoscopy (for CD)/colonoscopy (UC)
- Abdominal CT scan, MRI
- Biopsy of intestinal lining
- Stool for ova and parasites, calprotectin (released with bowel inflammation)

Nursing Interventions

- Administer pain medications as ordered.
- Obtain daily weights; maintain optimal nutritional balance, may need parental nutrition; administer nutritional supplements as ordered.
- Monitor I&O; maintain fluid and electrolyte balance.
- Administer blood products as ordered.
- Administer medications as ordered, such as anti-inflammatory agents, aminosalicylates, corticosteroids, biological therapies, immunomodulators, antibiotics if necessary.

Special Considerations

May need surgery in the long term; can be curative measure for UC, but not in CD

154 INFLAMMATORY BOWEL DISEASE—CROHN'S DISEASE AND ULCERATIVE COLITIS

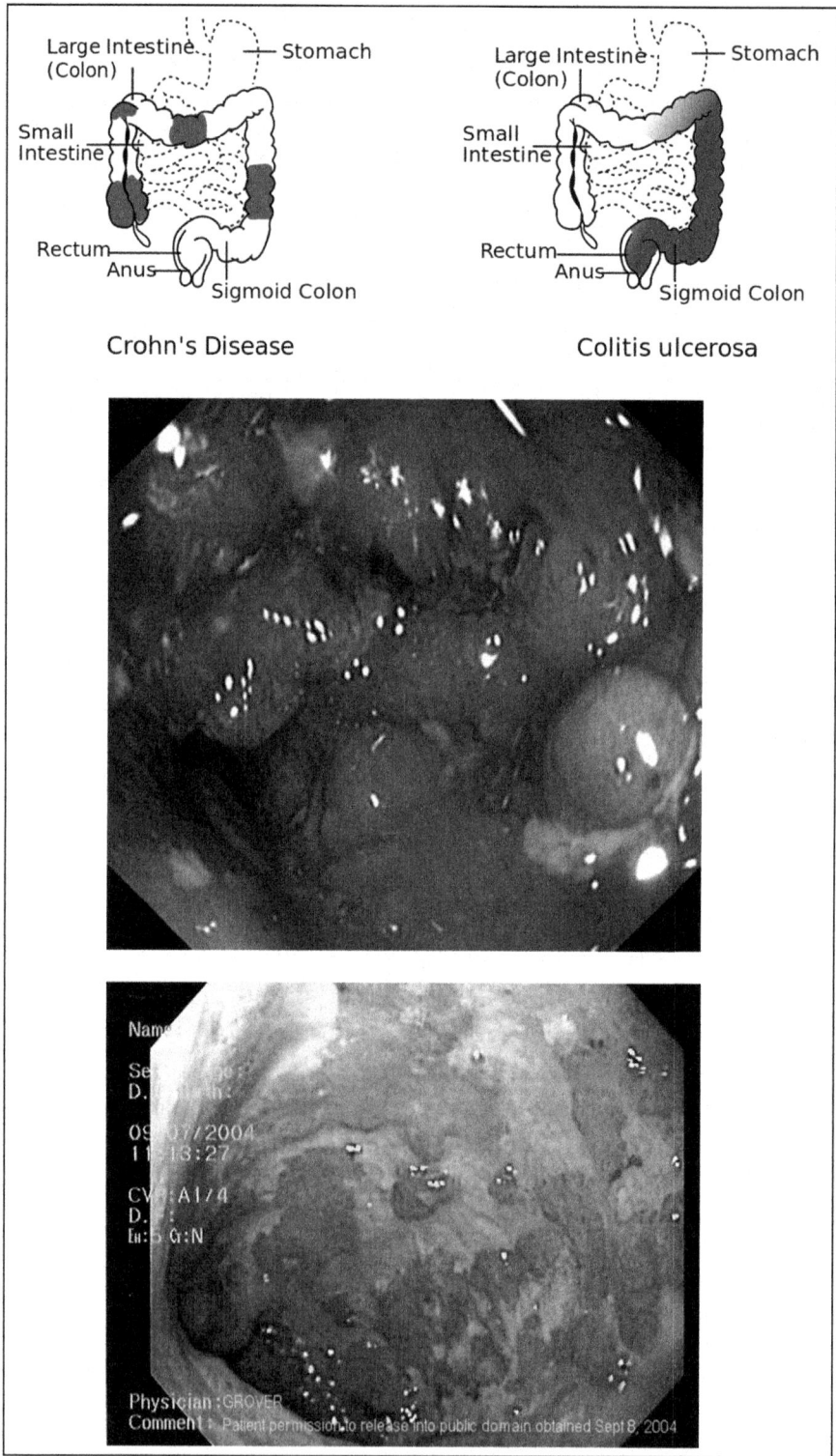

FIGURE 9.3: (A) Anatomical comparison of digestive tract with Crohn's disease and digestive tract with ulcerative colitis. **(B)** Endoscopic view of the bowel with Crohn's disease. **(C)** Endoscopic view of the bowel with ulcerative colitis

Source: **(A)** Courtesy of Samir, https://commons.wikimedia.org/wiki/File:Crohn%27s_Disease_vs_Colitis_ulcerosa.svg. **(B)** Courtesy of Bungi, https://commons.wikimedia.org/wiki/File:Sten%C3%B3za_%C4%8Dreva.jpg. **(C)** Courtesy of Samir, https://commons.wikimedia.org/wiki/File:Ulcerative_colitis.jpg.

Discharge Planning; Patient and Family Education

- Educate families on the importance of nutrition; maintain diet high in protein and carbohydrates, normal fat diet; may need TPN in severe cases.
- Discuss treatment options; may need surgery later in life with ostomy, refer to ostomy nurse.
- Offer support and resources to family.
- Refer to specialist in pediatric GI.

PEDIATRIC PEARLS

- *At risk for colon cancer*

INTUSSUSCEPTION

Description

- Condition in which the intestine slides or folds into itself causing an obstruction; medical emergency (Figure 9.4)
  - **Most common:** Ileocolic area, males, before two years of age, idiopathic; can be triggered by polyps, Meckel diverticulum, infection, cystic fibrosis, celiac disease
  - **Features:** Sudden abdominal pain in otherwise healthy infant/child in which they yell and clench their knees, irritable, vomiting, lethargy; infant or child is comfortable between acute episodes
  - **Key feature:** "Currant jelly-like" stools (stools are mixed with blood and mucous) and "sausage-like" mass in upper, middle abdomen
  - **Treatment:** Contrast air/barium enema can be used to reduce or push the intestine back into place with pressure or surgery
  - May recur especially in first 24 hours after treatment

Assessment

- Assess abdomen for nausea, vomiting, distention, pain, bloody stools.
- Note any masses in abdomen especially right upper quadrant (RUQ).
- Monitor for dehydration.

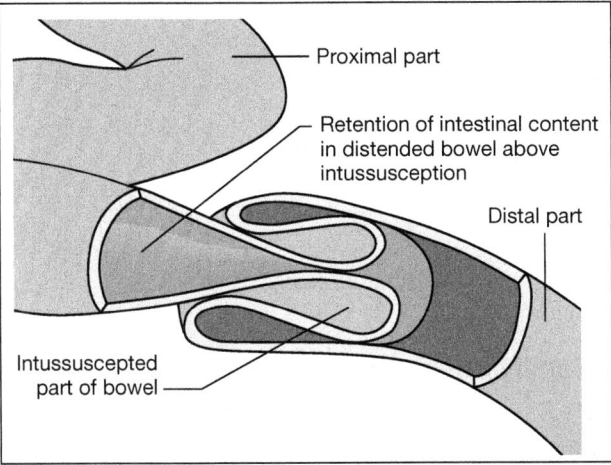

FIGURE 9.4: Intussusception of the bowel occurs when a distal segment of the intestine telescopes over a more proximal segment

Source: Reprinted from Tkacs, N. C., Hermann, L. L., & Johnson, R. L. (2020). *Advanced physiology and pathophysiology: Essentials for clinical practice* (1st ed.). Springer Publishing Company.

PEDIATRIC PEARLS

- If not treated, intussusception progresses to perforation → peritonitis → shock → death.

Diagnostics

- X-ray
- Contrast air or barium enema
- Ultrasound

Nursing Interventions

- Educate child and family on treatment.
- Administer antibiotics as ordered.
- Provide IV fluids if dehydrated.

Special Considerations

Diagnostic test can serve as treatment.

Discharge Planning; Patient and Family Education

- Provide emotional support to caregivers.
- Educate child and family on possible ostomy surgery.

MECKEL DIVERTICULUM

Description

- Congenital condition in which an outward pocket forms in the small intestine from a duct that did not close around seven weeks gestation; most common area is ileum
  - **Features:** Infants/children ≤ 2 years of age, males
  - **Treatment:** Surgery

Assessment

- Assess for abdominal pain/distention, fever, bloody stools, vomiting.
- **Monitor for complications:** Anemia, bleeding, obstruction.

Diagnostics

- Meckel scan (GI scintigraphy)
- Biopsy and pathology
- CT scan of abdomen

Nursing Interventions

- Educate caregivers on surgery; provide pre- and postoperative care.
- Administer blood transfusions for complications.

Discharge Planning; Patient and Family Education

- Provide emotional support to family.
- Discuss treatment and postoperative care.

NECROTIZING ENTEROCOLITIS

Description

- Acute GI infection with necrosis of the bowel; this is a medical emergency.
  - **Process:** Intestinal inflammation → ischemia → necrosis → septic shock → can lead to death
  - **At risk:** Premature infants, hypoxia in utero/asphyxia during delivery
  - **Prevention:** Breastfeeding, antenatal maternal corticosteroids, gradual initiation of feedings, antibiotics, and probiotics
  - **Treatment:** May need surgery to remove necrotic area

Assessment

- **Assess for GI issues:** Abdominal distention/tenderness, increased girth, decreased bowel sounds, visual "loops of bowel," vomiting (can be bilious), bloody stools.
- Note difficulty with feedings, increasing gastric residuals with naso-/oro-gastric tube feedings.
- **Monitor for worsening symptoms:** Temperature and cardiovascular instability, respiratory difficulties (apnea), lethargy.

Diagnostics

- Radiographs of abdomen and kidneys, ureters, bladder (KUB); shows dilated "loops of bowel" and gas bubbles made by bacteria; used to monitor disease progression and evaluate effects of treatment
- Blood cultures, C-reactive protein, coagulation studies (possible disseminated intravascular coagulation [DIC])
- Laboratory results: increased WBCs, metabolic acidosis

Nursing Interventions

- If suspect necrotizing enterocolitis (NEC), then discontinue feedings and contact healthcare clinician.
- Maintain infant NPO and gastric decompression started.
- Infuse IV fluids and TPN as ordered.
- Administer IV antibiotics, pain medications, blood products, as ordered.
- Monitor I&O.
- Once resolved, begin to feed infant as ordered; follow hospital protocol for advancing feedings.

PEDIATRIC PEARLS

- Immediately stop feedings if suspect NEC—need to rest bowel for healing.

Special Considerations

- Maternal infections and preeclampsia can predispose newborn to NEC.
- The lower the gestational age of the newborn, the higher the risk of NEC.

Discharge Planning; Patient and Family Education

- Provide emotional support to parents/caregivers.
- Educate parents/caregivers about ostomy care post-surgery if needed.
- **Discuss possible complications of NEC and surgery:** Short bowel syndrome and intestinal strictures.

PINWORMS (*ENTEROBIUS VERMICULARIS*) — HELMINTHIC INFECTION

Description

- Parasitic worm that invades and lives in the bowel
  - At night, adult female pinworm moves from rectum to perianal skin → lays eggs → dies → itching; child scratches at anus, has eggs in fingernails, then moves hands to mouth ingesting eggs, worms infest intestines and the process continues (usually takes about two weeks).
  - May be asymptomatic.
  - **Prevention:** Handwashing, short clean nails, not scratching egg area, avoid putting hands in mouth and biting nails.

Assessment

- Ask about insomnia, irritability at night.
- Assess for nighttime frequent pruritus of perianal and anal area.
- Inspect perianal area for worms (in morning), any marks from scratching.
- Note any "threads" from worms in undergarments or toilet.
- Assess for weight loss/failure to thrive.

Diagnostics

- **Identification of pinworms/eggs:** "Tape" test/adhesive cellophane tape "paddle"—eggs/worms stick to transparent tape when applied to perianal area at bedtime and/or upon awakening, look at tape via microscope; perform for at least three days in a row.

Nursing Interventions

- Educate parents/caregivers about tape tests.
- Administer medications as ordered.
- Educate family on frequent cleaning (using hot water) of linen, clothing, toilet seats, surfaces, not sharing items; pinworms can survive on surfaces for two to three weeks.

Special Considerations

Emphasize the importance of good handwashing to prevent infection.

Discharge Planning; Patient and Family Education

- Provide emotional support.
- Discuss recurrence/reinfection of pinworms and prevention strategies; instruct to shower (avoid baths which can leave eggs in water) in morning and daily to help get rid of eggs.
- Emphasize that all family members need to be tested and treated.
- Inform all caretakers including day-care centers and schools.

PYLORIC STENOSIS (HYPERTROPHIC)

Description

- Condition in which the pylorus muscle grows, increases in size (hypertrophy), and thickens, blocking the outlet where the feeding leaves the stomach, causing obstruction (Figure 9.5)
  - **At risk:** Genetics/family history, males
  - Signs and symptoms not apparent at birth; usually noted after the first week of birth; three weeks to four months of age

PYLORIC STENOSIS (HYPERTROPHIC)

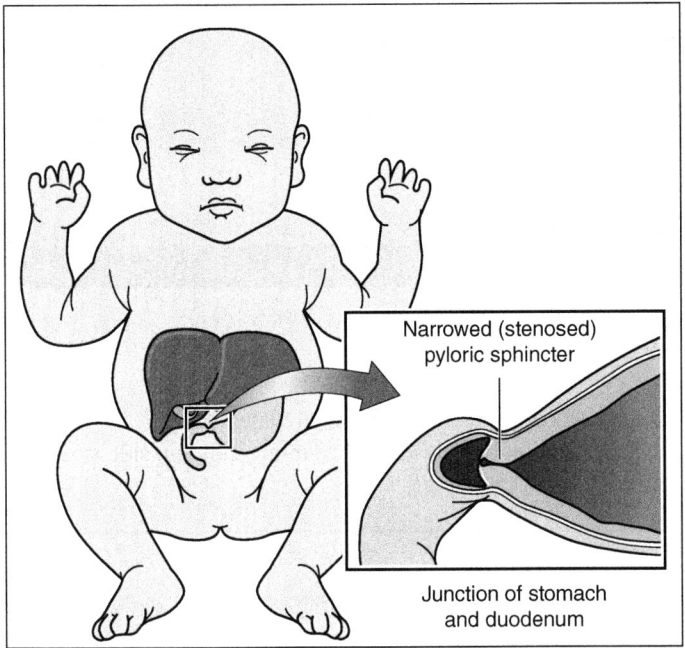

FIGURE 9.5: Pyloric stenosis
Source: Reprinted from Myrick, K., & Karosas, L. (2019). *Advanced health assessment and differential diagnosis* (1st ed.). Springer Publishing Company.

- **Features:** Emesis gets worse with obstruction, and infant has projectile (several feet away), nonbilious vomiting after feeding, infant appears "hungry/starving," weight loss/failure to thrive
- **Treatment:** Pyloromyotomy surgery to release the thick muscle fibers of the pylorus and open the gastric outlet between the stomach and intestines

PEDIATRIC PEARLS
- Projectile vomiting with every feeding can lead to complications such as metabolic alkalosis, dehydration, and malnutrition.

Assessment
- Assess for feeding intolerances, changes in bowel movements with fewer stools, constipation.
- Note an "olive-shaped" abdominal mass in RUQ.
- Assess for irritability and/or lethargy, complications.

Diagnostics
- Visible abdominal "peristalsis waves"
- Abdominal US
- Electrolytes

Nursing Interventions
- Monitor labs, electrolytes, I&O, dehydration.
- Administer IV fluids as ordered.
- Refer to surgeon.
- Provide pre- and postoperative care.

Special Considerations

Monitor for low blood sugar after surgery.

Discharge Planning; Patient and Family Education

- Educate parents/caregivers on treatment and care.
- Give emotional support to parents/caregivers.

VOMITING

Description

- Forceful, reflexive movement of stomach contents back up into mouth
  - Can be a single event or related to infectious agent or a medical diagnosis
  - **Prevention during feedings:** Keep head of bed elevated, turn infant/child on side/sitting up (right side), and remain supine

PEDIATRIC PEARLS

- Be alert for metabolic alkalosis in children with frequent vomiting of stomach acids.

Assessment

- Ask about activities before vomiting episodes; frequency, force, how often/when, color and contents of emesis, how much.
- Observe parents/caregivers during feedings and monitor infant/child for problems.
- Assess GI status, hydration status (daily weight, I&O).
- Assess neuro status.
- Inquire about other signs and symptoms not related to vomiting.

Diagnostics

Clinical features/presentation on assessment

Nursing Interventions

- Monitor for nausea.
- Administer ORT as ordered; offer small amounts at a time.
- If child not able to tolerate ORS, then administer IV fluids as ordered.
- Give antiemetics as needed, per prescription for appropriate age.
- Turn infant/child on side during vomiting episodes.

Special Considerations

Teach parents/caregivers the difference between vomiting and "wet burps/spitting up" (not due to a pathologic issue).

Discharge Planning; Patient and Family Education

- Educate families about promoting hydration using ORS (refer to Chapter 10).
- Suggest that pills and teas with ginger are safe for children over age 2; inform clinician if taking these.
- Inform parents/caregivers about turning infant/child on side during vomiting episodes.

BIBLIOGRAPHY

American Academy of Pediatrics. (2017). Acetaminophen dosage table for fever and pain. *Healthy Children*. https://www.healthychildren.org/English/safety-prevention/at-home/medication-safety/Pages/Acetaminophen-for-Fever-and-Pain.aspx

American Academy of Pediatrics. (2021). Diarrhea in children: What parents need to know. *Healthy Children*. https://www.healthychildren.org/English/health-issues/conditions/abdominal/Pages/Diarrhea.aspx

Centers for Disease Control and Prevention. (2020). *Pinworm infection FAQs*. https://www.cdc.gov/parasites/pinworm/gen_info/faqs.html

Centers for Disease Control and Prevention. (2018). *Inflammatory bowel disease (IBD)*. https://www.cdc.gov/ibd/what-is-IBD.htm

DynaMed. (2019, August 20). *Celiac disease*. EBSCO Information Services. Retrieved May 24, 2021, from https://www.dynamed.com/condition/celiac-disease

DynaMed. (2019, October 31). *Cleft lip and palate*. EBSCO Information Services. Retrieved May 24, 2021, from https://www.dynamed.com/condition/cleft-lip-and-palate

DynaMed. (2020, November 10). *Tracheoesophageal malformations*. EBSCO Information Services. Retrieved June 2, 2021, from https://www.dynamed.com/condition/tracheoesophageal-malformations

DynaMed. (2014, November 22). *Meckel diverticulum*. EBSCO Information Services. Retrieved June 29, 2021, from https://www.dynamed.com/condition/meckel-diverticulum

DynaMed. (2020, December 9). *Necrotizing enterocolitis*. EBSCO Information Services. Retrieved June 29, 2021, from https://www.dynamed.com/condition/necrotizing-enterocolitis-19

Hockenberry, M. J., Wilson, D., & Rodgers, C. C. (2019). *Wong's nursing care of infants and children* (11th ed.). Elsevier Inc.

Ricci, S. S., Kyle, T., & Carman, S. (2021). *Maternity and pediatric nursing* (4th ed.). Wolters Kluwer.

Silbert-Flagg, J., & Sloand, E. D. (Eds.). (2017). *Pediatric nurse practitioner certification review guide: Primary care* (6th ed.). Jones & Bartlett Learning, LLC.

KNOWLEDGE CHECK

1. A 20-month-old toddler is diagnosed with gastroenteritis. The caregiver reports that the child has shown signs of vomiting, diarrhea, and fever for the past 24 hours. The nurse assesses the child and finds mild dehydration. Which intervention is the most appropriate?

    A. Have the child drink sips of Pedialyte® frequently.
    B. Give the child apple juice in small amounts.
    C. Inform the caregiver that the child needs IV fluids.
    D. Administer anti-diarrheal medication to the child.

2. An infant diagnosed with pyloric stenosis has been vomiting for the past several days. On assessment, the nurse notes weight loss, dehydration, and changes in bowel movements. Which complication should the nurse be alert for?

    A. Metabolic acidosis
    B. Metabolic alkalosis
    C. Thrombocytopenia
    D. Hyperglycemia

3. A 2-month-old infant is seen in the pediatric urgent care clinic. The caregiver states that the infant has been projectile vomiting right after feeding and seems hungry afterward. The nurse should suspect which condition in the infant?

    A. Celiac disease
    B. Hirschsprung disease
    C. Intussusception
    D. Pyloric stenosis

4. A nurse is providing discharge teaching to caregivers of an infant diagnosed with a cleft lip and palate. Which instruction is appropriate for the care plan after surgical repair of the defects?

    A. Avoid breastfeeding the infant.
    B. Infant must use straw when drinking from a cup.
    C. Refer infant to speech therapy.
    D. Position infant prone immediately after repair.

5. Which factor is important in preventing infectious gastroenteritis in infants and children?

    A. Receiving *Rotavirus* vaccination
    B. Receiving *Influenza* vaccination
    C. Giving anti-diarrheal medication
    D. Attending day care

6. Which assessment findings should a nurse expect when caring for an infant diagnosed with intussusception?

    A. Weight loss and constipation
    B. Currant jelly-like stools and sudden abdominal pain
    C. Intermittent nausea and vomiting with pale stools
    D. Lack of appetite and ribbon-like stools

KNOWLEDGE CHECK

1. **Correct Answer: A) Have the child drink sips of Pedialyte® frequently.** The child diagnosed with gastroenteritis should be monitored for dehydration. This child has mild dehydration, not severe dehydration, therefore, ORT using nonsugary drinks with electrolytes is appropriate. It is important to give the child ORS in small frequent amounts. Apple juice contains sugar and will worsen diarrhea. The child will be hospitalized for severe dehydration if they cannot tolerate ORS and need IV fluids. Children under the age of two should not receive anti-diarrheal medications and caregivers should contact their clinician before giving any anti-diarrheal medications.

2. **Correct Answer: B) Metabolic alkalosis.** Pyloric stenosis causes projectile vomiting. Frequent vomiting causes the loss of stomach acids (gastric pH), leading to metabolic alkalosis. Presentation usually includes hypokalemic, hypochloremic metabolic alkalosis. Based on the presentation, metabolic acidosis, thrombocytopenia, and hyperglycemia are not expected.

3. **Correct Answer: D) Pyloric stenosis.** Pyloric stenosis is a condition in which the pylorus muscle increases in size (hypertrophy) and thickens, blocking the outlet where the feeding leaves the stomach, causing obstruction. The features of this condition are as follows: emesis gets worse with obstruction, infant has projectile, nonbilious vomiting after feeding, infant appears "hungry/starving," and weight loss/failure to thrive is observed. Due to the child's symptoms, pyloric stenosis is most likely. Celiac disease is characterized by steatorrhea, chronic diarrhea/constipation, abdominal distention/bloating, nausea/vomiting, and anorexia/weight loss leading to failure to thrive. Hirschsprung disease is characterized by small, ribbon-like stools distinct from diarrhea. Intussusception features sudden abdominal pain in an otherwise healthy infant/child, irritability, vomiting and lethargy. Between these episodes, the child patient is comfortable.

4. **Correct Answer: C) Refer infant to speech therapy.** A cleft lip is usually repaired around two to three months of life, a cleft palate is repaired around 9 to 12 months to avoid speech delays—long-term follow up with speech therapists are necessary to monitor speech development. Protect the sutures on the lip and place the infant supine, not prone immediately after repair. Avoid hard objects (e.g., a straw) in the mouth after a cleft palate repair. Keep incision site clean by rinsing with water after feedings and feed via syringe or cup during first postop day. After the first postop day, encourage breastfeeding. Decrease irritability and crying.

5. **Correct Answer: A) Receiving *Rotavirus* vaccination.** Gastroenteritis is an infection/inflammation of the stomach that can be acute and infectious. Rotavirus is the common infectious agent to gastroenteritis and prevention includes the Rotavirus vaccination. An *Influenza* vaccination will not prevent gastroenteritis in children. Signs and symptoms include abdominal pain, fever, nausea, vomiting, and diarrhea. Children are at risk if they attend day-care centers. Do not give anti-diarrheal medication to children, especially under two years of age without consulting a clinician.

6. **Correct Answer: B) Currant jelly-like stools and sudden abdominal pain.** Intussusception is a condition in which the intestine slides or folds into itself, causing an obstruction and is a medical emergency. It features sudden abdominal pain in an otherwise healthy infant/child in which they yell and clench their knees, irritability, vomiting, and lethargy. The infant or child is comfortable between acute episodes. Its key features are "currant jelly-like" stools (stools are mixed with blood and mucous) and a "sausage-like" mass in upper, middle abdomen. Weight loss can occur, but constipation is a sign of pyloric stenosis. Nausea and vomiting can occur, but they are not accompanied by pale stools. Pale stools are a sign of biliary atresia and hepatitis. Ribbon-like stools are a sign of Hirschsprung disease.

7. A caregiver brings their child into the primary care office with complaints of insomnia and intense itching at the perianal area. The nurse suspects a pinworm infestation. The nurse understands that which test can confirm the diagnosis of pinworms?

    A. Barium enema to remove the worms and eggs
    B. Blood test for parasites to determine treatment
    C. X-ray of abdomen to show worms in intestines
    D. Clear tape "paddle" test on anus at bedtime for the eggs to stick to it

8. A nurse is providing education to a caregiver with a child diagnosed with pinworms. Which statement by the caregiver demonstrates an understanding of the nurse's teaching about pinworms?

    A. "Our entire family should be tested and treated."
    B. "I can allow my children to take a bath together."
    C. "Pinworms cannot spread to others."
    D. "It is okay for my children to share clothes."

9. A nurse is caring for a child diagnosed with celiac disease. The caregiver asks about which foods the child can eat. The nurse suggests which food choices are most appropriate for a child with celiac disease?

    A. Cereal and milk
    B. Granola oat bars and carrots
    C. Cheese sticks and apples
    D. Corn and pasta

10. A nurse is caring for an 11-year-old child with abdominal pain. The nurse assesses for McBurney's point and suspects appendicitis. Which location of the abdomen does the nurse assess McBurney's point?

    A. Right Upper Quadrant (RUQ)
    B. Right Lower Quadrant (RLQ)
    C. Left Upper Quadrant (LUQ)
    D. Left Lower Quadrant (LLQ)

7. **Correct Answer: D) Clear tape "paddle" test on anus at bedtime for the eggs to stick to it.** At night, adult female pinworm moves from rectum to perianal skin, lays eggs and dies. Anus becomes itchy; child scratches at anus, has eggs in fingernails, then moves hands to mouth ingesting eggs. Worms infest intestines and the process continues (usually takes about two weeks). The adhesive cellophane tape "paddle"/"tape" test can identify pinworms as the eggs/worms stick to transparent tape when applied to perianal area at bedtime and/or upon awakening. This tape is viewed through a microscope. The other tests are not involved in the diagnosis of pinworms.

8. **Correct Answer: A) "Our entire family should be tested and treated."** All family members must be tested and treated to stop the spread of the pinworm infestation, as it can spread to others. Discuss recurrence/reinfection of pinworms and prevention strategies; instruct family members to shower alone (avoid baths which can leave eggs in water) in morning and daily to help get rid of eggs. Inform all caretakers including day-care centers and schools. Educate family on frequent cleaning (using hot water) of linen, clothing, toilet seats, and surfaces, and not sharing items. Pinworms can survive on surfaces for two to three weeks.

9. **Correct Answer: C) Cheese sticks and apples**. The child must be on a gluten-free diet. Cheese and fruit do not contain gluten. Many cereals, granola oat bars, and pastas contain gluten. Educate family on importance of maintaining the child on a gluten-free diet for lifetime especially avoiding wheat, rye, and barley products since they contain the protein gluten.

10. **Correct Answer: B) Right Lower Quadrant (RLQ)**. With appendicitis, the nurse assesses McBurney's point in the RLQ. The RUQ, left upper quadrant and left lower quadrant are all incorrect positions to evaluate McBurney's point.

CHAPTER 10

Genitourinary, Renal, and Reproductive Conditions

Maureen Fitzgerald and David Jack

INTRODUCTION TO THE PEDIATRIC RENAL SYSTEM AND KIDNEY FUNCTION

The genitourinary (GU) system is responsible for the elimination of body waste through the urinary/renal system. The nurse should be familiar with the various GU and reproductive disorders that children can experience due to fetal development, genetics, infection, and trauma, to name a few.

- Children have short urethras, especially females, placing them at increased risk for organisms to travel into the bladder.
- A child's kidney attains adult number of nephrons shortly after birth and continues to mature into early childhood; the kidney is less protected than in adults and at risk for injury.
- The kidney is less able to concentrate urine and reabsorb amino acids increasing risk of dehydration; an infant's average specific gravity is less than 1.010 compared with 1.010 to 1.030 for an adult.
- **Kidney functions:**
  - Blood detoxification
  - Fluid and electrolyte balance and acid/base balance
  - **Waste elimination:**
    - Aldosterone increases renal excretion.
  - **Blood pressure (BP) regulation by:**
    - Producing renin which stimulates angiotensin I production → angiotensin II production → peripheral vasoconstriction and aldosterone secretion
    - Aldosterone → sodium and water reabsorption → increases BP
- Reproductive organs are immature and hormonal changes in puberty may attribute to some conditions.

ACID/BASE BALANCE

Description

- The pH of the blood is controlled via three systems: chemical buffering, respiratory function, and renal function. These systems regulate the serum (regulation of H+) that determines pH, through the control of bicarbonate HCO_3 (buffer/base/alkaline) and $PaCO_2$ (acid).
  - Normal neutral serum pH values are 7.35 to 7.45.

- Less than 7.35 is acidosis, loss of HCO_3, or gain of CO_2, whereas serum blood levels greater than 7.45 alkalosis, gain of HCO_3, or loss of CO_2.
  - Normal serum $PaCO_2$ values are 35 to 45 (regulated by lungs).
  - Normal serum HCO_3 values are 22 to 26 (regulated by kidneys).
  - Normal PaO_2 values = 80 to 100 mmHg.

Assessment

- Begin by examining the pH.
  - Below 7.35 → acidosis, above 7.45 → alkalosis (these states are uncompensated).
  - If the pH is within normal range, the child's body may have compensated for the altered acid–base state.
- Next, examine the $PaCO_2$ level. Does it fall within range? What is the relationship with the pH (are they going in opposite directions)?
  - If pH ↓ $PaCO_2$ ↑ → Respiratory acidosis
  - If pH ↑ and $PaCO_2$ ↓ → Respiratory alkalosis
- Then, if pH and $PaCO_2$ are going in the same direction, look at the HCO_3 (metabolic problems go in the same direction).
  - If pH ↓ and $PaCO_2$ normal to ↓ and HCO_3 ↓ → metabolic acidosis
  - If pH ↑ and $PaCO_2$ normal to ↑ and HCO_3 ↑ → metabolic alkalosis
- Causes:
  - **Respiratory acidosis:** Respiratory acidosis is due to alveolar hypoventilation, which results in an increased $PaCO_2$ (e.g., respiratory insufficiency, failure, neuromuscular disease, airway obstruction); as PCO_2 rises, symptoms may include somnolence (sleepiness) from hypercarbia.
  - **Respiratory alkalosis:** Respiratory alkalosis is due to alveolar hyperventilation, which results in a diminished $PaCO_2$ (e.g., CNS: disturbances of the respiratory regulation, anxiety and panic attacks, fever); brief loss of consciousness due to the combination of hypocarbia-induced cerebral vascular vasoconstriction; and not eliminating the O_2 from the hemoglobin.
  - **Metabolic acidosis:** Metabolic acidosis is primary reduction in bicarbonate (HCO_3-; e.g., diarrhea, increased acid ingestion, salicylate poisoning, diabetic ketoacidosis, or kidney failure); signs in severe cases include nausea and vomiting, lethargy, and hyperpnea.
  - **Metabolic alkalosis:** Metabolic alkalosis is primary increase in bicarbonate (HCO_3-; prolonged vomiting, diuretic use, hypokalemia, renal impairment of HCO_3- excretion); signs in severe cases include headache, lethargy, and tetany.

ACUTE POSTSTREPTOCOCCAL GLOMERULONEPHRITIS

Description

- Acute poststreptococcal glomerulonephritis (APSGN) is an inflammation of the kidney tubules (glomeruli) that filter waste products from the blood, following a group A *Streptococcal* infection such as strep throat or, rarely, a skin infection (impetigo).
  - Antigen–antibody complexes become trapped in the glomerular capillary membranes, leading to inflammation and impaired glomerular functioning.
- Occurs more commonly in males and in children between the ages of 4 and 8 years.
- The prognosis for APSGN is good, with 95% patients making a full recovery.
  - Most clinical symptoms resolving spontaneously within 2 to 3 weeks after onset.
  - *Streptococcus* is not present in the kidney during the course of illness.

Assessment

- Assess for recent upper respiratory infection or streptococcal infection.
- Assess urine for:
  - **Color:** Gross hematuria; cloudy or smoky, tea-colored, or cola-colored
  - **Amount:** Decreased, oliguria, or anuria
  - **Protein:** Loss of protein in urine, proteinuria
- Assess for periorbital edema.
  - Facial edema that is worse in the morning and spreads downward to extremities and abdomen as the day progresses
- Assess for pallor, lethargy, anorexia.
- Assess and monitor for BP elevation and hypertension.
- May have vague reports of discomfort, headache, abdominal pain, dysuria.

Diagnostics

- Throat culture to identify possible *Streptococcus* infection, usually negative at the time of diagnosis.
- Urinalysis (UA) reveals protein, blood, red blood cells (RBCs), white blood cells (WBCs), or mixed cell casts, indicating renal failure.
- Urine specific gravity is elevated.
- Creatinine clearance test shows a low result, indicating a decreased glomerular filtration rate.
- Serum protein levels are decreased.
- Serum blood urea nitrogen (BUN) level creatinine level results are elevated.
- Electrolyte levels may be imbalanced with elevated serum potassium levels, decreased serum calcium levels, and metabolic acidosis.
- Antistreptolysin-O (ASO) level test titers are elevated.
  - The test may be performed twice, with samples collected about 2 weeks apart, for acute and convalescent titers. This is done to determine if the antibody level is rising, falling, or remaining the same.
  - ASO antibodies are produced about a week to a month after an initial strep infection.
  - The titer peaks at about 3 to 5 weeks after the illness and then tapers off but may remain detectable for several months after the strep infection has resolved.
  - Antideoxyribonuclease-B Titer (ADNase-B) may be done along with or following an ASO test.
- Serum C3 complement levels are decreased in acute stage of APSGN, but increase during recovery and return to baseline at 8 to 10 weeks after infection resolves.
- Renal ultrasonography reveals bilateral kidney enlargement.

Nursing Interventions

- Monitor intake and output (I&O), daily weight, weigh the child on the same scale with the same amount of clothing daily.
- Monitor vital signs (esp. the BP).
- Monitor neurologic status and observe for behavioral changes, implement seizure precautions if condition indicates.
- Encourage adequate nutritional intake:
  - Possible restriction of sodium and fluid.
  - Restrict foods high in potassium during periods of oliguria and anuria.
  - Provide small, frequent meals of favorite foods.
  - Avoid added salt and salty foods (e.g., pretzels and chips).
  - Consult with a nutritional therapist about low-sodium, low-potassium foods, and protein restrictions, as appropriate.

- Monitor for skin breakdown, elevate any edematous body parts.
- Dialysis may be required if the kidneys have stopped functioning.

Special Considerations

Evaluate and treat any complaints of sore throat or skin infections that could be streptococcal infections.

Discharge Planning; Patient and Family Education

- Ensure that the parents or caregivers are able to obtain the prescribed medications.
- Avoid the use of nonsteroidal anti-inflammatory drugs (NSAIDs) unless ordered by the healthcare clinician.
- Schedule UA at 2, 4, 8 weeks and 4, 6, and 12 months.
  - Microscopic hematuria may persist for up to 2 years and possibly longer with complete recovery.
  - Proteinuria may persist for up to 3 months.
- Schedule serum creatinine lab levels at 2, 6, and 12 months.
- BP monitoring at each visit.

CRYPTORCHIDISM (UNDESCENDED TESTES)

Description

- A condition where an infant is missing one or both testes in the scrotal sac; the teste(s) may still be found in the abdomen; it did not move down into the scrotal sac during fetal development.
  - Most common congenital GU anomaly
  - Can be absent
  - Undescended by 4 months of age or corrected premature age
  - **Risk factors:** Prematurity, small for gestational age (SGA), birth weight less than 2.5 kg

Assessment

Unable to palpate teste(s) in the scrotal sac

Diagnostics

May do imaging studies if unable to palpate both testes

Nursing Interventions

- Referral to pediatric urology and/or surgery if not descended by 6 months of age.
- **Orchiopexy:** Surgical treatment usually performed between 6 and 18 months.
- **Pre- and postoperative care:** One suture passes through testes and scrotum and attaches to thigh. Be sure that there is no tension on thigh suture to avoid suture breakage.

Special Considerations

Complications of undescended testes: inguinal hernia, testicular torsion and/or trauma, fertility issues, testicular cancer

Discharge Planning; Patient and Family Education

Postoperative care: See "Nursing Interventions" in this section; monitor for bleeding and infection.

DEHYDRATION

Description

- The World Health Organization (WHO) defines dehydration as a condition that results from excessive loss of body water, reduction of one's total body water content.
- Dehydration may also occur with insufficient intake of fluids.
- In children, these losses usually occur from vomiting or diarrhea.
  - Altered fluid balance where fluid losses exceed fluid intake.
- Children susceptible to dehydration due to increased metabolic rate, limited ability to communicate their needs or hydrate themselves, increased insensible loss, larger body surface area, inability to concentrate urine, and higher body water content when compared to adults.
  - Infants and children require proportionally greater volumes of water than adults to maintain their fluid equilibrium and are more susceptible to volume depletion.
- Specific causes of dehydration can be placed into three general categories: (a) decreased fluid intake; (b) increased fluid output (gastrointestinal [GI], renal, or insensible); or (c) fluid translocation (burns or ascites).
- In addition to total body water losses, electrolyte abnormalities may exist.
- Dehydration is classified according to:
  - **Percent of body weight loss:** Mild (3%–5%), moderate (6%–10%), and severe (more than 10%)
  - **Serum osmolarity:** Hyponatremic (sodium less than 130), isonatremic (sodium 130–150), or hypernatremic (sodium greater than 150)
    - Isonatremic (isotonic) is the deficiency of fluid and electrolytes in approximately equal proportions with a normal serum sodium level.
    - Hyponatremic (hypotonic) electrolyte loss is greater than fluid loss with a decreased serum sodium level, causing movement of water to move from extracellular to intracellular space possibly resulting in cerebral edema and/or seizures (e.g., watering down formula, water intoxication).
    - Hypernatremic (hypertonic) fluid loss is greater than electrolyte loss with an increased serum sodium level, causing movement of water to move from the intracellular to the extracellular space possibly resulting in neurologic changes, confusion, inability to concentrate, and motor tremors (e.g., diabetes insipidus, ketoacidosis, or excessive sweating).

Assessment

- Assess the quality and quantity of I&O, note any weight loss.
- Assess characteristics as in Table 10.1.
- Assess for highly concentrated urine.
- Assess for the presence of cool, dry, doughy skin with the presence of tenting, indicating poor skin turgor (see Figure 10.1).
- Assess for vomiting pattern after feedings.

Diagnostics

- UA demonstrates increased urine osmolarity and increased urine specific gravity.
  - Normal specific gravity of the urine in a child is less than 1.015 and infants less than 1.010. A specific gravity greater than 1.025 in any child is suggestive of dehydration and greater than 1.015 in infants as the infantile kidney can only maximally concentrate urine to 800 mOsm/L correlating to a specific gravity of about 1.020.
- Serum lab studies may reveal elevated HCO_3 due to a contraction alkalosis (increased HCO_3 reabsorption from the kidney due to solute loss).

DEHYDRATION

TABLE 10.1: Characteristics of Dehydration Levels

Dehydration %	Mild 3%–5%	Moderate 6%–10%	Severe >10%
Mental status	Normal	Listless, irritable	Altered mental
Heart rate	Normal	Increased	Increased
Pulses	Normal	Decreased	Thready
Capillary refill	Normal	Prolonged	Prolonged
Blood pressure	Normal	Normal	Decreased
Respirations	Normal	Tachypnea	Tachypnea
Eyes	Normal	Slightly sunken	Fewer tears
Fontanelle	Normal	Sunken	Sunken
Urine output	Normal	Decreased	Oliguric

Source: Adapted from Vega, R. M., and Avva, U. (2020). Pediatric dehydration. In *StatPearls* [Online]. StatPearls Publishing. https://www.ncbi.nlm.nih.gov/books/NBK436022/

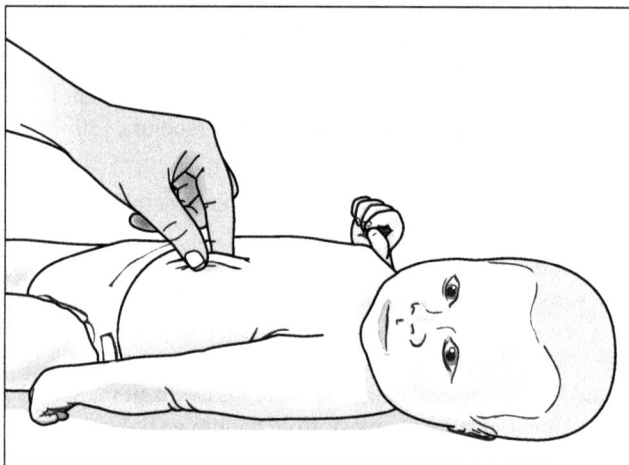

FIGURE 10.1: Assessment of skin turgor to assess dehydration
Source: Reprinted from Chiocca, E. M. (2021). *Advanced pediatric assessment* (3rd ed.). Springer Publishing Company.

Nursing Interventions

- Monitor strict I&O with hour totals for intake and output; record urine specific gravity measures.
- Promote fluid intake, encourage PO intake, if patient is vomiting, intravenous (IV) route is used.
- Perform a daily weight, same scale, time of day, and with the child naked or wearing the same clothes.
- Monitor vital signs; note signs of hypovolemia and intervene to prevent hypovolemic shock.
- Provide mouth care.
- Provide skin care, turn the child every 2 hours, and apply moisturizing lotion to the extremities and pressure points.
- Administer medications as directed, if child remains nauseated, administer ondansetron (Zofran).
  - Note that Zofran cannot be used under the age 6 months.

Special Considerations

- Dehydration can be severe enough to cause volume depletion, circulatory collapse, and hypovolemic shock.
- For severe dehydration and continued volume depletion, institute IV or IO (interosseous) resuscitation with a bolus (20 mL/kg) of isotonic normal saline (NS) or Ringer Lactate (RL).
- Multiple boluses may be needed for children in hypovolemic shock.

Discharge Planning; Patient and Family Education

- For mild to moderate dehydration, oral rehydration therapy (ORT) is recommended.
  - Administer ORT (e.g., Pedialyte®, Ricealyte®, Speedlyte®) to the child, 1 or 2 teaspoons (5 or 10 mL) of an ORS (oral rehydration solution) every few minutes. You can use a spoon or an oral syringe.
  - The WHO and the United Nations Children's Fund (UNICEF) recommend ORS and zinc as essential to clinical treatment of acute diarrhea.
  - If parents can't afford ORSs, they can use this recipe: ORS is 1 L of water, six teaspoons of sugar, and a half teaspoon of salt.
  - If the child still needs ORS after 24 hours, make a fresh solution.
  - Avoid fluids with high sugar content, tea, soda, fruit juice, Kool-Aid, Jello, and skim milk.
  - Older children may have water, ice chips, half-strength Gatorade, noncarbonated, decaffeinated soda, avoid high sodium foods such as broth and milk, introduce bland diet.
- A breastfed infant should continue to be nursed, even during rehydration, unless vomiting repeatedly.
- Stop giving formula to a formula-fed baby during rehydration and restart as soon as the baby can keep fluids down and isn't showing signs of dehydration.

PEDIATRIC PEARLS

- 90% of potassium is excreted by the kidney, do not add K+ to IV solution until satisfactory urinary output is established.

ENURESIS (INTERMITTENT NOCTURNAL INCONTINENCE)

Description

- Involuntary urination past the age of toilet training/bladder control in children ≥5 years of age, often during sleep (nocturnal); usually resolves by 7 years of age.
  - **Primary enuresis:** Child has not had voluntary bladder control or a satisfactory period of dryness; most common form.
  - **Secondary enuresis:** Urinary incontinence in children who previously demonstrated bladder control of at least 6 consecutive months; most often cause unknown
  - **Diurnal enuresis:** Loss of urinary control in the daytime.
  - **Nocturnal enuresis:** Nighttime bedwetting.
- Causes may include small size of bladder, deep sleeping, immature bladder muscle reflex, stress, and urinary tract infections (UTIs).

Assessment

- Determine toilet training age, enuresis onset, and frequency of enuresis episodes.
- Assess previous UTIs; elevated BP (renal abnormalities); and other possible causes (diabetes mellitus, bladder dysfunction, constipation).

ENURESIS (INTERMITTENT NOCTURNAL INCONTINENCE)

- Assess for urine-holding behaviors such as squatting, dancing, or running to the bathroom (diurnal enuresis).
- Assess for any fluids (amount and type) consumed before bedtime (nocturnal enuresis); be aware of urine odor on clothing or bedding.
- Assess for burning on urination and a sense of urgency (UTI).

Diagnostics

- To rule out UTI, GU abnormalities/obstructions, and monitor kidney function:
  - Obtain UA and culture and sensitivity (see Pediatric Skill 10.1).
  - Complete blood count including BUN and creatinine.
  - May need renal ultrasound/vesicoureterogram.

PEDIATRIC SKILL 10.1: URINE SPECIMEN COLLECTION

- **Bladder catheterization** performed the same as in adults: most accurate test identifies bacterial content in urine of child less than 2 years of age; sterile specimen for urine culture.
- **Clean-catch urine specimen:** Do not use first-voided urine (including after a nap) for sample due to urinary stasis; collected midstream for routine UA, not sterile specimen.
- **Bagged, urine collection:** Place urine bag securely around genitals before the anal sphincter, so that stool does not enter the bag and contaminate the specimen. Tuck the bag downward inside the diaper to avoid leakage. Instruct caregivers not to remove the urine bag. Check the collection bag frequently for urine.

Nursing Interventions

- Instruct child and caregivers to set a fixed voiding schedule with frequent toileting approximately four to seven times per day, especially before bedtime.
- Encourage increasing amounts of fluids consumed during day to increase frequency of the urge to void; limit fluids after dinner; avoid high-sugar and caffeine-based drinks especially before bedtime.
- Discourage use of diapers and pull-ups which may decrease motivation.
- Suggest behavioral training with an enuresis alarm or at bedtime; administer desmopressin (DDAVP; antidiuretic hormone) nasal spray to decrease volume of urine at night, if ordered (alternate nares, should not be used in children with hyponatremia).

Special Considerations

- Treatment varies with underlying cause or coexisting conditions.
- High rate of spontaneous resolution.

Discharge Planning; Patient and Family Education

- Provide emotional support and positive reinforcement to family; educate that enuresis is common; important to educate families that enuresis is no one's fault and always avoid punishment for bedwetting.
- Enuresis may be a source of shame and embarrassment which can interfere with socialization with peers; associated with low self-esteem.
- Keep a voiding diary or calendar of dry and wet episodes.

EPISPADIAS AND HYPOSPADIAS

Description

- Congenital anomalies with an abnormal opening of the urethra
- **Epispadias:** Urethra located on dorsal surface of penis (see Figure 10.2)
- **Hypospadias:** Urethra located on ventral surface of penis

Assessment

- Observe urination direction.
- Assess tip of penis for signs and symptoms (s/s) of infection.

Diagnostics

Clinical features upon inspection of the location of the urethral meatus

Nursing Interventions

- Maintain clean area of urination to prevent infection.
- **Postoperative care:** Monitor I&O, assess for bleeding, infection, pain, and bladder spasms.

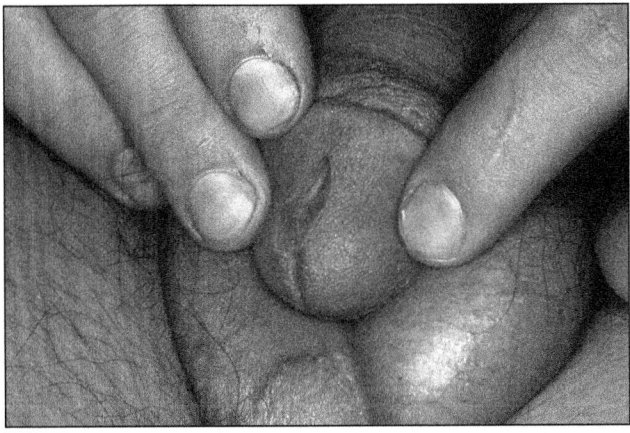

FIGURE 10.2: Epispadias
Source: Courtesy of Centers for Disease Control and Prevention/Gavin Hart, MD.

Special Considerations

Children with these conditions are not circumcised; will have surgical correction between 6 and 18 months of life; may need foreskin for repair.

Discharge Planning; Patient and Family Education

- Teach incision care and use of double-diapering technique if stent placement; may be sent home with catheter; educate on proper urine catheter care.
- Avoid tub baths, straddle toys for about 2 weeks until incisions heal or stents are removed.
- Educate caregivers on the importance of completing antibiotics as instructed.
- Encourage child to drink plenty of fluids.
- Contact clinician for s/s infection.

HEMOLYTIC UREMIC SYNDROME

Description

- An acute renal disease characterized by acute renal failure, hemolytic anemia, and thrombocytopenia.
  - Kidney injury that occurs in response to RBCs being destroyed and blocking the kidney's filtering system
- Hemolytic uremic syndrome (HUS) is the most common cause of acute kidney injury in children.
- HUS is most commonly caused by a particular strain of *Escherichia coli* (*E. coli*; *E. coli* O157:H7); commonly found in petting zoos and ingestion of undercooked meats.
  - Produces toxins that can enter the bloodstream and destroy the RBCs.
  - Glomeruli become clogged with the damaged RBCs and prevent the kidney from functioning.

Assessment

- Assess for a medical and family history; may be predisposed to inherited HUS.
- Assess for prodromal symptoms such as headache, fever, chills, GI upset, abdominal pain, vomiting, and diarrhea that may be bloody.
- Assess for oliguria, albuminuria, and/or blood in the urine.
- Assess for signs of anemia such as fatigue, weakness, fainting, pallor.
- Assess for possible bruising and seizures.
- Assess electrolyte imbalance such as hyperkalemia, hyponatremia, hypocalcemia, anemia, elevated BUN, and metabolic acidosis.
- Assess EKG for cardiac arrhythmias.

Diagnostics

- **24-hour urine:** A high urine albumin-to-creatinine ratio indicates that the kidneys are leaking large amounts of albumin into the urine.
- Urine dipstick for blood and protein.
- Stool sample can show the presence of *E. coli* O157:H7.
- Renal biopsy.

Nursing Interventions

- Monitor I&O and obtain daily weights.
- Monitor fluid and electrolyte balance, replacements as needed.
- Limit fluid intake as prescribed, monitor IV fluid therapy.
- Monitor vital signs for hypertension complication.
- Prepare for dialysis if indicated.

Special Considerations

Handle gently to prevent further bruising.

Discharge Planning; Patient and Family Education

- Teach prevention:
  - Cooking meat to an internal temperature of at least 160°F
  - Avoiding unpasteurized milk, juice, and cider
  - Washing foods before eating
  - Cleaning utensils and food surfaces often

- Keeping children out of pools if they have had diarrhea
- Washing hands well after using the restroom and after changing diapers
■ Some children may need to follow a low-salt diet to help prevent swelling and high BP.

HYDROCELE

Description

■ A hydrocele is the accumulation of fluids around the testicle.
■ Classified as communicating and noncommunicating (see Figure 10.3).
- **Communicating:** Patency between the scrotal sac and the peritoneal cavity allows peritoneal fluids to collect in the scrotum, especially with eliciting a Valsalva maneuver.
- **Noncommunicating:** Imbalance between the secreting and absorptive capacities of scrotal tissue, or an obstruction of lymphatic or venous drainage in the spermatic cord.

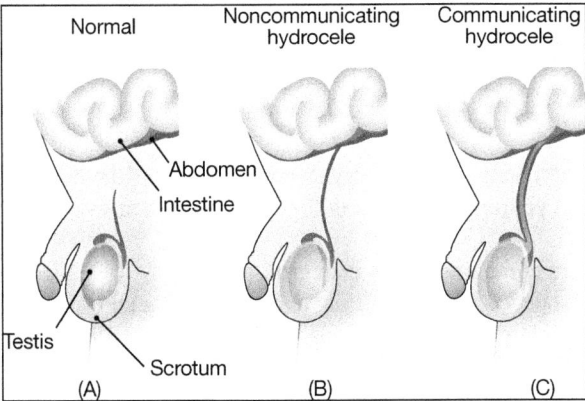

FIGURE 10.3: Hydrocele

Source: Reprinted from Gawlik, K. S., Melnyk, B. M., and Teall, A. M. (2021). *Evidence-based physical examination: Best practices for health and well-being assessment* (1st ed.). Springer Publishing Company.

■ Most common cause of painless scrotal swelling.
■ Commonly resolves spontaneously; however, a communicating hydrocele can become indirect inguinal hernia, with potential for incarceration.

Assessment

■ Assess for painless swelling of one or both testicles.
■ Assess for complaints of heaviness of a swollen scrotum.
■ Assess for scrotum to become softer and smaller upon positioning the child supine.

Diagnostics

■ Physical examination with ultrasound.
■ Transillumination may help to differentiate a hydrocele from a hernia.
■ Abdominal radiography distinguishes a hydrocele from an incarcerated hernia.

Nursing Interventions

■ Application of heat or cold compresses to the scrotum.
■ Place a rolled towel between the child's legs and elevate the scrotum to help reduce severe swelling.

Discharge Planning; Patient and Family Education

- Avoid tub baths postoperatively for 5 to 7 days.
- Signs and symptoms of infection and the need to notify a healthcare clinician if any occur.

PEDIATRIC PEARLS
- Transillumination is not reliable for establishing the final diagnosis.

NEPHROTIC SYNDROME

Description

- Nephrotic syndrome is a condition where the glomerular membrane of the kidney allows protein (specifically albumin) to pass into the urine.
  - Results in decreased serum osmotic pressure (hypoalbuminemia), marked proteinuria, edema, and hyperlipidemia.
  - Due to the decrease in colloidal osmotic pressure, fluid shifts from intravascular space to interstitial space resulting in pronounced edema.
- It can be primary, secondary, or congenital.
  - **Primary idiopathic:** Primary minimal change nephrotic syndrome (MCNS) is the most common type of idiopathic nephrotic syndrome, accounting for 90% of children with nephrotic syndrome.
  - Idiopathic nephrotic syndrome is more common in boys than girls.
  - **Secondary nephrotic syndrome:** Associated with glomerular damage due to a known cause such as an underlying disease or infection (e.g., diabetes, lupus, malaria, IgA vasculitis).
  - **Congenital nephrotic syndrome:** Inherited by an autosomal recessive gene and presents within the first few weeks of life.
- Peak incidence is between 2 and 3 years of age.
- The disorder may be self-limiting, poorer prognosis with congenital type.

Assessment

- Assess for weight gain.
- Assess for edema; most common presenting symptom and physical finding (e.g., lower extremities, face and periorbital regions, scrotum or labia, and abdomen).
- Assess urine for color and quantity looking for decreased, dark, foamy, and frothy appearance.
  - Microscopic hematuria
  - Massive proteinuria
  - Elevated urine specific gravity
- Assess for serum hypoalbuminemia and/or signs of hypovolemia.
  - BP within the expected reference range or slightly below
- Assess serum electrolytes, note particularly potassium which is lost in the urine.
- Irritability, lethargy, and fatigue.
- Anorexia, malnutrition, diarrhea.

Diagnostics

- Single first-morning urine that demonstrates proteinuria (greater than 40 mg/m² per hour).
  - A high urine albumin-to-creatinine ratio indicates that the kidneys are leaking large amounts of albumin into the urine.

- 24-hour urine collection may be performed looking at albumin excretion (proteinuria: 3 g protein is diagnostic).
- Serum albumin level is decreased (less than 30 g/L), whereas cholesterol, phospholipid, and triglyceride levels are elevated.
- Kidney ultrasound may reveal enlarged kidney/s.
- Kidney biopsy may be indicated for a child who has signs and symptoms of systemic disease.

Nursing Interventions

- Monitor I&O and urine for protein.
- Monitor skin for edema and breakdown, abdominal girth daily, and turn every 2 hours.
  - Avoid restrictive bandages.
  - Warm compress to periorbital sites and elevate the head of the bed (HOB).
  - Consider scrotal support.
- Monitor daily weight at the same time of day, using the same scale and amount of clothing.
- Monitor for signs of infection.
- Cluster care to promote rest periods.
- Promote nutritional intake, low cholesterol/saturated fat, and limit the use of salt during edematous phase.
  - Allow for protein intake of 1 to 2 g/kg/d.
  - Fluid restrictions may need to be implemented if the child is hyponatremic or demonstrates severe edema.
- Administer corticosteroids (prednisone therapy) and diuretics as prescribed.
- Offer reassurance during the edematous phase that may alter child's/family's perception of body image.

Special Considerations

Since the treatment plan usually have these children on corticosteroid therapy, monitoring for and prevention of infection is a top priority.

Discharge Planning; Patient and Family Education

- Ensure that the parents or caregivers are able to obtain the prescribed medications and reinforce to complete the entire prescription.
- Monitor for adverse effects of corticosteroids, if appropriate, including weight gain, cushingoid effects, and growth suppression.
- Inform parents and caregivers to report any signs of infection.
- Inform parents and children of possible relapses.
- Inform parents and caregivers to check the child's weight, and dipstick urine every morning and keep a log.
- Inform parents to maintain a low sodium, possible fluid restriction diet while the child is edematous and until proteinuria subsides, then resume normal diet.

PEDIATRIC PEARLS

- Prognosis with MCNS pathology is very good, with most patients going into remission following corticosteroid treatment.
  - **Remission:** Urine albumin absent or trace for three consecutive early morning specimens

PYELONEPHRITIS INFECTION (KIDNEY INFECTION)

Description

- UTIs of the upper urinary tract that involve the kidneys, renal pelvis, and ureters.
- Caused by a bacterial UTI that has spread from the bladder to the kidneys.
- Infection involves the renal parenchyma, which is generally associated with systemic signs of inflammation.
- The bacteria triggers inflammation, and the kidneys respond by producing more urine, which leads to dehydration.
    - *Escherichia coli* is responsible in most cases.
- Repeat acute kidney infections can ultimately lead to the need for a kidney transplant.
    - In infants, complications can include sepsis and meningitis.

Assessment

- Assess for fever (38.5°C and over); infants and children under the age of 2 may be afebrile in presentation.
- Assess for urinary symptoms, symptoms of urgency, frequency, and pain with urination.
- Assess urine for color and odor, looking for strong, foul-smelling urine which may contain blood.
- Assess for stomach, low-back, flank pain; a unilateral mass can usually be palpated.
- Assess for costovertebral angle (CVA) tenderness.
- Assess for enuresis.
- Assess for poor feeding, a decreased change in appetite, anorexia, vomiting, and/or diarrhea.

Diagnostics

- Microscopic urine analysis for WBCs and bacterial count; refer to Pediatric Skill 10.1.
- Urine dipsticks for nitrites and/or leukocyte esterase are a common indicator of infection.
- Urine culture and sensitivity report will determine antibiotic treatment choice.
- Serum creatinine and BUN levels may be elevated.
- Helical CT or intravenous urography (IVU).
- Technetium-99 m–dimercaptosuccinic acid (DMSA) scanning; routine use is not generally recommended due to the radiation dose.
- Procalcitonin (PCT), a precursor of calcitonin, produced by the thyroid gland and released during bacterial infections, is a new promising marker of renal parenchymal involvement.
- Voiding cystourethrogram (VCUG) is recommended only if hydronephrosis, scarring, or other anomalies are detected at ultrasound.

Nursing Interventions

- Administer prescribed IV antimicrobial medication.
- Increase fluid intake to flush organism from the urinary tract system, consider clear liquids such as water and cranberry juice.
    - Monitor I&O.
- Encourage patient to verbalize concerns, use active listening to provide support and acceptance, use patient questions as an opportunity to provide relevant information and educate the patient on condition.

Discharge Planning; Patient and Family Education

Ensure that the parents or caregivers are able to obtain the prescribed medications and reinforce to complete the entire prescription.

PEDIATRIC PEARLS

- Infants and children with a urine analysis that is positive for leukocyte esterase or nitrite should be cultured.

TESTICULAR TORSION

Description

- Testicular torsion is the sudden rotation of the testicle, specifically the spermatic cord, around its axis in the inguinal canal or below (see Figure 10.4).
- Testicular torsion is a urologic emergency; the acute rotation results in compromised blood flow to and from the testicle, which puts the testicle at risk for necrosis.
- Affects the left testicle more frequently than the right testicle.

Assessment

- Assess for a hard scrotal mass that does not transilluminate.
- Assess for discolored or bruised hemiscrotum with swelling, affected testicle lies horizontally.
- Assess for a high-riding testicle due to spermatic cord shortening.
- Assess for acute-onset, severe, constant testicular or scrotal pain, one-sided with duration less than 24 hours.
  - Children may wake up at night with scrotal pain from cremasteric contraction.
- Assess for nausea and vomiting.
- Assess for Prehn sign, pain increases with scrotum elevation, absent cremasteric reflex.
- Assess for symmetrical scrotum presentation.

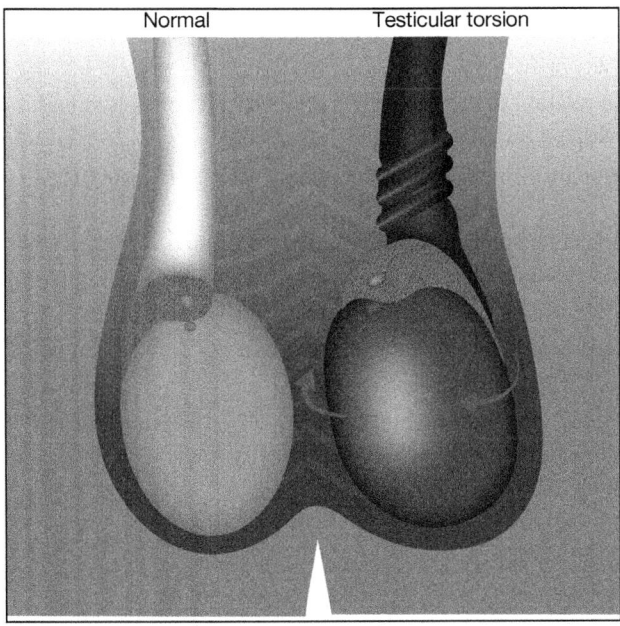

FIGURE 10.4: Testicular torsion

Source: Reprinted from Gawlik, K. S., Melnyk, B. M., and Teall, A. M. (2021). *Evidence-based physical examination: Best practices for health and well-being assessment* (1st ed.). Springer Publishing Company.

Diagnostics

- Doppler ultrasonography
- TWIST Score assessment: https://pedemmorsels.com/testicular-workup-for-ischemia-and-suspected-torsion-twist-score/

Nursing Interventions

- Prepare for possible surgery.
- Promote comfort.
- Apply ice bag to the scrotum to reduce edema.

Discharge Planning; Patient and Family Education

- Avoidance of strenuous activity until cleared by clinician.
- Ensure child wears protective scrotal cup during contact sports until cleared by clinician.

PEDIATRIC PEARLS

- Early examination is crucial because testicular necrosis can occur after 6 hours.

URINARY TRACT INFECTION (LOWER URINARY TRACT INFECTION OR CYSTITIS)

Description

- UTIs occur when bacteria, and sometimes viruses and fungi, invade the urinary tract, through which the body removes wastes and excess water.
- Common in the first year of life, the incidence of UTI decreases as the child gets older and urethra lengthens.
- More prevalent in girls than boys, related to urethra location (closer to the anus) and size of urethra (shorter in girls than in boys).
  - Proximity of the female urethra in relation to the anus poses a greater risk of contamination by incorrect proper wiping hygiene following a bowel movement.
- UTIs may also be caused by poor hygiene, urinary stasis, irritation of urethra from bubble bath, limited oral intake.
- In children 2 to 24 months of age, a UTI is the presence of bacteria on UA and at least 10,000 colony-forming units per mL from a catheter specimen, and 50,000 colony-forming units/mL of a uropathogen from the urine culture.
  - Commonly caused by a single gram-negative enteric bacterium, such as *Escherichia coli*, *Klebsiella*, *Proteus*, *Enterobacter*, *Pseudomonas*, or *Serratia*
- Assess for history of vesicoureteral reflux (VUR) which is a condition in which the urine flows backward from the bladder to one or both ureters and occasionally to the kidneys leading to inflammation, possible infection, and renal scarring.

Assessment

- Dependent on child's age, irritability, fatigue, lethargy, may/may not have fever.
- Assess the number of UTIs per year as UTIs can reoccur.
- Assess urine for color, odor, and quantity looking for cloudy, foul-smelling urine.
- Assess urine for increased pH and presence of hematuria, enuresis.
- Assess micturition pattern for increase in frequency, urgency, and quantity of urine.

URINARY TRACT INFECTION (LOWER URINARY TRACT INFECTION OR CYSTITIS)

- Assess for dysuria, burning, stinging upon urination, palpable bladder.
- Assess toileting practices for proper front-to-back wiping and hand hygiene practices.
- Assess frequency and duration of tub baths and use of bubble bath liquids.

Diagnostics

- Microscopic urine analysis for RBCs, WBCs, and bacterial count; refer to Pediatric Skill 10.1.
- Urine dipstick may be positive for blood, WBC, and nitrates.
- Urine culture and sensitivity report will determine antibiotic treatment choice.
- Serum creatinine and BUN levels may be elevated.
- Micturating cystourethrogram (MCUG) may be used as an imaging study may demonstrate congenital anomalies, such as VUR, predisposing the child to recurrent UTIs.
- Bladder scan can show residual urine and incomplete bladder emptying (see Pediatric Skill 10.2).

PEDIATRIC SKILL 10.2: USE OF BLADDER SCANNER

- A bladder scan uses a noninvasive, portable ultrasound device that provides a virtual 3D image of the bladder and the volume of urine retained within the bladder.
- Some scanners may have an operator login in the system to validate authorized users. Turn the scanner on and select your patient's sex. If your patient is a woman who has undergone a hysterectomy, use the male setting.
  - Scanning is contraindicated in large abdominal wounds and pregnancy.
- Place patient supine and apply conducting gel midline on the patient's abdomen, approximately 3 cm above the pubic bone.
- Aim probe toward the direction of the bladder, make sure the probe button is facing the patient's head directly and tilt the probe slightly toward the patient's tailbone so the scan clears the pubic bone.
- Press the scan button; when you find the ideal ultrasound bladder image, press the probe button again. When you hear a "beep," the calculation is finished. The result of urine volume will be displayed.
- An audio alert may signal when the scan is completed and the urine volume will be displayed.
- Wipe off ultrasound gel.

Nursing Interventions

- Administer prescribed antibiotics.
- Increase fluid intake to flush organisms from the urinary tract system; consider clear liquids such as water and cranberry juice.
  - Avoid bladder irritants such as carbonated beverages and those that contain caffeine.
  - Monitor I&O.
- Good bathroom habits, with frequent opportunities to micturate; girls should demonstrate wiping from front to back after using the toilet to reduce exposure of the urethra to UTI-causing bacteria in the stool.
- Frequent diaper changes in infants; cotton underwear for children as cotton underwear is less likely to encourage bacterial growth near the urethra than nylon or other fabrics.
- For adolescent girls, encourage voiding after having intimate relationships.

Special Considerations

Low-dose prophylactic antibiotic that may be recommended for 6 to 12 months for children with recurrent UTIs

Discharge Planning; Patient and Family Education

Ensure that the parents or caregivers are able to obtain the prescribed medications and reinforce to complete the entire prescription.

PEDIATRIC PEARLS

- The American Academy of Pediatrics (AAP) Subcommittee on UTI stresses that prompt treatment should be started less than 48 hours after onset of symptoms to improve clinical outcomes.

VARICOCELE

Description

- Abnormal dilation of the veins in the scrotum (pampiniform plexus) resulting from ineffective function of the valves in the testicular veins.
- Varicoceles usually become evident around adolescence due to elevated blood flow to the scrotum during puberty and are more common on the left side of the scrotum.
- Generally caused by incompetent or congenitally absent valves at the juncture of the testicular vein and renal vein.
- Varicoceles may lead to overheating of the testes and lead to lower sperm production and function.
- In the majority of situations, varicoceles cause no problems and are harmless.

Assessment

- Although the majority present asymptomatically, assess for feeling of "heaviness" or aching pain on the affected side that worsens with sitting, standing, and physical activity; increases during the day; and relieved by lying down.
- Assess for a visible mass.
- Assess for palpable small mass in the scrotum when the adolescent is upright.
- Assess for possible testicular tenderness or "bag of worms" feel, as describing the look and feel.

Diagnostics

- Can be found through self-testicular examination
- High-resolution color-flow Doppler ultrasonography
  - Signs of varicoceles on ultrasound are veins that are wider than 3 millimeters with blood flowing the wrong way with during a Valsalva maneuver.
  - Ultrasonography confirms the size of the testicles and is helpful in identifying if the left testicle is growing more slowly than the right.

Nursing Interventions

- Placement of scrotal support (athletic supporter) to relieve discomfort.
- Allow the patient to verbalize feelings related to the condition and its potential effect on fertility. Provide support and encouragement, answer any questions, and provide clear explanations.
- If indicated and concern for fertility, prepare the adolescent physically and emotionally for surgery.
  - Treat the adolescent's pain, as needed and ordered, using nonpharmacologic (such as ice packs to the surgical area), pharmacologic, or a combination of approaches.
  - Perform routine postoperative care.

Discharge Planning; Patient and Family Education

- Assess the patient's and family's understanding of the diagnosis, treatment, follow-up, and warning signs for which to seek medical attention.
- Instruct adolescent and family regarding activity recommendations and restrictions:
  - Wait for 48 hours after surgery to shower or bathe.
  - Avoid straddling and riding activities for 6 to 8 weeks.
  - Return to normal nonstrenuous activities after postoperative day 2.
  - Return to more strenuous activities in about 2 weeks following surgery.

BIBLIOGRAPHY

Baskin, L. S. (2020). Hypospadias: Management and outcome. *UpToDate*. Retrieved November 14, 2020, from https://www.uptodate.com/contents/hypospadias-management-and-outcome

Cooper, C. S., & Docimo, S. G. (2019). Undescended testes (cryptorchidism) in children: Clinical features and evaluation. *UpToDate*. Retrieved November 14, 2020, from https://www.uptodate.com/contents/undescended-testes-cryptorchidism-in-children-clinical-features-and-evaluation

Fox, S. (2019). *Testicular workup for ischemia and suspected torsion (TWIST) score*. https://pedemmorsels.com/testicular-workup-for-ischemia-and-suspected-torsion-twist-score/

Morello, W., La Scola, C., Alberici, I., & Montini, G. (2016). Acute pyelonephritis in children. *Pediatric Nephrology*, *31*, 1253–1265. https://doi.org/10.1007/s00467-015-3168-5

National Center on Birth Defects and Developmental Disabilities, Centers for Disease Control and Prevention. (2019). *Facts about hypospadias*. https://www.cdc.gov/ncbddd/birthdefects/hypospadias.html

Tapia, C., & Bashir, K. (2020). Nephrotic syndrome. In *StatPearls* [Online]. StatPearls Publishing. https://www.ncbi.nlm.nih.gov/books/NBK470444/

Tu, D. T., & Baskin, L. S. (2020). Nocturnal enuresis in children: Management. *UpToDate*. Retrieved December 16, 2020, from https://www.uptodate.com/contents/nocturnal-enuresis-in-children-management

Vega, R. M., & Avva, U. (2020) Pediatric dehydration. In *StatPearls* [Online]. StatPearls Publishing. https://www.ncbi.nlm.nih.gov/books/NBK436022/

KNOWLEDGE CHECK

1. A nurse is caring for a child who is experiencing enuresis. What would the nurse most likely expect to assess for in the child?

   A. Frequent bedwetting
   B. Abdominal pain
   C. Irritability
   D. Fever and chills

2. A nurse is assessing an infant's GU system. Which finding would the nurse document as normal?

   A. Undescended testes
   B. Urine specific gravity of less than 1.010
   C. Urethral opening on ventral surface of penis
   D. Urethral opening on dorsal surface of penis

3. A nurse is caring for an infant with hypospadias. Which statement by the parents indicates the need for further teaching?

   A. "My son's condition means the urethra is located on the ventral surface of the penis."
   B. "He will need to be circumcised before being discharged from the hospital."
   C. "After surgery, my son will not be able to play with straddle toys."
   D. "We will be sure that our child completes the entire course of antibiotics."

4. A nurse is caring for a 50 kg child with dehydration. What rate should the nurse set the infusion pump for the child's daily maintenance fluid requirements?

   A. 2,100 mL/hr
   B. 125 mL/hr
   C. 90.5 mL/hr
   D. 87.5 mL/hr

5. Which assessment finding would the nurse expect in a patient diagnosed with nephrotic syndrome?

   A. Urine specific gravity of less than 1.010
   B. Dipstick protein of 1+
   C. Hyperlipidemia
   D. Weight loss

6. The nurse is caring for a 6-year-old child with acute glomerulonephritis. Which finding should the nurse expect over the course of the illness?

   A. Rising ASO titers
   B. BP 100/60
   C. Prednisone therapy
   D. Scrotal support

7. The nurse is teaching a parent group on ways to avoid contracting HUS. Which of the following teaching points should the nurse include?

   A. Avoid unpasteurized milk, juice, and cider
   B. Cook meat to an internal temperature of at least 100°F
   C. Use plastic pants if a child has diarrhea and wants to go swimming
   D. Defrost meat on the counter

KNOWLEDGE CHECK

1. **Correct Answer: A) Frequent bedwetting.** Enuresis is defined by continued urinary incontinence past the age of toilet training in children ≥5 years of age often during sleep. Abdominal pain, irritability, and fever and chills are not clinical manifestations of enuresis.

2. **Correct Answer: B) Urine specific gravity of less than 1.010.** The kidney is less able to concentrate urine and reabsorb amino acids increasing risk of dehydration; an infant's average specific gravity is less than 1.010 compared with 1.010 to 1.030 for an adult. Undescended testes describe cryptorchidism. A urethral opening on the ventral surface of the penis describes hypospadias. A urethral opening on the dorsal surface of the penis describes epispadias.

3. **Correct Answer: B) "He will need to be circumcised before being discharged from the hospital."** Do not allow for circumcision; will have surgical correction in the first year of life and may need foreskin for repair. The definition of hypospadias is the urethra is located on the ventral surface of the penis. Avoid tub baths, straddle toys for about 2 weeks after surgery, until incisions heal or stents are removed. Educate caregivers on the importance of completing antibiotics as instructed.

4. **Correct Answer: D) 87.5 mL/hr**

    Steps: 100 mL × the 1st 10 kg = 1,000 mL
    50 mL × the 2nd 10 kg = 500 mL
    20 mL × the remaining 30 kg = 600 mL
    Total = 1,000 + 500 + 600 = 2,100 mL/d
    Hourly infusion rate = 2,100/24 hours = 87.5 mL/hr

5. **Correct Answer: C) Hyperlipidemia.** Hyperlipidemia would be seen as there is increased hepatic synthesis of proteins and lipids with nephrotic syndrome. The child would exhibit 2+ or greater and a higher urine specific gravity due to the inability of the kidneys to filtrate the urine. The child would most likely experience weight gain due to the decreasing colloidal osmotic pressure in the capillaries leading to edema.

6. **Correct Answer: A) Rising ASO titers.** ASO antibodies indicate that there was a previous strep infection, which is the causative agent to APSGN. The BP of 100/60 is in the expected range of a 6-year-old child and is not reflective of hypertension that could be a complication of APSGN. Both Prednisone therapy and scrotal support would be more consistent with nephrotic syndrome.

7. **Correct Answer: A) Avoid unpasteurized milk, juice, and cider.** Unpasteurized milk, juice, and cider should be avoided as it can carry harmful bacteria. Cooking meat to an internal temperature of 160°F assists with destruction of *E. coli* O157:H7 which is the causative organism to many of the cases of HUS. Children should not be allowed to swim, regardless of plastic pants if they have diarrhea as this could lead to water contamination with *E. coli*. Meat should be defrosted in the microwave or refrigerator.

8. A child is evaluated in the emergency department for vomiting and diarrhea and subsequently is diagnosed with mild dehydration. The nurse anticipates the plan of care to include:
    A. Fluid restriction
    B. A 20 mL/kg NS bolus infusion
    C. Prednisone therapy
    D. ORS
9. The nurse is evaluating the following arterial blood gas (ABG) for acid/base imbalance. The values are pH = 7.29, $PaCO_2$ = 50, HCO_3 = 24. What conclusion should the nurse come to regarding the analysis? The blood gas analysis reveals:
    A. Respiratory acidosis
    B. Respiratory alkalosis
    C. Metabolic acidosis
    D. Metabolic alkalosis
10. Which of the following statements by a 17-year-old female patient with a UTI indicates that additional patient teaching is necessary?
    A. "I will add more coffee and tea to my diet to help me urinate more."
    B. "I'll make sure to remember to wipe from front to back after going to the bathroom."
    C. "I will drink more water every day."
    D. "I will wear cotton underwear instead of nylon underwear."

KNOWLEDGE CHECK

8. **Correct Answer: D) ORS.** ORSs are indicted to replace fluid and electrolytes in children with mild to moderate dehydration. The nurse should not restrict fluids, as the goal is to replace fluid and electrolyte loss; and if the child is nauseated, introduce fluids slowly 2 to 5 mL every 2 to 3 minutes or 5 to 10 mL every 5 minutes. A fluid bolus of 20 mL/kg infusion would be considered for a child presenting with severe dehydration who may be severely volume depleted and at risk for hypovolemic shock. Corticosteroid therapy is not indicated for mild dehydration.

9. **Correct Answer: A) Respiratory acidosis.** Note that the pH is below the 7.35 to 7.45 range and that the $PaCO_2$ is above the 35 to 45 range, going in the opposite direction of each other; hence this ABG is indicative of respiratory acidosis without compensation. The bicarbonate level (HCO_3) is within normal limits.

10. **Correct Answer: A) "I will add more coffee and tea to my diet to help me urinate more."** Caffeinated beverages such as coffee and tea are bladder irritants and should be avoided when a patient has a UTI. Instead, the patient should increase her intake of clear liquids such as water and cranberry juice in order to flush the organism from her urinary tract system. Girls should wipe from front to back to reduce exposure to UTI-causing bacteria. Cotton underwear is recommended as it is less likely to encourage bacterial growth than nylon.

CHAPTER 11

Musculoskeletal Conditions

David Jack and Maureen Fitzgerald

INTRODUCTION

A variety of alterations in musculoskeletal development and usage can impact children and their mobility and independence. Some of the disorders can result from a neurologic insult, while others the result of a genetic dysfunction or structural anomaly that may be present at birth or discovered at some point during childhood or adolescence. Many neuromuscular and musculoskeletal disorders are chronic and result in disabilities. The pediatric nurse caring for these children takes an active role in the management of these disorders.

INTRODUCTION TO PEDIATRIC MUSCULOSKELETAL SYSTEM

- The development and maintenance of skeletal muscle and bone mass is critical for movement, health, and issues associated with the quality of life.
- Bones serve as an ion bank for important elements such as calcium and magnesium.
- Bone length occurs in the epiphyseal plates; when the epiphyses close, then growth stops.
  - Trauma or damage to the epiphyseal plates may result in disrupted growth.
  - See fractures in Chapter 19.
- Skeletal muscles contribute to bone mechanics through contraction and relaxation.

DEVELOPMENTAL HIP DYSPLASIA

Description

- Hip joint develops abnormally in utero; the hip joint does not work correctly due to the malalignment of the femoral head and the acetabulum.
- Three types of hip dysplasia depending on severity, location of femoral head, and joint stability.
  - **Subluxation:** Partial dislocation; femoral head located in acetabulum but can only be partially dislocated on exam.
  - **Dislocatable:** Dislocation of hip can occur during examination but is reducible.
  - **Dislocation:** No connection between the femoral head and the acetabulum.
  - **Dysplasia:** The acetabulum is flat, not cup shaped for the femoral head to fit in the hip joint.
- **At risk:** Breech presentation in utero, oligohydramnios, congenital ligamentous laxity, genetic factors, first-born White infants, 80% of cases are girls (may be due to maternal hormones affecting laxity of ligaments).
- Unilateral or bilateral.

DEVELOPMENTAL HIP DYSPLASIA

- **Complications:** Avascular necrosis of the femoral head, femoral nerve palsy, limited range of motion (ROM), frequent hip instability, differences in leg length, and osteoarthritis.

Assessment

- Assess newborn for risk factors listed previously.
- Perform lower extremity newborn assessments for hip abduction and adduction.
    - **Barlow's sign:** Femoral head pops out of hip joint/acetabulum (dislocates) = + positive
    - **Ortolani's sign:** + Positive sign when the femoral head is placed into (reduces) or out of the acetabulum (can hear a sound or feel the "click"/"clunk"); limited abduction; examiner's fingers are manipulating the hip joint (Figure 11.1)
- **Observe for knee asymmetry, Galeazzi sign (Allis sign):** Infant supine with knees and hips flexed and feet touching surface, ankles touching buttocks; the shorter (lower) limb is the limb with hip dysplasia (Figure 11.2).
- Assess for unequal thigh and/or gluteal skin folds, both prone and supine positions of infant; the affected limb presents with skin folds lower than the opposite side (Figure 11.3).
- If not detected in the newborn period, assess for limp in child due to femur shortening, and limited hip (affected hip) abduction; contracture of hip muscles may occur.

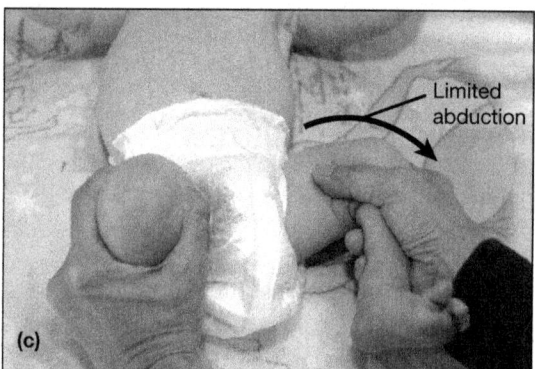

FIGURE 11.1: Ortolani maneuver to assess for developmental hip dysplasia

Source: Reprinted from Tkacs, N. C., Herrman, L. L., and Johnson, R. L. (2020). *Advanced physiology and pathophysiology: Essentials for clinical practice*. Springer Publishing Company.

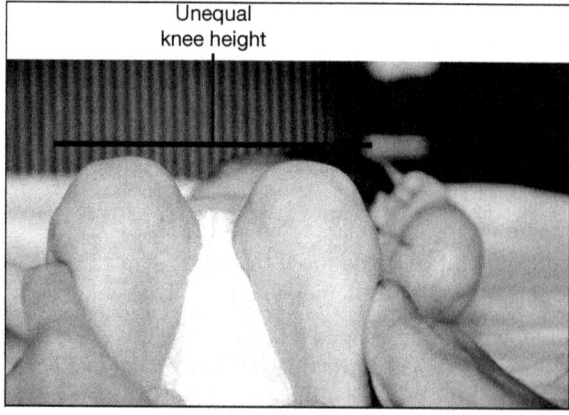

FIGURE 11.2: Developmental dysplasia of the hip

Source: Reprinted from Tkacs, N. C., Herrman, L. L., and Johnson, R. L. (2020). *Advanced physiology and pathophysiology: Essentials for clinical practice*. Springer Publishing Company.

DEVELOPMENTAL HIP DYSPLASIA

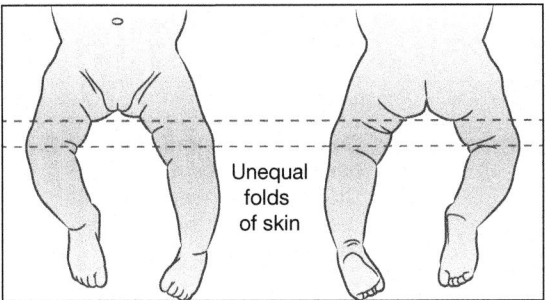

FIGURE 11.3: Asymmetrical thigh and gluteal folds
Source: Reprinted from Tkacs, N. C., Herrman, L. L., and Johnson, R. L. (2020). *Advanced physiology and pathophysiology: Essentials for clinical practice*. Springer Publishing Company.

Diagnostics

- Clinical features assessed during first newborn examination
- Radiographs after 6 months of age
- Ultrasound

PEDIATRIC PEARLS

- Early identification in newborn is key to promote a positive outcome in the infant.

Nursing Interventions

- If infant diagnosed <6 months of age, then place infant in Pavlik harness to keep hip joint abducted and flexed for normal growth and development
- If infant diagnosed after 6 months of age, then will need surgery to keep the hips in the joint
  - Child in hip spica cast after surgery for approximately 3 months, then brace until normal development of acetabulum and femoral head

Special Considerations

Treatment goal: Keep the hip joint connected/reduced by sustaining the femoral head inside the acetabulum for normal growth and development.

Discharge Planning; Patient and Family Education

- Educate caregivers on the proper use of the Pavlik harness (Table 11.1); emphasize the need for harness for 3 months.
- Encourage breastfeeding while in Pavlik harness.
- Teach postoperative care if child has surgery, including cast care.

TABLE 11.1: Care of Child With Developmental Dysplasia of the Hip in a Pavlik Harness

DO	DON'T
• Keep child in harness at all times including at bath time—first 2 weeks and then per clinicians orders • The child will sleep on their back in the harness	• Do not change strap measurements—only clinicians adjust straps
• When the clinician says the child can be out of the harness, then bathe the child during that time period • Diaper changes occur with the harness on	• Do not use heat when drying harness—it can shrink and then the appropriate sizing is incorrect

(continued)

TABLE 11.1: Care of Child With Developmental Dysplasia of the Hip in a Pavlik Harness (*continued*)

DO	DON'T
• Assess for signs/symptoms of skin breakdown especially groin area, behind knees • Keep skin clean and dry	• Do not remove markings on the harness with spot cleaner—Clean the harness with mild detergent and then let the harness air dry
• Dress the infant in an undershirt and long knee socks to maintain skin integrity	• Do not remove the harness unless instructed by the clinician
• The clinician will mark on the harness where the straps go when placing infant in harness	
• Notify clinician if you notice infant's lower extremities/feet are swollen or blue in color, the harness seems too small, or a rash or skin infection, or if you do not see the child moving their legs in the harness	

DUCHENNE MUSCULAR DYSTROPHY

Description

- Duchenne muscular dystrophy (DMD) is a genetic disorder characterized by progressive muscle degeneration and weakness.
- Caused by alteration/absence of a protein called dystrophin that helps keep muscle cells intact.
  - Characterized by progressive symmetrical wasting of skeletal muscles
  - Children become wheelchair-bound by age 12 and death usually occurs by the late teens or early 20s
- DMD symptom onset is in early childhood, usually between ages 2 and 3 years old.
- Males are primarily affected, however, in rare incidences, females can have the disorder.

Assessment

- Assess for inheritance pattern, X (sex)-linked recessive inheritance.
- Assess for progressive muscle weakness, delays in motor development.
- Assess for frequent falling, clumsiness, and a possible waddling gait.
- Gower sign/maneuver when rising from a sitting or supine position; getting up from the ground, the child assumes the hands-and-knees position and then climbs to standing by "walking" hands progressively up shins, knees, and thighs (Figure 11.4).
- Assess for enlarged calves as the result of fat infiltration into the muscle (pseudohypertrophy).
- **Posture changes:** Lordosis, scapular winging or flaring when raising the arms.

Diagnostics

- Urine creatinine and serum creatine kinase levels are elevated.
- Muscle biopsy confirms the diagnosis.
- An electromyogram shows abnormal muscle movements.
- Cardiac screening and pulmonary function tests may be implemented.

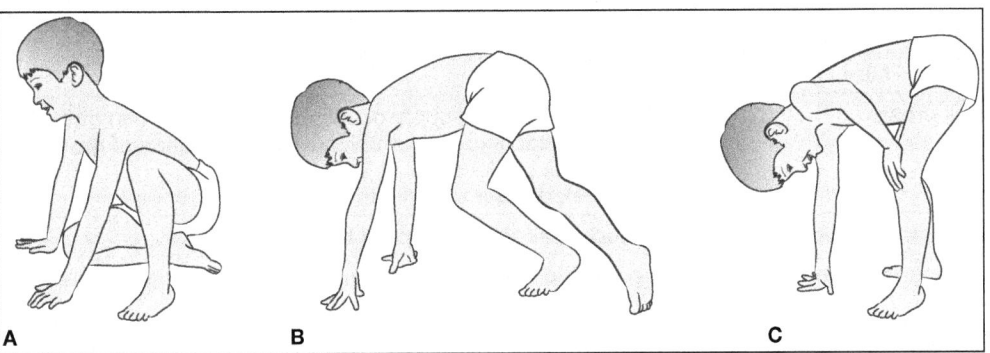

FIGURE 11.4: Gower sign. **(A)** First the child sits, then **(B)** shifts the body weight to hands and knees, then **(C)** uses his hands to "climb up" to stand

Source: Reprinted from Chiocca, E. M. (2019). *Advanced pediatric assessment.* Springer Publishing Company.

Nursing Interventions

- Symptom management, as there is no cure.
- Encourage the child to remain independent, perform passive ROM and stretching exercises, and reinforce the physical therapy regimen.
- Encourage coughing and deep-breathing exercises to aid in the prevention of respiratory illness.
- Provide the child with splints, braces, grab bars, overhead slings, high-top shoes, and foot board to keep body aligned and joints and tendons flexible.
- Provide a low-calorie, high-protein, high-fiber diet.
- Encourage the child (as age appropriate) and family to verbalize their concerns and feelings; allow time for them to process information.

PEDIATRIC PEARLS

- Eteplirsen (Exondys 51) is a new medication that sometimes increases muscle strength in patients with DMD.

Special Considerations

Treatment goal: Promote independence and activity for as long as possible.

Discharge Planning; Patient and Family Education

- Educate child and family on the importance of coughing and deep-breathing exercises, and signs and symptoms of respiratory tract infections.
- Emphasize the need for a high-fiber diet with adequate fluid intake to prevent constipation.
- Stress the need to avoid long periods of bed rest and inactivity, conduct active/passive ROM routinely.

LEGG–CALVÉ–PERTHES DISEASE (PERTHES)

Description

- Legg–Calvé–Perthes disease is a condition where there is avascular necrosis of the femoral head that can result in multiple fractures. As bone is reabsorbed, there could be complete collapse of the femoral head.
- Commonly affects boys ages 4 to 7 years but can occur as late as 12 years.
- May have a hereditary aspect with possible type-2 collagen gene defects.
- Exact cause is unknown, self-limiting process.
- Table 11.2 lists the four phases.

LEGG–CALVÉ–PERTHES DISEASE (PERTHES)

TABLE 11.2: Four Phases of Legg–Calvé–Perthes Disease

Phase	Description
1) Necrosis	• Disruption of blood supply occurs, causing infarction of the femoral capital epiphysis and leading to cessation of growth of the ossific nucleus • The infarcted bone softens and dies
2) Fragmentation	• The body reabsorbs infarcted bone
3) Reossification	• Osteoblastic activity takes over, reestablishing the femoral epiphysis
4) Remodeling	• The new femoral head reshapes during growth, becoming enlarged or flattened

Assessment

- Assess for family history of the disorder.
- Assess for **limp** that becomes progressively worse, aggravated by activity and relieved by rest.
- Assess for hip pain or pain referred to the knee.
  - May complain of pain and stiffness in the hip
- Assess for restricted hip abduction and internal rotation.
- Assess for slight shortening of the affected leg.

Diagnostics

- Serial hip radiography every 3 to 4 months confirms the diagnosis.
  - Findings vary according to the stage of the disease; changes might not be evident on radiography until 1 to 2 months after symptoms start.

Nursing Interventions

- Maintain splints, cast, or abduction bracing which can remain in place for 6 to 18 months.
  - May require traction for immobilization
- Nonweight bearing until re-ossification occurs; this relieves pressure from the head of the femur and increases blood flow to the area, preventing degeneration.
- Collaborate with physical therapy to provide or assist with ROM exercises, as appropriate.
- Provide emotional support to the child and family; allow the child to verbalize feelings and concerns.

PEDIATRIC PEARLS

- Exposure to secondhand smoke may also increase the child's risk of Perthes disease, although the exact reasons why are not known.

Special Considerations

- **Expectations regarding effects of the condition:**
  - After 18 to 24 months of treatment, most children return to daily activities without major limitations.

Discharge Planning; Patient and Family Education

- Consult with physical therapy and teach child and family how to use crutches and/or walker.
- Teach family regarding activity restrictions, including weight-bearing restrictions.

NURSEMAID'S ELBOW (RADIAL HEAD SUBLUXATION)

Description

- Nursemaid's elbow is a dislocation of the head of radius in the child's elbow.
  - Can occur when a child is pulled up too hard by their hand or wrist; a forceful longitudinal traction is applied to the extended and pronated forearm.
    - Other causes can include rolling over in an unusual way, stopping a falling child by grabbing their arm, swinging a young child by their arms during play, playing rough, or getting dressed.
  - Usually occurs in children under 5 years old.

Assessment

- Assess for reports of pain in the forearm.
- Assess for refusal to use the affected extremity, unwillingness to flex the elbow.
- Assess for holding the arm in a position of comfort at the side with the elbow extended and forearm and wrist pronated, there is no evidence of swelling or deformity with radial head subluxation (RHS).

Diagnostics

- Nursemaid's elbow is a clinical diagnosis and typically does not require radiographs.
- Radiographic images may be required if fracture of elbow is suspected, in which the reduction maneuver is contraindicated (see "Nursing Interventions").
- If the history or examination is not consistent with RHS, or if significant swelling, ecchymosis, or deformity is present, fracture or other etiology/conditions should be considered.

Nursing Interventions

- Manual closed reduction via either hyperpronation or supination–flexion maneuvers leads to regained function of the arm and relief of pain.
  - Maneuver produces a "click."
- If symptoms do not immediately abate, then short-term immobilization with a cast, splint, or sling may be warranted.

PEDIATRIC PEARLS

- Analgesia and anesthesia are rarely needed, and occasionally the elbow will slip back into place on its own.

Special Considerations

Radiograph if presentation is inconsistent with a RHS history

Discharge Planning; Patient and Family Education

- Educate on prevention.
  - Do not lift a child by a single arm, such as from their wrist or hand.
  - Do not swing children by their hands or forearms.

OSGOOD-SCHLATTER DISEASE (OSTEOCHONDRITIS)

Description

- Osgood-Schlatter disease is a condition where there is inflammation of the area just below the knee where the tendon from the patella (patellar tendon) attaches to the tibia.
  - Commonly affects boys between the ages of 10 and 15 who play games or sports that include frequent running and jumping.
  - Occurs during growth spurts, may occur unilaterally or bilaterally.
  - Exact cause is unknown.

Assessment

- Assess for intermittent knee pain; pain is generally over the tibial tubercle.
  - Pain that worsens with running, jumping, squatting, and ascending or descending stairs
- Assess for risk factors, growth spurts.
- Assess for soft tissue swelling over the tibial tubercle, palpable firm mass.
- Symptoms are relieved with rest.

Diagnostics

Radiography film of the knee; may show epiphyseal closings, soft tissue swelling, and/or calcification or thickening of the patellar tendon

Nursing Interventions

- Apply ice for 20 minutes every 2 to 4 hours, if ordered.
- Plaster cast or splint; may require immobilization.
- Avoidance of exercises that demand quadriceps contraction.
- Apply protective pad over the tibial tubercle.
- Encourage the child to verbalize feelings related to the condition and activity restriction; suggest ways to continue participation in sports activity without involving the affected extremity, such as attending practice to support other team members.

Special Considerations

- Expectations regarding effects of the condition:
  - Signs and symptoms will gradually diminish with time and rest and usually resolve within 1 year.
  - Discomfort may continue for 2 to 3 years, until the growth plate closes.

Discharge Planning; Patient and Family Education

- Self-limiting disorder, but can last for up to 3 years
- In severe cases, immobilization for 6 to 8 weeks
- Rehabilitation exercises

OSTEOGENESIS IMPERFECTA (BRITTLE BONE DISEASE)

Description

- Osteogenesis imperfecta (OI) is a genetic connective tissue disease in which bones are thin, poorly developed, and easily fractured.
  - Primarily a heterogeneous, autosomal dominant disorder of the connective tissue affecting bones, ligaments, and sclera with different degrees of presentation; there are at least 19 recognized forms of OI.
    - Involves mutations in the *COL1A1* or *COL1A2* gene
  - Equal presentation in both male and female genders.

Assessment

- Assess for family history of OI.
- Assess for bones that break with no known cause or from very minor trauma.
- Assess for bone pain, and/or deformity such as bowlegs and scoliosis.
- Assess for growth and developmental delays, short stature, triangular facial structure.
- Assess for bluish-grey brittle teeth (dentinogenesis imperfecta), a blue, purple, or gray tint to their sclera, and thin skin that bruises easily.
- Assess for hearing loss related to otosclerosis; this most often occurs in the third decade of life.
- Assess for increased laxity of the ligaments of the joints.

Diagnostics

- Prenatal ultrasound studies may reveal characteristic findings such as fractures or bowing of the long bones.
- Radiographs can show fractures or healed breaks; abnormal healing with bone thickening, curved or altered in shape with repeated improper healing.
- DNA testing to identify the collagen gene mutation.
- A skin culture shows reduced quantity of fibroblasts.

Nursing Interventions

- Gentle handling to prevent further fractures.
- Apply splints or maintain casting of fractures.
- Apply orthotics.
- Provide a diet that is nutritious, well-balanced with adequate amounts of calcium, vitamin D, and phosphorus.
- Administer bisphosphonates medications to prevent bone fractures, and growth hormone to increase linear growth.
- Implement falls precautions.
- Handle the infant or child gently and position using appropriate supports to reduce the risk of fractures.

Special Considerations

Meticulously gentle handling in all childcare activities to prevent further fractures

Discharge Planning; Patient and Family Education

- Educate family on safe handling of the child.
- Ensure a padded, soft environment.
- Monitor for any signs of fracture.

SCOLIOSIS

Description

- An abnormal lateral (sideways) curvature of the spine ÷10° (Figure 11.5)
- Three types (idiopathic, neuromuscular, congenital); 70% idiopathic—unknown etiology; family history common
- Occurs often before and/or during growth spurts in adolescence, 10–18 years old (mainly in girls); screening performed by school nurse, primary care clinician during well visits
- Usually asymptomatic, rarely causes pain
- **Features:** Uneven hips (waistline), scapula (shoulder height), ribs, arm length
- Progression of disease ends with growth increases
- **Complications in severe form:** Respiratory and cardiovascular problems

Assessment

- Assess for asymmetry in features listed previously; perform Adam's Forward Bend test (see "Diagnostics") and use an inclinometer for curve rotation.
- Assess for risk factors, growth spurts.

Diagnostics

- Usually detected during screenings at school or in primary care office
- **Adam's Forward Bend test:**
  - Ask child to stand with knees and feet together and then bend forward at hips to touch toes with hands dangling down.
  - Clinician stands behind child and assesses from the neck down to the ribs for symmetry; notes any hump on upper back.
  - If suspicion of scoliosis, then x-rays will be ordered to determine the degree of curvature.

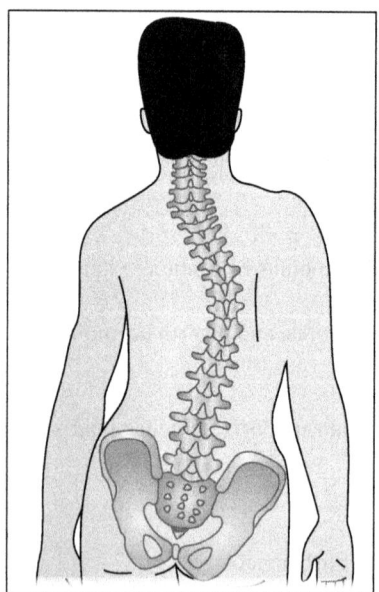

FIGURE 11.5: Lateral curvature of spine in scoliosis

Source: Reprinted from Gawlik, K. S., Melnyk, B. M., and Teall, A. M. (2020). *Evidence-based physical examination*. Springer Publishing Company.

TABLE 11.3: Degrees of Curvature of the Spine and Treatment

Curvature of spine	Treatment
≤25°	• Monitor and follow-up care • Possible brace use
25–45°	• Consider brace use
>45°–50°	• Spinal surgery: fusion, rods, and bone grafting
>75°	• Monitor for pulmonary complications due to lung expansion restriction • Surgery

Nursing Interventions

- Discuss treatment with child and family (Table 11.3).
- Emphasize the importance of follow-up care and appointments.
- **Brace wearing:** Wear cotton shirt under brace, bathe when allowed to take off brace, monitor skin integrity; put brace on after bathing, ensuring skin is dry.
- Provide psychologic support with brace use as this can cause body image issues.
- Perform pre- and postoperative care; ensure log rolling of patient after surgery to keep spine straight.

PEDIATRIC PEARLS

- Monitor for blood loss after spinal fusion surgery.

Special Considerations

Treatment goal: Prevention of further curvature and complications

Discharge Planning; Patient and Family Education

- Educate child and family on treatment strategies; dependent on degree and/or severity of curvature.
- Emphasize brace wearing for at least 18 hours per day to prevent progression of scoliosis.

SLIPPED CAPITAL FEMORAL EPIPHYSIS

Description

- Slipped capital femoral epiphysis (SCFE) is a condition in which a child's hip (the top part of the femur, or ball of the ball and socket joint of the hip) slips through the growth plate.
- Most common hip disease in adolescents.
- Classified as two types: stable and unstable:
  - **Stable:** Child or adolescent can still walk on the leg and bear weight.
  - **Unstable:** Patient cannot walk or bear weight.
- Early detection and treatment lead to a more favorable prognosis.
  - Complications may include failure of the joint to heal, avascular necrosis, and/or osteoarthritis.
  - May be unilateral or bilateral.
- Unknown cause; SCFE is more common in boys than it is in girls.
- Commonly occurs during a growth spurt; risk factors include overweight/obese, males and puberty.

Assessment

- Assess for history of hip, thigh, or knee pain unrelieved by rest.
- Assess for risk factors, growth spurts.
- Assess for intermittent limp or altered gait, decreased ROM, or inability to bear weight.
- Affected leg may be outwardly rotated, obligate external rotation is noted with hip flexion.

Diagnostics

Radiography film of the pelvis: shows a displaced femoral neck from the seat of the acetabulum

Nursing Interventions

- Maintain immobilization or traction until surgery occurs, if ordered.
  - Provide care for the child in traction, use logrolling techniques to turn the child in bed.
- Maintain proper body alignment and posturing; assist with quadriceps-setting exercises of the affected extremity to prevent muscle atrophy.
- Perform assessment of the neurovascular status of the affected extremity; compare it with the unaffected extremity.

Special Considerations

Treatment goal: Weight loss/management to prevent further stress on the bones

Discharge Planning; Patient and Family Education

- Educate child and family on treatment and activity limitation (based on stage of healing).
  - Nonweight bearing until cleared to use crutches.
- Monitor the opposite hip since the condition may reoccur on the other hip.

TALIPES EQUINOVARUS CONGENITA (CONGENITAL CLUBFOOT)

Description

Congenital condition where the foot and lower extremity do not form properly; referred to as clubfoot because of shape of leg and foot turned inward (adduction); not able to contact surface in standing position; more common in males (Figure 11.6)

Assessment

- Assess for abnormal feet and lower leg deformity; rigid, difficult to manipulate into "normal" place (limited dorsiflexion).
- Assess for risk factors, breech position.

Diagnostics

Clinical features; may obtain x-rays

PEDIATRIC PEARLS

- Early identification in newborn is key to promote a positive outcome in the infant.

Nursing Interventions

- Treatment includes serial casting of lower leg and foot (weekly to biweekly), braces, special shoes.
- Educate caregivers about treatment and the length of time, approximately 3 to 6 months.

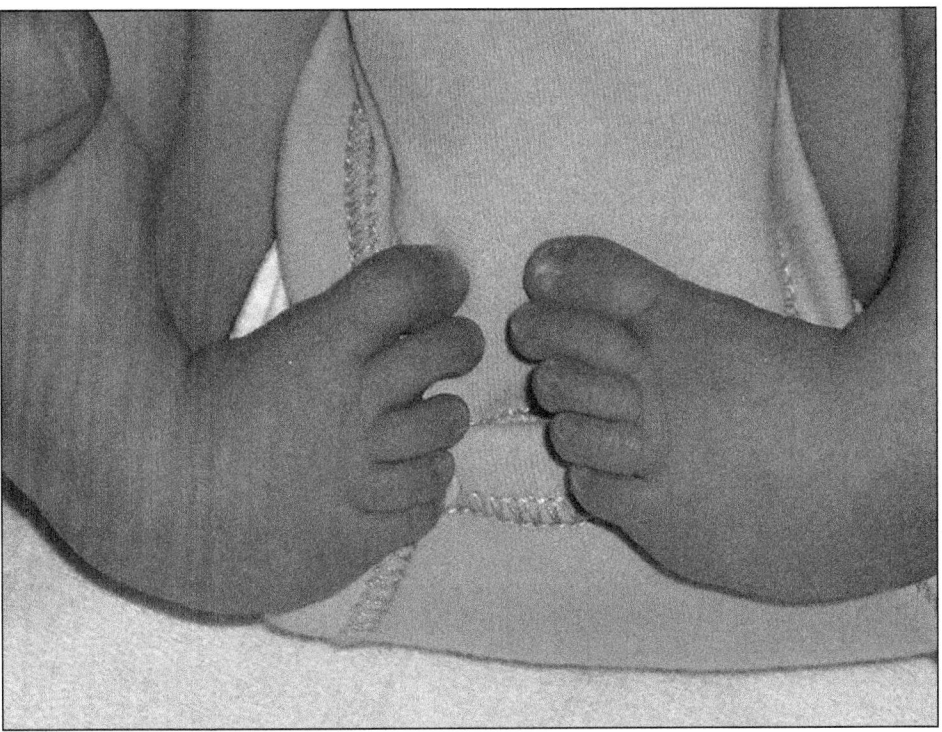

FIGURE 11.6: Talipes equinovarus (true clubfoot)

Source: Reprinted from Tkacs, N. C., Herrman, L. L., and Johnson, R. L. (2020). *Advanced physiology and pathophysiology: Essentials for clinical practice.* Springer Publishing Company.

- Refer to orthopedics; may need surgery if casting is not effective.
- Provide emotional support to parents.

Special Considerations

Treatment goal: Normal, functioning foot and lower extremities

Discharge Planning; Patient and Family Education

- Emphasize the need for serial casting and follow-up appointments.
- Cast care education.

BIBLIOGRAPHY

Dixon, A., Clarkin, C., Barrowman, N., Correll, R., & Osmond, M. (2014). Reduction of radial-head subluxation in children by triage nurses in the emergency department: A cluster-randomized controlled trial. *CMAJ, 186*(9):E317–E323. https://doi.org/10.1503/cmaj.131101

DynaMed. (2020, August 21). *Adolescent idiopathic scoliosis.* EBSCO Information Services. Retrieved June 28, 2021, from https://www.dynamed.com/condition/adolescent-idiopathic-scoliosis

Johnson, M. (2019). Nursemaid's elbow reduction. *Advanced Emergency Nursing Journal, 41*(4), 330–335.

Ricci, S. S, Kyle, T., & Carman, S. (2021). *Maternity and pediatric nursing* (4th ed.). Wolters Kluwer.

Silbert-Flagg, J., & Sloand, E. D. (Eds.). (2017). *Pediatric nurse practitioner certification review guide: Primary care* (6th ed.). Jones & Bartlett Learning, LLC.

Tkacs, N. C., Herrman, L. L., and Johnson, R. L. (2020). *Advanced physiology and pathophysiology: Essentials for clinical practice.* Springer Publishing Company.

KNOWLEDGE CHECK

1. A nurse is assessing a preschool-aged child for developmental dysplasia of the hip (DDH). Which of the following assessment screening motions should the nurse include?

    A. Ortolani sign
    B. Barlow sign
    C. Psoas sign
    D. Trendelenburg sign

2. A 2-year-old child is admitted to the pediatric unit with a fractured humerus and a diagnosis of OI. On physical examination of this child, the nurse also assesses this child to have which of the following clinical manifestations?

    A. Muscular pseudohypertrophy
    B. Bluish-grey brittle teeth
    C. Waddling gait
    D. Knock knees

3. A nurse who works with overweight children monitors them carefully for signs and symptoms of which of the following musculoskeletal disorders?

    A. DMD
    B. Legg–Calvé–Perthes
    C. SCFE
    D. Talipes equinovarus

4. A nurse is caring for a child who is suspected of having Legg–Calvé–Perthes disease. Which of the following diagnostic tests would most likely be indicated to confirm this disorder?

    A. Radiographs
    B. Genetic testing
    C. Goniometer measures
    D. Bone biopsy

5. A nurse is caring for a 13-year-old girl who has been fitted to wear a brace for her structural scoliosis. Which of the following statements demonstrate the teen's understanding regarding use of the brace?

    A. "I only have to wear my brace at night."
    B. "I'm glad that I can take my brace off whenever I get tired."
    C. "I'm going to take the brace off when I go to the homecoming dance."
    D. "I'll look forward to taking off my brace to take my bath every day"

6. The nurse is caring for a patient who has returned from surgery to correct their scoliosis and has undergone Harrington rod instrumentation along with a spinal fusion. Which of the following has the highest priorities?

    A. Comfort level
    B. Dietary needs
    C. Physical therapy needs
    D. Understanding of the procedure

KNOWLEDGE CHECK

1. **Correct Answer: D) Trendelenburg sign.** The Trendelenburg sign assesses for DDH. The preschooler bears weight on the affected leg while holding on to something for balance. The nurse observes from behind for abnormal downward tilting of the pelvis on the unaffected side. The Ortolani and Barlow tests are useful for assessing hip stability in the newborn. A palpable "clunk" during either maneuver is considered a strongly positive sign for dislocation of the hip. By 8 to 12 weeks of age, the Ortolani and Barlow tests are no longer useful, regardless of the status of the femoral head. At this age, capsule laxity decreases and muscle tightness increases. The Psoas sign, evidenced by right lower quadrant (RLQ) pain with extension of the right hip or with flexion of the right hip against resistance, indicates a possible inflamed appendix.

2. **Correct Answer: C) Bluish-grey brittle teeth.** The signs and symptoms of OI can include blueish-grey brittle teeth, bowed legs, blue-tinted sclera, bone pain, developmental delays, short stature, triangular facial structure, possible hearing loss, and skin that bruises easily. Muscular pseudohypertrophy and waddling gait are consistent with a DMD presentation and diagnosis. Knock knees is not a symptom of OI.

3. **Correct Answer: C) SCFE.** Orthopedic disorders, including genu valgum, SCFE, and tibia vara, are observed more commonly in children with obesity. Excess weight in young children can cause bowing of the tibia and femurs; the resulting overgrowth of the proximal tibial metaphysis is called Blount disease. DMD is an inherited disorder where there is an alteration/absence of a protein called dystrophin. Legg–Calvé–Perthes disease is a condition where there is avascular necrosis of the femoral head which appears to be idiopathic or have some genetic predisposition. Talipes equinovarus is a congenital condition where the foot and lower extremity do not form properly.

4. **Correct Answer: A) Radiographs.** A child with Legg–Calvé–Perthes presents with necrosis of the femoral head and can be diagnosed by radiographs (x-rays) of the hip and pelvis. Legg–Calvé–Perthes is not a genetically passed disorder so there is no indication for genetic testing or counseling. Goniometry is used to evaluate ROM but does not specifically identify Legg–Calvé–Perthes. A bone biopsy is used to diagnose cancer, infection, and other bone disorders; it is not indicated to diagnose Legg–Calvé–Perthes.

5. **Correct Answer: D) "I'll look forward to taking off my brace to take my bath every day."** The brace should be removed for 1 hour every 24 hours for hygiene and skin care. The wearing of the brace at night would be true only following radiographic studies indicating that the spine has bone marrow maturity, and the adolescent has been weaned from the 24-hour requirement, neither of which have happened yet. The patient stating that she can take the brace off when she gets tired, or that she can take it off when going to a dance both indicate poor understanding of the brace's therapeutic intent. Although physical appearances at social events with peers are significant, the brace should not be excluded during these times.

6. **Correct Answer: A) Comfort level.** Instrumentation and spinal fusion surgery causes considerable pain. The child may require significant pain management to control the pain of the invasive surgery and promote optimal healing. The nurse needs to assess for, monitor, and manage the child's pain adequately. This may be accomplished by utilizing opioids given via a patient-controlled analgesia (PCA) pump. Assessment for pain, pain medication, and evaluation will be essential in the postoperative period. Typically, immediately after the surgery, the adolescent will not be taking anything by mouth but will advance diet as tolerated once conscious and alert. Physical therapy is not the priority in the immediate postoperative period. Assessment of the adolescent's understanding of the procedure is a preoperative nursing responsibility.

KNOWLEDGE CHECK

7. A nurse is completing preoperative teaching with an adolescent client who is scheduled to receive spinal instrumentation for scoliosis. Which of the following information should the nurse include in the teaching?

    A. "You will be discharged the same day of surgery."
    B. "You will need to receive blood."
    C. "You will have minimal pain."
    D. "You will not be able to eat until a few days after surgery."

8. The mother of a 4-month-old infant who is in the Pavlik harness device is questioning her ability to correctly change the child's diaper while the infant is in the traction device. Which of the following actions should the nurse use to determine the mother's competency in changing the diaper?

    A. Request a home health nurse to visit the mother after discharge.
    B. Have the mother demonstrate changing the diaper while the child is in the device.
    C. Have the mother verbalize the steps in changing the diaper while the child is in the harness.
    D. Instruct the mother to remove the brace with each diaper change.

9. A hip spica cast is placed on a 12-month-old for the treatment of DDH. Which nursing actions should take priority following the application of the hip spica cast?

    A. Keeping the cast clean and dry
    B. Covering the perineal area
    C. Performing neurovascular checks
    D. Elevating the cast

10. The nurse is caring for a teenage child who is in traction prior to surgery for SCFE. He has been in the hospital for 2 weeks now and complains that he feels isolated. Which response by the nurse would be most appropriate?

    A. "I know it is dull being in the hospital, but you need to remain immobile for 2 more weeks."
    B. "If there are no complications, you only have 2 more weeks to remain here."
    C. "Let's come up with things to do like hobbies, games, and friends to visit."
    D. "If you resist your treatment, your condition will only get worse."

7. **Correct Answer: B) "You will need to receive blood."** Spinal instrumentation surgery for correction of scoliosis can have a lengthy surgery period with blood loss that requires blood replacement. Generally, patients who undergo instrumentation for scoliosis will be hospitalized for approximately 1 week. Patients who have spinal instrumentation surgery usually experience intense pain that require PCA (PCA medication pump) for pain management. Patient's postoperative recovery may include a regular diet to advance diet as tolerated.

8. **Correct Answer: B) Have the mother demonstrate changing the diaper while the child is in the device.** Having the mother demonstrate the diaper change in front of the nurse prior to discharge allows the nurse to directly observe the mother's method and comfort level. The mother may need to be reshown how to change the diaper and be given several opportunities to increase her confidence. Requesting a home health nurse to visit, is a further means of evaluation but does not provide immediate feedback and is not advised. Verbalizing the steps for diaper change would allow the nurse to assess the mother's understanding, but would not observe the psychomotor task involved with the diaper change. It is inappropriate to remove the traction device with each diaper change.

9. **Correct Answer: C) Performing neurovascular checks.** Neurovascular checks are always a priority in the assessment of newly applied cast to ensure that circulation and neurologic function is maintained. Keeping the cast clean and dry, covering the perineal area, and elevating the cast are all nursing actions appropriate for a child with a newly applied spica cast, however, the neurovascular assessment is critical in the prevention of complications and injury, and therefore must be prioritized.

10. **Correct Answer: C) "Let's come up with things to do like hobbies, games, and friends to visit."** After 2 weeks in traction, a teenager can become easily bored and isolated from usual peer interaction. The most helpful intervention would be to engage the help of the teen to develop a list of hobbies, games, perhaps books, and other activities that they would enjoy. The nurse should also encourage visitation and phone calls from friends. Telling the adolescent that he needs to remain immobile or telling him that he has only 2 more weeks do not address the adolescent's issue. Telling the adolescent that his condition will worsen if he resists is threatening and inappropriate.

CHAPTER 12

Endocrine and Metabolic Conditions

Joseph Cipriano and Molly Powell

INTRODUCTION

The endocrine system working in conjunction with the nervous system controls and regulates metabolic function throughout the body. The endocrine system is made up of endocrine glands, hormones, and receptors. The endocrine glands that produce specific hormones are the pituitary gland (Figure 12.1), thyroid gland, parathyroid gland, adrenal gland, pancreas, thymus, pineal gland, ovaries, and testes. A hormone is chemical substance produced by endocrine glands that causes metabolic changes that may affect most cells in the body or target organs.

Each of the hormones is released into the bloodstream and regulated by either negative or positive feedback. Negative feedback occurs when the production of a certain hormone decreases when the

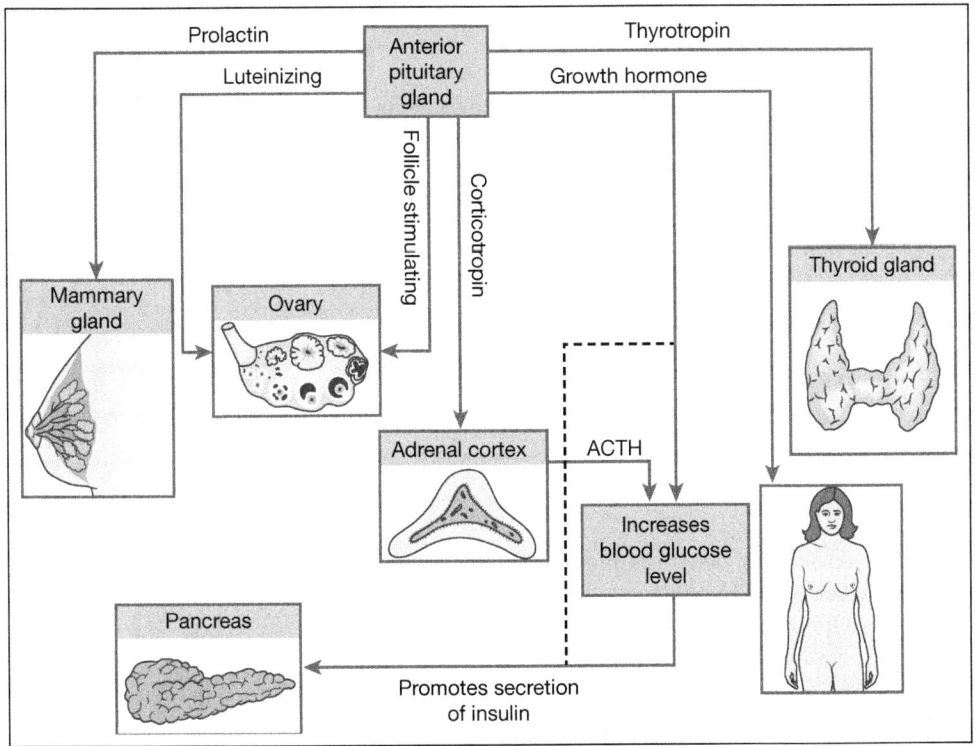

FIGURE 12.1: Anterior pituitary gland hormone secreted and their target organs

Source: Reprinted from Slota, M. C. (2018). *AACN core curriculum for pediatric high acuity, progressive, and critical care nursing* (3rd ed.). Springer Publishing Company.

concentration of that hormone increases in the bloodstream. For example, the thyroid-stimulating hormone (TSH) will stop production once sufficient levels of T_4 and T_3 are reached in the bloodstream. Positive feedback occurs less frequently in the body and occurs when the production of the hormone increases as the concentration of the hormone increases in the blood stream. An example of positive feedback is the production of oxytocin. During labor, pressure increased on the cervix stimulating oxytocin to be released in turn increasing uterine muscle contractions.

ADRENAL DISORDERS

ACUTE ADRENAL CRISIS

Description

- A critical deficiency of mineralocorticoids and glucocorticoids
- Rare in nature, caused by adrenal insufficiency from trauma (difficult labor, infection, or abrupt withdrawal of exogenous sources of cortisone)

Assessment

- **Early Signs/Symptoms**
  - Assess for abdominal pain, diarrhea, and nausea and vomiting.
  - Assess for headache, irritability, and weakness.
- **Other Signs/Symptoms**
  - Assess for sepsis shock.
    - Decreased blood pressure, shallow respirations, weak peripheral pulses
    - Circulatory collapse
- **Newborn Signs/Symptoms**
  - Assess for cyanosis.
  - Assess for high fevers.
  - Assess for tachypnea.
  - Assess for seizure.

Diagnostics

- Diagnosis often made by clinical manifestations.
- Improvement with cortisol therapy confirms diagnosis.

Nursing Interventions

- Administer replacement corticosteroids, fluids, and/or antibiotics in the presence of sepsis.
- Vital signs taken every 15 minutes.
- Seizure precautions.
- Monitor response to fluids and corticosteroid replacement.

Special Considerations

Rapid ingestion of fluids may induce vomiting; monitor serum electrolytes.

Discharge Planning; Patient and Family Education

Educate the child and family, paying attention to the psychosocial needs since acute adrenal crisis can be sudden and potentially life-threatening in nature.

ADRENAL DISORDERS: CHRONIC ADRENOCORTICAL INSUFFICIENCY (ADDISON'S DISEASE)

PEDIATRIC PEARLS

- Prompt recognition of signs and symptoms are imperative due to circulatory collapse, coma, and death.

CHRONIC ADRENOCORTICAL INSUFFICIENCY (ADDISON'S DISEASE)

Description

- Rare in children, chronic adrenocortical insufficiency involves the hormones cortisol and aldosterone.
- Decreased levels can reduce hepatic glucose output leading to hypoglycemia and reduce stomach enzymes causing vomiting and diarrhea.
- Decreased levels of aldosterone can lead to electrolyte imbalances due to sodium and water loss and potassium retention in the kidneys which can lead to heart dysrhythmias and hypotension.
- 90% of adrenal tissue must be nonfunctioning before signs and symptoms are manifested, therefore the onset of symptoms is gradual.

Assessment

- **Signs/Symptoms**
  - Assess for craving salty foods.
  - Assess for dehydration, vomiting, and diarrhea.
  - Assess for fatigue, muscle weakness, hypotension, and possible seizure activity.
  - Note presence of hyperpigmentation (bronzed) in the creases of hands, elbows, and knees.
  - Assess for hypoglycemia and weight loss.
- Monitor for electrolyte imbalances.
- Monitor for EKG changes.

Diagnostics

- Lab studies
  - Definitive testing made by checking plasma adrenocorticotropic hormone (ACTH) elevated in response to corticotropin stimulation
- Imaging
  - X-rays to show decrease in heart size and adrenal calcifications
  - Abdominal ultrasound to show adrenal gland abnormalities
  - CT scan to show the size and shape of the pituitary gland or abnormalities

Nursing Interventions

- Administer cortisone and hydrocortisone due to mineralocorticoid effect.
- Maintain fluid and electrolyte balance.

Special Considerations

Sudden termination of the drug or inability to ingest orally can result in acute adrenal crisis.

Discharge Planning; Patient and Family Education

- Explain that corticosteroid therapy will be lifelong.
- Advise patient and family members that during times of stress (infection, trauma, injury, emotional upset), dosage of corticosteroid therapy may need to be increased as must as three times their normal dose.
- Teach parents to keep an emergency kit containing a prefilled hydrocortisone syringe for use in time of an adrenal crisis. Patients and family members should be able to demonstrate injection method.

PEDIATRIC PEARLS

- Cortisone has a bitter flavor and may present a challenge. Try flavoring the medication or mixing it with chocolate milk or juices.

CUSHING SYNDROME

Description

- Although rare in children, Cushing syndrome results from excessive circulating cortisol with multiple etiologies.
    - Pituitary gland secreting excess ACTH causing the adrenal glands to hypersecrete corticosteroids
    - Adrenal tumor
    - Excessive use of exogenous corticosteroids (e.g., prednisone)

Assessment

- **Signs/Symptoms:**
    - Bruises easily
    - Central obesity
    - Dorsocervical fat pad (buffalo hump)
    - Hirsutism
    - Red abdominal striae
    - Round facies (moon face)
- Plot growth curve, often a gradual progression and not as recognizable as with infants.
    - Lack of height growth with weight gain is a common presentation.

Diagnostics

- Prepare to obtain the following lab tests:
    - 24-hour urinary free cortisol (UFC)
    - Late-night salivary cortisol
    - Low-dose dexamethasone-suppression test (DST; 1 mg overnight or 2 mg/d over 48 hours)
    - Fasting blood glucose
    - Serum electrolyte levels to check for hypokalemia
- Prepare child for CT or MRI imaging studies to check for presence of tumor on the pituitary or adrenal glands.

Nursing Interventions

- Treatment depends on cause, prepare patient and family for surgery if ordered.
  - **Adrenal tumors:** Adrenalectomy
  - **Pituitary tumors:** Transsphenoidal surgical (TSS) resection of pituitary tumor or radiation therapy
- Monitor for postoperative complications.
  - Due to the sudden withdrawal of cortisone, observe for signs of hypotension and increase in body temperature.
  - Alert the clinician of any shock-like symptoms observed.

Special Considerations

If patient undergoes pituitary surgery, treatment for panhypopituitarism will be needed. Replacement of key hormones such as growth hormone (GH), thyroid hormone (TH), antidiuretic hormone (ADH), and steroids are needed.

Discharge Planning; Patient and Family Education

- Postsurgery, teach patient and family to take replacement therapy with food to reduce gastric irritation.
- Instruct to inform their clinician during times of illness or increase in stress which may need a temporary increase dosage of hormone replacement therapy.

PEDIATRIC PEARLS

- Assess for control of chronic conditions such as asthma and inflammatory bowel disease (IBD) due to treatment with corticosteroids.

CONGENITAL ADRENAL HYPERPLASIA

Description

- Failure of the adrenal gland to produce cortisol, a steroid hormone that regulates a wide range of vital processes throughout the body including metabolic and immune response.
- Aldosterone and androgens (testosterone) can be affected by the lack of cortisol production.
- Autosomal recessive disorder.
- 21-hydroxylase deficiency leads to two types of congenital adrenal hyperplasia (CAH):
  - **Simple virilizing:** Cortisol deficiency caused by a deficiency of 21-hydroxylase increases corticotropin which produces excess androgens leading to early or inappropriate male characteristics.
  - **Salt-losing:** 21-hydroxylase is absent producing salt wasting cortisol precursors. This can lead to an acute adrenal crisis.

Assessment

- **Signs/Symptoms**
  - Females
    - Assess infants for ambiguous genitalia, enlarged clitoris, labial fusions.
    - During puberty, females develop male characteristics including hirsutism, acne, deep voice, and failure to menstruate.

- Males
  - Assess infants; no abnormalities are usually seen.
  - During puberty, male features include deeper voice and enlarged penis with frequent erections.
- Both males and females may grow taller prior to their peers but will have early closure of the epiphyseal plate.

Diagnostics

- Abnormal serum lab results
  - Elevated hormone levels
  - Elevated serum 17-hydroxyprogesterone levels (a precursor of cortisol)
  - Elevated serum 17-ketosteroids
  - Hyponatremia seen in salt-losing CAH

Nursing Interventions

- Administer intramuscular (IM) cortisone or hydrocortisone.
- Administer IM hormones.
- Provide emotional support and therapeutic communication to the family of the newborn with ambiguous genitalia.
- Prepare female child and family for genital surgery typically completed between ages 1 to 3.

Discharge Planning; Patient and Family Education

- Advise family that lifelong steroid replacement therapy will be needed.
- Parents need to recognize signs and symptoms of dehydration in salt-losing CAH.
- Encourage parents to obtain genetic testing due to autosomal recessive disorder if they want to conceive children in the future.

PEDIATRIC PEARLS
- Adrenal crisis in the first week of life is suggesting of salt-losing CAH.

PHEOCHROMOCYTOMA

Description

- Catecholamine tumor secreting epinephrine and norepinephrine hormones from the chromaffin cells in the adrenal medulla
- Usually rare in pediatrics, average age of presentation between 11 to 13 years old with males having a 2:1 ratio over females
- Can be caused by an inherited autosomal dominant gene mutation

Assessment

- **Signs/Symptoms:**
  - Assess for constipation and weight loss.
  - Assess for hyperglycemia, hypertension, and tachycardia.
- Assess in severe cases for heart failure and stroke.

Diagnostics

- Draw plasma free metanephrines (metanephrine and normetanephrine) as ordered.
- Obtain 24-hour urinary fractionated metanephrines as ordered.
  - Teach patients to avoid foods high in vanillin (coffee, nuts, chocolate, bananas, citrus fruits, and vanilla) 48 hours prior to collection of urine to ensure catecholamine levels are reliable.
- CT or MRI of the abdomen and pelvis are ordered by the clinician to visualize the adrenal tumor.
  - Some clinicians advocate for MRI due to radiation exposure with the CT.

Nursing Interventions

- Preoperative nursing interventions
  - Patients are usually admitted 24 to 36 hours prior to surgery.
  - Administer intravenous (IV) fluids as ordered to prevent hypotension during surgery.
  - Administer alpha-blockers, beta-blockers, and some cases, a tyrosine hydroxylase inhibitor.
- Postoperative nursing interventions
  - Monitor for hypoglycemia that can occur postoperatively due to rebound hyperinsulinism from a reduction of catecholamines.
  - Persistent hypertension is possible postoperatively.
    - Monitor blood pressure, if hypertensive crisis occurs; blood pressure and heart rate should be measured every 2 to 5 minutes until the patient stabilizes.
    - Provide a calm environment to reduce hypertensive episodes.
  - Keep the room cool since postoperative adrenal gland secretions cause diaphoresis, change clothing and linens as needed.

Special Considerations

Do not palpate mass which can stimulate server hypertension and tachyarrhythmias.

Discharge Planning; Patient and Family Education

- Educate that the patient's activities need to be adjusted without being overly strenuous or physically demanding during the postoperative period.
- If the pheochromocytoma is due to autosomal-dominant transmission, encourage other family members to be tested.

PEDIATRIC SKILL 12.1

- Obtaining a 24-hour urine sample
  - Upon waking, have the patient void in the toilet; do not collect this sample.
  - For the next 24 hours, collect each void in the provided container, storing the container either on ice or kept cool in the refrigerator. Ensure the cap is closed securely.
  - The next morning upon waking, collect the urine for the final time.

PEDIATRIC PEARLS

- Tumors secreting epinephrine cause tachycardia and require a beta-blocker.

PANCREATIC DISORDERS

TYPE 1 DIABETES

Description

- Autoimmune in nature.
- Result of pancreatic beta-cell destruction.
- **Insulin deficiency:** Complete lack of insulin secretion from the pancreas.
- Symptoms may appear suddenly.

Assessment

- Signs/Symptoms (usually occur before the onset of puberty)
  - Rarely obese, usually present with weight loss.
  - Assess for polyuria, polydipsia, polyphagia.
  - Assess for blurred vision.
  - Assess for nonhealing skin infections/wounds.
  - **Diabetic Ketoacidosis (DKA):** Lack of glucose in the body leads to excess ketones, buildup of acid. The body begins to break down muscle for energy.
    - Fruity smelling breath
    - Lethargy
    - Stupor
    - Increased respirations and heavy breathing
    - Vomiting

Diagnostics

- Lab studies
  - **Hemoglobin A1C (Hgb A1C):** ≥6.5%, greater diagnostic accuracy in type 2 diabetes mellitus (DM). Fasting plasma glucose or random plasma glucose should be used in combination to confirm.
  - **Fasting plasma glucose:** ≥126, should be repeated to confirm.
  - **Random plasma glucose:** ≥200 mg/dL
    - Usually well above 200 mg/dL in type 1 DM
  - **Oral glucose tolerance test:** ≥200 mg/dL 2 or more hours after ingesting glucose solution 1.75 g/kg (no more than 75 g). Rarely used for diagnosis in children.

Nursing Interventions

- Adequate hydration, oral or IV fluids depending on care setting
- Insulin therapies
  - Rapid-acting
    - **Onset:** 15 minutes
    - **Peak:** 1 hour
    - **Duration:** 3 hours

- Short-acting
  - **Onset:** 30 minutes
  - **Peak:** 2 hours
  - **Duration:** 8 hours
- Intermediate-acting
  - **Onset:** 2 hours
  - **Peak:** 8 hours
  - **Duration:** 16 hours
- Long-acting
  - **Onset:** 2 hours
  - **Peak:** None
  - **Duration:** 18 to 24 hours

- **Subcutaneous insulin injection**
  - Safe sites for children and adolescents (inject areas with highest amount of adipose tissue)
    - Outer thighs
    - **Back of arms:** One to two inches above the elbow
    - **Abdomen:** One to two inches around the umbilicus
    - Top-lateral buttocks
  - Important to rotate among and within injection site areas to reduce hypertrophy and scarring

- **Sick Day Rules**
  - Education on insulin adjustment during sick days should be taught at time of diagnosis, reviewed annually with family and patient to reduce potential complications.
  - Dose adjust, but do not stop administering insulin.
  - More frequent blood glucose and ketone monitoring to adjust insulin dose.
  - Monitor and maintain hydration.
  - Address underlying illness.

Special Considerations

Honeymoon phase in type 1 DM: With initiation of insulin therapy, pancreas may secrete small amounts of endogenous insulin. May last anywhere from 1 week to a full year. Insulin therapy is necessary throughout this phase.

Discharge Planning; Patient and Family Education

- Follow-up with primary care and endocrinology.
- Educate patient and family on signs and symptoms of hypo- and hyperglycemia.
- Blood glucose monitoring.
  - **Finger sticks:** Usually four times daily; fasting and 2 hours postprandial breakfast, lunch, and dinner
  - Continuous blood glucose monitoring
  - Need for repeat Hgb A1C every 3 months

PEDIATRIC PEARLS
- Insulin infusion pump is rapid-acting insulin only.

TYPE 2 DIABETES

Description

- Insulin resistance.
- Impaired function pancreatic beta-cell function.
- Increased association with being overweight, obesity, hypertension, and hyperlipidemia.
- Symptoms may appear gradually.

Assessment

- **Signs/Symptoms**
- **More likely to occur around, during, or after the onset of puberty**
  - **Obesity:** Body mass index (BMI) ≥95th percentile for age.
  - Assess for acanthosis nigricans.
  - Assess for polyuria, polydipsia, polyphagia.
  - Assess for blurred vision and fatigue.
  - Assess for nonhealing skin infections/wounds.
  - **Hyperosmolar hyperglycemic syndrome:** Rare occurrence, less than 1%.

Diagnostics

- Lab studies
  - **Hgb A1C:** ≥6.5%, greater diagnostic accuracy in type 2 DM. Fasting plasma glucose or random plasma glucose should be used in combination to confirm.
  - **Fasting plasma glucose:** ≥126, should be repeated to confirm.
  - **Random plasma glucose:** ≥200 mg/dL
  - **Oral glucose tolerance test:** ≥ 200 mg/dL 2 or more hours after ingesting glucose solution 1.75 g/kg (no more than 75 g). Rarely used for diagnosis in children.

Nursing Interventions

- Adequate hydration oral or IV depending on setting, needed in acute phase
- Education on dietary and lifestyle modifications
  - Weight management and increased activity
  - Balance of calorie intake and output
  - Preplanned timing of meals and snacks
  - Carbohydrate intake consistency for meals and snacks
  - Prioritize foods with good nutritional content

Special Considerations

Often occurs with other comorbid conditions: hypertension, obesity, hyperlipidemia.

Discharge Planning; Patient and Family Education

- Follow-up planning with primary care and endocrinology
- Need for repeat Hgb A1C every 3 months
- Medication management oral versus insulin therapy and potential side effects
- Signs and symptoms of hypo- and hyperglycemia

PARATHYROID DISORDERS

HYPOPARATHYROIDISM

Description

- Parathyroid hormone (PTH) is secreted by the parathyroid gland and works by a negative feedback loop based on the serum calcium levels.
- Congenitally may be caused by a deficiency in PTH by underdevelopment or absence of the parathyroid gland.
- Secondary causes by accidental removal or destruction of the parathyroid gland during a thyroidectomy.
- PTH is responsible for regulation of calcium release from the bones, absorption of calcium from the intestines, and conversation of calcium in the kidneys.

Assessment

- **Signs/Symptoms:**
  - Arrhythmias
  - Anxiety
  - Muscle hypertonia
  - Brittle nails
  - Dry skin
  - Fatigue
  - Paresthesia
  - Poor dentition due to teeth decay or tooth loss
  - Weakness
  - Seizures
  - Laryngospasms
- Observe for Chvostek sign.
  - Hyperirritability of the facial nerve occurring when the facial nerve branches are tapped
- Observe for Trousseau sign.
  - Spasmic contractions of the muscles of the hands and feet trigged after blood pressure cuff is inflated

Diagnostics

- Based on clinically on signs and symptoms and abnormal lab values including:
  - Hyperphosphatemia
  - Hypocalcemia
  - Hypomagnesaemia
- EKGs may be ordered due to prolonged QT intervals due to hypocalcemia.

Nursing Interventions

- Administer calcium as ordered.
  - IV calcium needs to be given slowly as the solution is irritating and can cause thrombosis.
  - Educate patient that flushing of the skin is common during the infusion.
- Administer vitamin D as ordered to promote calcium absorption.
- Tracheostomy kit should be readily available due to risk of laryngospasm and stridor.

- Safety precautions put into place due to risk seizure activity.
- Consult dietician or educate family on diet high in calcium and low in phosphorus.
  - High-calcium foods include green leafy vegetables, fortified orange juice, and breakfast foods.

Discharge Planning; Patient and Family Education

- Educate patient and family on signs and symptoms of hypocalcemia and when to call their healthcare clinician.
- Advise parents to only take the prescribed doses of calcium and vitamin D; some families may shop for over-the-counter (OTC) preparations to save money but may not be the correct strength needed.
- Educate that serum calcium levels will need monitoring throughout the year.

PEDIATRIC PEARLS

- Central nervous system (CNS) signs and symptoms are exaggerated during times of stress or infection.
- Remember calcium and phosphorous levels have an inverse relation.

HYPERPARATHYROIDISM

Description

- Occurs when the parathyroid makes too much PTH causing high levels of serum calcium in the body.
- Most common cause due to benign tumors of the parathyroid gland.
- Secondary causes include renal disease and low vitamin D levels.
- If left untreated can lead to osteopenia or osteomalacia and renal calculi.

Assessment

- Assess for joint pain, fractures, and muscle weakness.
- Assess for nausea, vomiting, and abdominal pain.
- Assess for weight loss and fatigue.
- Assess for headaches, hallucinations, and depression.
- Assess for flank/kidney pain and frequent urination.

Diagnostics

- Based on clinical manifestations and abnormalities in serum lab values
  - Hypercalcemia
  - Hypophosphatemia
  - Low vitamin D levels
  - Elevated PTH levels
  - Abnormal renal functions
- Imaging studies to check for parathyroid tumor
  - Ultrasound is most common test used for diagnosis.
  - Sestamibi scan may be used; this is where radioactive agent is injected into the veins that travels to an overactive parathyroid gland.
- Bone density scans to check for osteoporosis or osteomalacia
- EKGs for cardiac dysrhythmias

Nursing Interventions

- Prepare patient and family for possible surgery if the cause is from a parathyroid tumor.
- Administer high levels of vitamin D to promote calcium reabsorption.
- Ensure safe environment due to risk of bone fractures with fall.
- Monitor for signs of dehydration due to polyuria.
- Promote restful environment to avoid fatigue.

Discharge Planning; Patient and Family Education

- Postsurgical care education for families at discharge.
- Continue to take vitamin D and calcium at home to promote bone health.

PEDIATRIC PEARLS

- Sestamibi scans take approximately 2 hours to complete and that patient may complain of metallic taste in their month with injection but resolves within minutes.

PITUITARY DISORDERS

HYPERPITUITARISM

Description

- Overproduction of GH resulting giantism, an exaggerated bone growth, and abnormal height before the epiphyseal plate closes.
- Very rare condition with about 100 reported causes to date.
- Hypersecretion of GH after the epiphyseal plate closes is referred to as acromegaly seen in adults.

Assessment

- Signs/Symptoms:
  - Extreme height
  - Large hands and feet
  - Projection of the jaw
  - Excessive sweating
  - Headaches
- Monitor growth curve for rapid height increase.
- Mean onset of rapid growth is 13 years old.

Diagnostics

- X-rays to check bone age
- Serum insulin-like growth factor 1 (IGF-1)
- MRI to check for pituitary adenomas or hyperplasia

Nursing Interventions

- Given this is an extremely rare condition, emotional support for the patient and family is needed.
- Prepare child and family for surgery to remove adenoma.
- Observe for signs of diabetes insipidus a potential surgical complication.

Discharge Planning; Patient and Family Education

- Advise on emotion support group given the rarity of hyperpituitarism.
- Educate family on risk of premature cardiovascular disease and increased risk of DM.

PRECOCIOUS PUBERTY

Description

- The hypothalamic–pituitary–gonadal axis is activated early stimulating the secretion of gonadotropin-releasing hormone (GnRH) causing a secretion of luteinizing hormone (LH) and follicle-stimulating hormone (FSH) making puberty occur before age 8 in females and before 9 in males.
    - Production of secondary sex characteristics
        - **In females:** FSH causes the ovaries to produce estrogen.
        - **In males:** FSH causes tests to develop sperm and LH causes the production of testosterone.
- Due to early activation of puberty, rapid growth will occur, but epiphyseal plates will close earlier causing short stature in adulthood.
- Most causes are idiopathic but can be caused by hypothalamic tumors, infection, radiation, and head trauma.

Assessment

- **Signs/Symptoms**
    - **Females:** Breast development, axillary and pubic hair, early onset of menses
    - **Males:** Penis and testicular enlargement, chest, pubic and axillary hair, deep voice

Diagnostics

- Abnormal lab values
    - Serum FSH, LH, estradiol, and testosterone
- X-ray
    - Check for bone age by looking at epiphyseal closure.
- **Additional imagining:**
    - Some clinicians may choose to obtain an MRI of the brain.

Nursing Interventions

- Provide emotional support.
- Using therapeutic communication, ascertain any concerns regarding body image.
- Administer LH IM as ordered to slow progression of puberty.

Discharge Planning; Patient and Family Education

- Encourage open communication with family and patient due to feelings of body image issues and peer bullying/teasing.
- Teach family how to correctly administer LH IM every 4 to 12 weeks as directed.
- Advise family that patient should be treated as their chronological age with regards to clothing, activities, and sports.

DIABETES INSIPIDUS

Description

- Excessive large amounts of dilute urination with excessive thirst due to a decreased amount of ADH being released from the posterior pituitary gland
- Causes
  - **Central diabetes insipidus (DI):** Neoplasm, surgical removal of the pituitary gland, head trauma
  - **Nephrogenic DI:** X chromosome inherited disorder; polycystic kidney disease; electrolyte disorders (hypercalcemia, hypokalemia); nephrotoxic drugs (lithium, amphotericin B)

Assessment

- **Signs/Symptoms**
  - Polyuria
  - Polydipsia
  - Enuresis

Diagnostics

- Fluid restriction trials.
  - Hold all fluids to observe for concentration of urine; in patient with DI, the fluid restriction trial will have no effect on concentrating the patient's urine.
- IV vasopressin trial should correct polydipsia and polyphagia.

Nursing Interventions

- Obtain strict intake and output.
- Measure weight daily.
- Monitor for electrolyte imbalances.
- Administration of vasopressin may be IV or nasal.

Discharge Planning; Patient and Family Education

- Educate patient and family that treatment is with vasopressin is lifelong.
- Encourage the older child to participate in care and administration of vasopressin.
- Advise to make school personnel aware of diagnosis for self-administration of vasopressin and also bathroom privileges.

PEDIATRIC PEARLS

- Fluid restriction trials require close monitoring of the patient to avoid obtaining water from other sources such as toilet bowls.

THYROID DISORDERS

HYPOTHYROIDISM

Description

- TSH is secreted in the pituitary gland stimulating the production of TH in the thyroid located in the neck.
- Deficiency in TH results in the diagnosis of hypothyroidism.
- TH regulates metabolic processes in the body and contributes to maintaining heart rate, digestion, bone growth, muscle and reproductive functions.
- Causes:
  - Congenital hypothyroidism where the gland fails to develop before birth.
  - Acquired hypothyroidism from an autoimmune disorder causing decrease in thyroid function.
  - Other causes occur from having the thyroid gland surgically removed or destroyed via radiation therapy.

Assessment

- **Signs/Symptoms**
  - Fatigue
  - Constipation
  - Dry skin
  - Goiter
  - Cognitive decline or mental impairment
- **Infants (Figure 12.2)**
  - Impaired growth
  - Lack of cry or hoarse cry

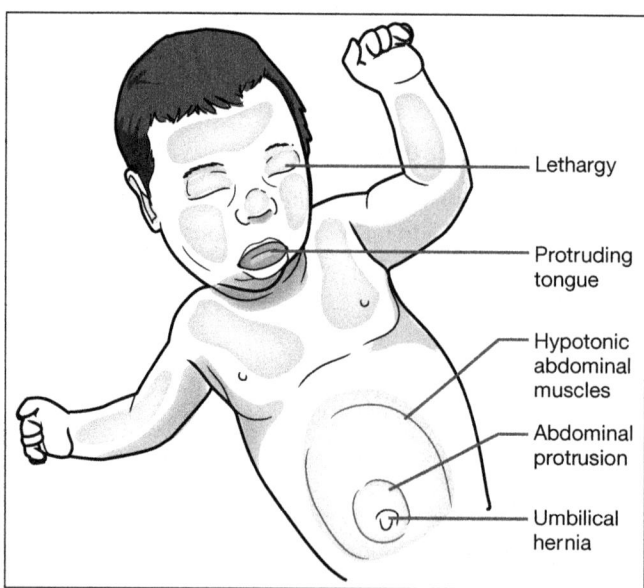

FIGURE 12.2: Congenital hypothyroid infant

Source: Reprinted from Chiocca E. M. (2019). *Advanced pediatric assessment*. Springer Publishing Company.

- Feeding problems
- Protruding abdomen
- Macroglossia
- Monitor growth curve

Diagnostics

- Based on clinical presentation and abnormal thyroid lab panel
  - High TSH
  - Low thyroxine (T_4)
  - Antithyroid antibodies present
- Ultrasound to check for hypertrophy of the thyroid gland

Nursing Interventions

- Infants born with large goiter may require surgery due to risk of airway obstruction, hyperextension of the neck helps facility breathing.
- Administer thyroid replacement doses; nurses should note that children metabolize TH more quickly than an adult; therefore, pediatric doses are typically higher.
- Infants born with congenital hypothyroidism should be positioned on their side to prevent airway obstruction.
- Provide emotional support to family if cognitive decline is noted in the patient.

Discharge Planning; Patient and Family Education

- Educate family that thyroid monitor will need to occur periodically throughout the year.
- TH replacement medication needs to be given on an empty stomach first thing in the morning.
- Teach parents to check child's pulse rate to check for tachycardia which is a sign of overdose in medication.
- Refer families to community groups if child exhibits mental decline for support.

HYPERTHYROIDISM

Description

- Often referred to as Graves' disease; caused by autoantibodies that stimulate the growth of the thyroid and overproduction of TH.
- Incidence of hyperthyroidism rises during puberty.
- Female incidence higher over males.
- Genetics strongly influence predisposition of hyperthyroidism.

Assessment

- **Signs/Symptoms:**
  - Restlessness
  - Tachycardia
  - Hyperactivity
  - Inattentiveness
  - Insomnia
  - Weight loss
  - Exophthalmos
  - Goiter
  - Tremor
  - Fine hair

- Thyroid storm is severe and life threatening. Signs/symptoms include:
  - Delirium
  - Diarrhea
  - Hyperthermia
  - Hypertension
  - Tachycardia
- Monitor growth curve for weight loss.
- Inquire about change in academic performance due to inattentiveness.
- Ask about sleep cycle.

Diagnostics

- Serum lab test confirming low or diminished levels of TSH and increased levels of free T4
- Ultrasound to confirm the presence of goiter or thyroid hypertrophy

Nursing Interventions

- Administer antithyroid medication and monitor for side effects such as rash, fever, and arthralgias. Monitor for labs for changes in liver function and agranulocytosis.
- Prepare child and family for surgery if antithyroid treatment option fails.
- Provide a nonstimulating environment that promotes rest.
- Instill eye drops as needed due to exophthalmos and risk of dryness.
- Offer therapeutic communication due to patient irritability as a result of the hyperthyroid process.
- Restrict activities until thyroid levels return to acceptable levels.

Discharge Planning; Patient and Family Education

- Educate that monitoring of thyroid will be lifelong with more frequent monitoring being required until puberty is reached.
- Parents should be aware of signs and symptoms of hypothyroidism due to risk of overdose with antithyroid medication.

BIBLIOGRAPHY

American Diabetes Association. (2021). *Professional practice committee: Standards of medical care in diabetes*. https://care.diabetesjournals.org/content/44/Supplement_1/S1

Avillion, A. (2016). *Disorders of the endocrine system: Anatomy, physiology and current treatment initiatives*. https://s3.amazonaws.com/EliteCME_WebSite_2013/f/pdf/ANCCFL10ESI16B.pdf

Barthel, A., Benker, G., Berens, K., Diederich, S., Manfras, B., Gruber, M., Kanczkowski, W., Kline, G., Kamvissi-Lorenz, V., Hahner, S., Beuschlein, F., Brennand, A., Boehm, B., Torpy, D., & Bornstein, S. (2018). *An update on Addison's disease*. Georg Thieme Verlag KG.

Delahanty, L. M. (2020). Nutritional considerations in type 2 diabetes mellitus. *UpToDate*. Retrieved April 30, 2021, from https://www.uptodate.com/contents/nutritional-considerations-in-type-2-diabetes-mellitus

Fleming, L., Van Riper, M., & Knafl, K. (2017). Management of childhood congenital adrenal hyperplasia—An integrative review of the literature. *Journal of Pediatric Health Care, 31*(5), 560–577. https://doi.org/10.1016/j.pedhc.2017.02.004

Hockenberry, M. J., Wilson, D., & Wong, D. L. (2013). *Wong's essentials of pediatric nursing*. Elsevier/Mosby.

Jain, A., Baracco, R., & Kapur, G. (2020). Pheochromocytoma and paraganglioma: An update on diagnosis, evaluation, and management. *Pediatric Nephrology (Berlin, West), 35*(4), 581–594. https://doi.org/10.1007/s00467-018-4181-2

Klein, D. A., Emerick, J. E., Sylvester, J. E., & Vogt, K. S. (2017). Disorders of puberty: An approach to diagnosis and management. *American Family Physician, 96*(9), 590–599. PMID: 29094880.

Laffel, L., Limbert, C., Phelan, H., Virmani, A., Wood, J., & Hofer, S. E. (2018). International Society for Pediatric and Adolescent Diabetes [ISPAD] Clinical Practice Consensus Guidelines: Sick day management in children and adolescents with diabetes. *Pediatric Diabetes, 19*(Suppl. 27), 193–204. https://doi.org/10.1111/pedi.12741

Levitsky, L. L, & Misra, M. (2020). Epidemiology, presentation, and diagnosis of type 1 diabetes mellitus in children and adolescents. *UpToDate*. Retrieved April 30, 2021, from https://www.uptodate.com/contents/epidemiology-presentation-and-diagnosis-of-type-1-diabetes-mellitus-in-children-and-adolescents

McCulloch, D. K. (2019). Classification of diabetes mellitus and genetic diabetic syndromes. *UpToDate*. Retrieved April 30, 2021, from https://www.uptodate.com/contents/classification-of-diabetes-mellitus-and-genetic-diabetic-syndromes

Peard, L., Cost, N., & Saltzman, A. (2019). Pediatric pheochromocytoma: Current status of diagnostic imaging and treatment procedures. *Current Opinion in Urology*, *29*(5), 493–499. https://doi.org/10.1097/MOU.0000000000000650

Rushworth, R. L., Torpy, D. J., & Falhammar, H. (2019). Adrenal crisis. *The New England Journal of Medicine*, *381*(9), 852–861. https://doi.org/10.1056/NEJMra1807486

Sbardella, E., Pozza, C., Isidori, A. M., & Grossman, A. B. (2019). Endocrinology and adolescence: Dealing with transition in young patients with pituitary disorders. *European Journal of Endocrinology*, *81*(4), R155–R171. https://doi.org/10.1530/EJE-19-0298

Wassner, A. J. (2017). Congenital hypothyroidism. *Clinics in Perinatology*, *45*(1), 1–18. https://doi.org/10.1016/j.clp.2017.10.004

Witchel, S. F. (2017). Congenital adrenal hyperplasia. *Journal of Pediatric and Adolescent Gynecology*, *30*(5), 520–534. https://doi.org/10.1016/j.jpag.2017.04.001

KNOWLEDGE CHECK

1. A nurse is educating a mother of a newborn diagnosed with congenital hypothyroidism. On assessment, the newborn has a protruding abdomen, macroglossia, and soft anterior fontanels. The nurse knows further teaching is needed with the mother states which of the following:

   A. "I will increase feedings to 4 to 6 oz every 2 hours due to soft fontanels."
   B. "I will place my baby on her side when sleeping to ensure a patent airway."
   C. "My child may require higher thyroid replacement doses than adults."
   D. "My newborn needs to have vitamin D drops because I am breastfeeding."

2. A nurse working in the ED has just received a 7-year-old female patient who presented with fatigue, paresthesia in her hands, and increased anxiety. While taking the patient's vitals, the nurse observes a spasmatic contraction of the arm while the blood pressure cuff is being inflated. The nurse correctly identifies this as which of the following signs?

   A. Chvostek sign and the patient likely has hypothyroidism
   B. Trousseau sign and the patient likely has hyperthyroidism
   C. Trousseau sign and the patient likely has hypothyroidism
   D. Chvostek sign and the patient likely has hyperthyroidism

3. The nurse working at a pediatric endocrine unit recognizes the following sign or symptom is consistent with a diagnosis of Cushing disorder.

   A. Laryngospasms
   B. Scoliosis
   C. Hirsutism
   D. Hippocratic facies

4. The nurse is taking care of an 11-year-old male patient who is being worked up for pheochromocytoma. The nurse is about to conduct the admission assessment. Which assessment practice would be contraindicated given this diagnosis?

   A. Conduct a thorough abdominal assessment with deep palpation to check for a mass
   B. Obtain the patient's weight and plot on growth curve to check for weight loss
   C. Conduct a thorough cardiac assessment; check for hypertension and EKG changes
   D. Do not palpate the abdomen due to possibility of a mass which can stimulate server hypertension and tachyarrhythmias

5. A nurse working in a newborn nursery is caring for a 2-day-old female infant, whose mother had a difficult labor. Upon morning assessment, the nurse suspects acute adrenal crisis when they observe which of the following sign or symptom?

   A. Erythema toxicum rash
   B. Mild fever
   C. Tachypnea
   D. Lack of cry

6. A nurse is caring for an 8-year-old male whose parents report increase in thirst and frequent urination over the past week. The clinician has ordered fluid restriction trials which have failed to concentrate the patient's urine. The nurse anticipates which of the following orders from the clinician?

   A. Collect 24-hour urinary fractionated metanephrines
   B. Administer nasal vasopressin
   C. Check serum 17-hydroxyprogesterone levels
   D. Administer oral corticosteroids

KNOWLEDGE CHECK

1. **Correct Answer: A) "I will increase feedings to 4 to 6 oz every 2 hours due to soft fontanels."** The anterior fontanels should be soft, therefore increasing feedings is not needed due to the child not being dehydrated. The nurse knows that a newborn with hypothyroidism needs to be placed on their side due to macroglossia to ensure a patent airway. Vitamin D drops are recommended for newborns who are breastfeeding. Children metabolize TH more quickly than an adult. As a result, pediatric doses are typically higher.

2. **Correct Answer: C) Trousseau sign and the patient likely has hypothyroidism.** Trousseau sign results in spasmatic contractions of the arm or legs within 3 minutes of the blood pressure cuff being inflated. This is a sign of hypothyroidism due to hypocalcemia. Chvostek sign is when there is a hyperirritability of the facial nerve due to hypocalcemia seen in hypothyroidism.

3. **Correct Answer: C) Hirsutism.** Patients with Cushing disorder will have the following signs or symptoms: easily bruised, central obesity, dorsocervical fat pad (buffalo hump), hirsutism, red abdominal striae, and round facies (moon face). Laryngospasms are seen in congenital hypothyroidism. Hippocratic facies and scoliosis are not indicative of Cushing disorder.

4. **Correct Answer: A) Conduct a thorough abdominal assessment with deep palpation to check for a mass.** The nurse should recognize that a patient being evaluated for pheochromocytoma should not have abdominal palpation due to the risk of stimulation of a hypertensive crisis and tachyarrhythmias. The nurse should obtain a weight and plot against the growth curve to check for weight loss which is seen in patient with pheochromocytomas. The nurse should also conduct a thorough cardiac assessment including blood pressures to check for hypertension and EKG monitoring for tachyarrhythmias.

5. **Correct Answer: C) Tachypnea.** Tachypnea, high fever, cyanosis, weakness, vomiting or feeding problems, dry skin and lips, and seizures are all signs of acute adrenal crisis in newborns, likely precipitated by a difficult labor. A lack of cry is seen in infants with hypothyroidism. Erythema toxicum appears as red blotches with small white "pimple" in the center (onset 2–3 days) and is an expected finding.

6. **Correct Answer: B) Administer nasal vasopressin.** The nurse should administer nasal vasopressin to concentrate the urine of a patient with diabetes insipidus. Collecting 24-hours urinary fractionated metanephrines will likely be ordered in a patient with pheochromocytoma. Patients being worked up for congenital adrenal hyperplasia will have orders for obtaining serum 17-hydroxyprogesterone levels a precursor to cortisol. If the patient had Addison's disease, then the nurse would anticipate an order to administer oral corticosteroids.

7. A mother says to the nurse of a newly diagnosed type 2 diabetic 16-year-old patient, "This is horrible, I don't want my son to have to go on insulin forever! I've been trying to get him to lose weight and stop eating so much sugar. I'm so fearful of the needles, I won't be able to help him." What is the best response by the nurse?

    A. "Your son is 16 and if he would have lost weight like you told him, then he wouldn't need to go on insulin."
    B. "Type 2 diabetics have options such as oral medications and insulin. The clinician will be able to discuss these options with you and your son."
    C. "Unfortunately, the beta cells in your son's pancreas are destroyed and insulin is the only option at this time."
    D. "You will get over the fear of needles. It will be just fine."

8. A mother brings her newborn in for a 1-month-old well-care visit and states, "She is such a good baby, she never cries but I think she is just about the same weight as she was at discharge from the hospital although her belly seems to always look full, isn't that strange?" The nurse would be on heightened alert for which of the following potential disorders?

    A. CAH
    B. Type 1 DM
    C. Hypothyroidism
    D. Hyperthyroidism

9. A father brings his 11-year-old daughter into the clinic with complaints of facial hair, weight gain, and a red line across her abdomen. He states that her asthma has not been controlled recently and he keeps taking her to different pulmonologists, "but they just keep giving her prednisone." What is an appropriate response by the nurse?

    A. "Your daughter is going through early puberty, and I would suggest continuing the prednisone as ordered by the pulmonologist."
    B. "It is important that today I ask the clinician for lab work to check your daughter's parathyroid level which could be the cause of her facial hair."
    C. "Your daughter likely has an overproduction of GH that is causing these symptoms."
    D. "I suspect your daughter may have Cushing disorder from the excess prednisone. I will alert the clinician of her uncontrolled asthma and continued use of steroid therapy."

10. A nurse is working in the ED who just received a newly diagnosed type 1 diabetic 14-year-old male patient whose father brought him in asking for him to be drug tested. The father tells the nurse, "His breath smells different, and he is very lethargic today. I don't like these new friends he is hanging out." The nurse notices rapid, heavy breathing on the physical exam. Which of the following interventions will the nurse initiate?

    A. IV fluid rehydration due to risk of DKA
    B. Administer antidiabetic medications by mouth as ordered
    C. Start a peripheral IV and push 50% dextrose
    D. Ask the patient for a urine drug sample

7. **Correct Answer: B) "Type 2 diabetics have options such as oral medications and insulin. The clinician will be able to discuss these options with you and your son."** The nurse should provide therapeutic and informative communication. Type 2 diabetic patients are either insulin-resistant or have impaired insulin section, but their beta cells are not destroyed like in type 1 diabetic patients. Saying that the son wouldn't need to go on insulin if he lost weight and dismissing the fear of needles do not address the mother's concerns and do not promote therapeutic communication.

8. **Correct Answer: C) Hypothyroidism.** The nurse should be on heightened alert that this newborn could have hypothyroidism. Parents think the child is being a "good baby" because they don't cry but this is a sign of congenital hypothyroidism. The child also needs to be evaluated for poor weight gain and a protruding abdomen which are more signs of hypothyroidism. The patient presentation doesn't indicate type 1 DM, CAH, nor hyperthyroidism.

9. **Correct Answer: D) "I suspect your daughter may have Cushing disorder from the excess prednisone. I will alert the clinician of her uncontrolled asthma and continued use of steroid therapy."** The child has hirsutism, weight gain, and abdominal striae which are all signs of Cushing disorder secondary to the continued use of prednisone, a corticosteroid due to the child's uncontrolled asthma. The nurse needs to alert the clinician of these findings. It is not likely that the patient's symptoms are indicative of early puberty, imbalanced parathyroid level, nor overproduction of GH.

10. **Correct Answer: A) IV fluid rehydration due to risk of DKA.** The child is a newly diagnosed type 1 diabetic who is likely in DKA, a dangerous complication of uncontrolled blood glucose. The initial intervention should be initiating IV fluids. Type 1 diabetics cannot take antidiabetic medications by mouth because their beta cells in the pancreas do not produce insulin and will need supplemental insulin to lower their glucose levels. Pushing 50% dextrose is not indicated at this time as the patient's blood glucose levels are elevated and not low. The patient's symptoms are not consistent with drug abuse and further education on the patient's type 1 diabetic condition will be needed for the father at discharge.

CHAPTER 13

Wounds, Burns, and Dermatologic Conditions

DiAnn Ecret

INTRODUCTION TO PEDIATRIC WOUNDS, BURNS, AND DERMATOLOGIC CONDITIONS

- **Pediatric Anatomy and Physiology**
  - **Function of skin:** Perception of touch, pain, pressure, heat, and cold
    - Temperature regulation; barrier to evaporative water loss; metabolic production of vitamin D; immunologic protection; overall cosmetic appearance
  - Largest organ of the body, consisting of three layers
    - **Epidermis:** Thin outer layer of skin.
      - Contains flat keratin, nonnucleated cells, which provides protein production. Contains melanocytes, which provides skin pigmentation and color and Langerhans cells that initiate immune response.
    - **Dermis:** Middle layer of the skin that is much thicker than the epidermis.
      - The dermis consists of connective tissue, allowing for stretching and contraction of the skin. Contains collagen, hair follicles, sebaceous glands, sweat glands, eccrine glands, lymph channels, mast cells, vascular supply, nerves, and muscles.
      - Helps to regulate temperature and blood pressure.
      - The skin's response to hypersensitivity reactions occurs with the mast cells in the dermis.
    - **Subcutaneous Tissue:** The third layer of the skin connects the dermis to muscle beneath the skin. The fat layer in the subcutaneous tissue helps to insulate the body during cold temperatures.
- **Nursing Process Review for the Pediatric Patient**
  - Assessment of the pediatric patient's skin
    - **Skin Assessment Newborn**
      - Largest organ but is very thin and fragile. The stratum corneum of the epidermis is 30% thinner than an adult's epidermis.
      - Contains less subcutaneous fat. Children experience more rapid heat loss. Newborns have a difficult time with temperature regulation and experience increased absorption of topical medications.

- Increased risk for water loss, increased risk of irritation and inflammation than adult skin. Skin becomes stronger, retains more water, and decreases the risk for bacteria susceptibility as the newborn grows.
- **Comprehensive Pediatric Assessment focus**
- Skin
  - Inspect size, shape, type, location, color, imperfections, elevations, or depressions.
  - **Palpate:** temperature, turgor, texture, moisture, and edema.
  - Assess for pain.
- Hair
  - Inspect color, cleanliness, texture, distribution, nits, lice.
  - **Palpate:** Symmetry, temperature, texture of scalp, moisture, pain.
  - Assess for alopecia (hair loss): unusual or rapid, hereditary, friction, rubbing, traction, or stress.
- Lesions
  - **Primary:** Macule, papule, vesicle, plaque, pustule
    - **Macular rash:** Flat, color changes in circumscribed areas, not palpable, up to 1 cm in size
    - **Papular rash:** Circumscribed, elevated solid lesion, accentuated with oblique lighting, up to 1 cm in size
    - **Vesicular rash:** Raised circumscribed lesions with intact filled clear fluid, up to 1 cm in size
    - **Plaque:** Circumscribed, elevated, plateau-like, solid lesion, greater than 1 cm in size
    - **Pustule:** Circumscribed, elevated lesions, filled with purulent fluid, less than 1 cm in size
  - **Secondary:** Fissure, scale, scar, ulcer, and atrophy
    - **Fissure:** Linear, breaks within the skin surface, often painful
    - **Scale:** Occurs with increased shedding or accumulation of stratum corneum, abnormal keratinization, and exfoliation
    - **Scar:** Permanent fibrotic skin changes that develop as consequences of tissue injury; Scars can be hypertrophic, atrophic, sclerotic
    - **Ulcer:** Full thickness loss of epidermis with damage into dermis, heals with scarring
    - **Atrophy:** Localized shrinking of the skin, which results in paper-thin, wrinkled skin with easily visible vessels
- **Inspect:** Describe characteristics, erythema, excoriation, secondary infection manifestations. Identify location of lesion and describe the distribution and size. Palpate lesion for temperature, induration. Measure the dimensions of the lesion.
- **Pain:** Assess for pain, determine intensity by utilizing a pediatric appropriate pain scale.
- **Family History:** Assess family history of chronic skin conditions and allergies.

ACNE

Description

- Chronic localized inflammatory disorder of pilosebaceous hair follicles that frequently occurs during adolescence from increased production of androgen hormones. The pilosebaceous hair follicles are obstructed by comedones and become an ideal location for bacterium and localized inflammation. Common location of acne: face and trunk.
  - Commonly affects children and adults, age 12 to 25 years old. Occurs in males and females; however, severe acne is more common in male adolescents. Manifestations occurring before age 8 indicates early puberty.

Assessment

- **Location:** Face, upper chest, shoulders, and back
- Careful evaluation of family history and genetic predisposition
- **Type:**
  - **Closed comedones:** Whiteheads or flesh-colored papules with tiny follicular openings.
  - **Open comedones:** Blackheads, where the follicular head is enlarged and with a dilated follicular opening.
  - As inflammation increases, papules and pustules develop.
  - Nodules are larger areas of inflammation, including more than one hair follicle.
  - Cysts are compressible nodules without inflammation.
  - Scars may occur with healing and may be pitted, atrophied, hypertrophic, or keloid. Severity of acne may be classified as mild, moderate, moderately severe, or severe.
    - 1. **Mild:** Noninflammatory
    - 2. **Moderate:** Inflammatory with papules, pustules, and comedones. May have mild symptoms on back and chest
    - 3. **Moderately severe:** Inflammatory, numerous papules, numerous comedones, localized cysts. May have a few localized cysts and nodules. Increasing symptoms located on face, chest, and back
    - 4. **Severe:** Nodular and cystic acne on face, back, and chest; may have symptoms of numerous cystic lesions, comedones, papules, and pustules on face, back, and chest

Diagnostics

Assessment of skin

Nursing Interventions

- Assess family history, caregiver's, and adolescent's knowledge about etiology, treatment, care, and use of home therapies.
- Document type, severity, and distribution.
- Instruct skin care, proper hygiene, nutrition, and treatment of acne.
  - Teach skin care, frequent handwashing, washing affected areas with mild, non-oil-based soap twice a day, pat dry.
  - Avoidance of abrasive cleaners and astringent products.
  - Avoidance of use of products that contain oil-based products.
  - Teach adolescent documentation or self-journaling or diary use to include skin care, dietary intake, menses for females, and use of treatment interventions.
  - Provide education regarding medication use that includes the action of medication, side effects, dosage, and method of application.
  - Provide emotional and psychological support and resources.

Special Considerations

- Avoid picking and squeezing acne.
- Instruct decreased use of foods that have low nutritional value and are greasy.
- Avoid hats or headgear that can irritate skin and exacerbate acne.
- Wear protective clothing from sun and cold windy weather. Skin sensitivity to heat, sun, and cold.
- Carefully assess emotional distress, low self-esteem, impact on perceptions of embarrassment, depression, anxiety, and social withdrawal.
- If acne is severe and unresponsive to treatment, then isotretinoin (Accutane) may be considered; be aware of teratogen, contraindicated in pregnancy. Females need pregnancy tests, consent forms, and monthly labs.

Discharge Planning; Patient and Family Education

- Adolescents and families will verbalize understanding of interventions, medications, and teaching.
- Educate that medication will make acne worse at first and then see improvement in 4 to 8 weeks.

BURNS

Description

- Most commonly caused by exposure of skin to extreme heat sources but can also be caused by exposure to extreme cold, chemical exposure, electricity, and radiation to skin.
- Tissue destruction depends upon intensity of source, the duration in contact with source, conductivity of source, and the rate that the heat source disperses through the tissue.
- Thermal, scalding liquid burns are the most common in infants younger than 3 years of age.
- Thermal, scalding, or contact with hot appliances, such as ovens and irons, are the most common burns in preschool-aged children.
- Thermal burns, playing with matches, and lighters are the most common in school-aged children; additionally, electrical and chemical burns are common in school-aged children because of their curiosity and experimentation.
- Thermal burns, chemical burns, and radiation burns are common in adolescents from sunbathing, risk taking behavior with open fires, camping, and drug and alcohol use.
- Child abuse should be evaluated with any suspicious lesion or repeated injury.

Assessment

- **Determine type and source of injury:** Thermal, electrical, chemical, radiation.
- Assess total body surface area (TBSA); may utilize a chart (Figure 13.1) such as the Lund and Browder chart. Must account for differences in pediatrics related to the head and legs: the percentage body surface area (BSA) of the head and neck of an infant is twice the size of an adult, and the percentage BSA of the lower extremities is smaller, but as the child grows, the legs BSA percentage increases. Around 14 years of age, BSA-weight is comparable to adults.
- Assess the depth of injury.
  - Superficial (first-degree burns)
    - Damage to epidermis, erythema, dry, no blister formation (e.g., sunburn). Heals in 5 to 10 days without scarring

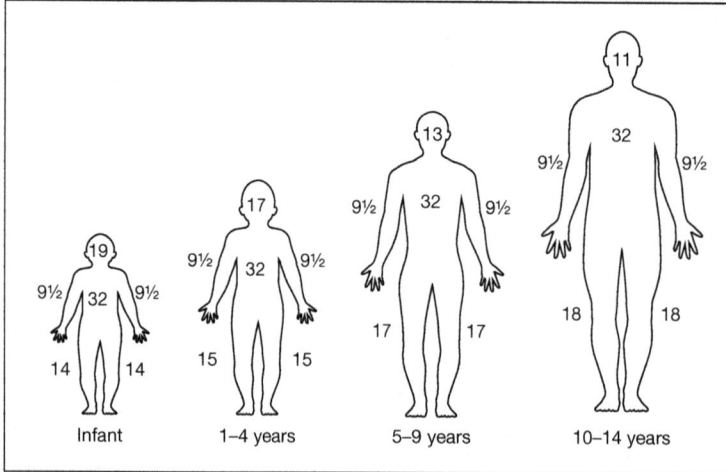

FIGURE 13.1: Total body surface area percentages

Source: Adapted from Cuccurullo, S. (2019). *Physical medicine and rehabilitation board review* (4th ed.). Springer Publishing Company.

- Partial thickness (second-degree burns)
  - Superficial partial thickness dermal burn; includes the epidermis and part of the dermis.
  - Wounds are painful, moist, red, with evidence of blistering. Heals in 14 to 21 days with varying levels of scarring.
  - Partial thickness deep dermal burn includes damage to epidermis and parts of deep dermal layers of the skin.
  - Resembles full thickness burns, except that sweat glands and hair follicles remain intact.
  - Mottled, red with waxy white areas. Heals beyond 21 days and is associated with increased scarring.
- Full thickness (third-degree burns)
  - Involve the entire epidermis and dermis, also extending into the subcutaneous tissue; nerve endings, sweat glands, and hair follicles are included in damage.
  - Color includes red, tan, waxy white, brown, or black. Appearance is thick, dry, and leathery; require surgical excision and grafting.
- Full thickness burns (fourth-degree burns)
  - Involves entire epidermis, dermis, subcutaneous tissue, muscle facia, and bones, appears dull, dry, ligaments, bone, tendon exposure possible; require surgical excision and grafting.

Diagnostics

- Wound cultures
- Complete blood cell count (CBC) with differential
  - Risk for infection and sepsis
- Basic metabolic panel (BMP)
  - Fluid and electrolyte abnormalities

Nursing Interventions

- **Airway:** Support airway.
  - Maintain patent airway.
  - Assess for inhalation injury.
    - Singed soot in nares, mouth
    - Hoarseness, difficult swallowing, copious secretions, stridor
- **Breathing:** Elevate head of bed, administer supplemental humidified oxygen.
  - Assess for difficult breathing.
    - Monitor rate and depth of respirations, nasal flaring, adventitious breath sounds, and audible wheezing, stridor.

PEDIATRIC PEARLS
STOP THE BURNING PROCESS

- Remove burning clothes and jewelry.
- Apply cool water to injury, never apply ice.
- Flush chemical burns with large volumes of water.
- Cover burn with clean sheet or cloth.
  - Prevent hypothermia and infection.

- **Circulation:**
  - Fluid resuscitation as per the Parkland formula and American Burn Association (2–4 mL/kg/TBSA).
  - Expect large fluid shifts to occur during the first 24 hours after a large TBSA burn; monitor for shock.
  - Monitor hemodynamic stability and urinary output; daily weights; monitor electrolytes especially sodium and potassium.
- **Asepsis:**
  - Maintain strict aseptic technique with all wound care; limit visitors.
  - Maintain protective environment; reverse isolation.
  - Patient is at risk for infection and sepsis.
  - Use patient equipment/no sharing of patient blood pressure cuff.
  - Administer antibiotics as ordered, carefully monitor peak and trough levels.
- **Pain:**
  - Administer all pain medications prior to wound care and via the intravenous (IV) route.
  - Provide supportive and restful environment; monitor effectiveness of comfort measures.
  - Provide psychological support and nonpharmacologic modes of pain control.

Special Considerations

- Prevention
  - Keep matches and lighters out of reach of children.
  - Never leave children unattended around a grill, indoor/outdoor fire; turn pot handles in when cooking on the stove.
  - Maintain home hot water temperature below 120 °F/48.9 °C; be sure to check temperature of bath water before child gets in.
  - Keep heated hair devices, such as curling irons, out of reach of children.
  - Keep working fire extinguisher in the home and instruct understanding of use.
  - Installation and use of home fire alarms, carbon dioxide alarms.

Discharge Planning; Patient and Family Education

- Educate families on burn prevention and care of burns at home; apply topical antimicrobial cream to open burns/wounds (Silver Sulfadiazine).

PEDIATRIC PEARLS

- Do not use Silver Sulfadiazine cream on children less than 2 months old or children with a Sulfa allergy, and do not apply to face due to hyperpigmentation.

- Offer emotional and psychological support as needed; body image and behavioral issues can occur.
- Educate families on burn injury, treatments, pain management, wound care, and infection prevention; emphasize to families the importance of understanding the signs and symptoms of wound infection and when to call clinician.
- Offer resources.
- Discuss with families that the child may need long-term rehabilitation and surgeries.
- Encourage adequate nutritional status.

DERMATOLOGIC CONDITION: BACTERIAL SKIN INFECTIONS—CELLULITIS

Description

- Inflammation caused by bacteria that enters through the skin and releases bacterial toxins into the subcutaneous tissue.
- The most common etiologic pathogen is either *Staphylococcus aureus* or *Streptococcus* bacterial species.
- Be alert for signs and symptoms related to the eye (periorbital cellulitis).

Assessment

- Acute onset of localized swelling, warmth, redness, and pain. Cellulitis is also frequently associated with systemic manifestations of fever, chills, and sweating.
- Regional lymph node enlargement.

Diagnostics

- History and physical assessment
- Culture and sensitivity of wound drainage

Nursing Interventions

- Elevate affected area; apply cool moist packs to site every 2 to 4 hours.
- Rest and immobilization of affected area.

Special Considerations

- IV antibiotics and hospitalization may be required with systemic manifestations.
- Ask the adolescent about body piercings.

DERMATOLOGIC CONDITION: BACTERIAL SKIN INFECTIONS—IMPETIGO

Description

- The most common bacterial skin infection in children; very contagious.
- Caused by *Staphylococcus aureus* or beta-hemolytic *Streptococcus pyogenes*. These normal organisms colonize on the skin's surface and enter with a break in the skin's surface.

Assessment

- Assess impetigo lesions for papules, vesicles, erosion, serous fluid, and characteristic honey-colored crust formation.
- Assess for widespread erythema, edema, and pain. Skin may be moist, red with scaled appearance. Extension of blistering can occur.

Diagnostics

- Can be diagnosed through physical appearance and symptoms of lesions.
- Diagnostic gram stains and bacterial cultures can be obtained to diagnose organisms.

Nursing Interventions

- Soak crusted lesions with cool compress or Burow solution; need to remove them before applying antibiotic ointment.

- Instruct parents to clean lesions with warm soap and water, apply topical antibiotic ointment and provide oral antibiotics as prescribed.
- Instruct frequent handwashing, avoidance of touching lesions.
- Prevent sharing of towels and clothing; highly contagious.
- Cover wounds to decrease exposure and spread of lesions.
- Educate caregivers on keeping child's nails short to reduce risk of secondary infections.
- Instruct parents to notify the primary care clinician when impetigo symptoms worsen.

Special Considerations

- Community-acquired methicillin-resistant *Staphylococcus aureus* (CA-MRSA)
  - Can cause aggressive soft tissue infections in children.
  - Prior skin infections can increase risk.
  - Manifestations include furuncles or abscesses.
  - Assess for redness, localized swelling that does not resolve, increase warmth to touch, purulent drainage, lesions that invade deeper tissue than impetigo.
  - Cover wounds at all times, instruct the importance of risk for respiratory transmission.
  - Household surfaces must be frequently cleaned with diluted bleach solution.
  - Decontamination of bed linens.
  - Educate parents and adolescents to take full course of prescribed antibiotics.
  - Educate parents and adolescents on importance to regularly clean equipment, take frequent showers with soap and hot water after close-contact sporting competitions.

DERMATOLOGIC CONDITION: CONTACT DERMATITIS—DIAPER RASH

Description

- **Irritant contact dermatitis:** One of the most common causes in infants from 9 to 12 months of age and toddlers.
- Primary reaction to urine, feces, moisture, and friction.
- Urine increases wetness and pH of skin. Increasing abrasions and causing irritation. Feces increases irritation and formation of ammonia with urine.
- Diapers made of plastics, clothing dye, and/or soap irritants may increase irritation to skin.

Assessment

- **Contact dermatitis:** Assess exposure location, develops within a few hours of contact and peaks within 24 hours. Rash quickly resolves when irritant is removed.
- Secondary infections caused by *Candida albicans* can occur. *Candida albicans* rash includes bright red plaques, sharp margins that can increase risk for rupture and can scale. Additional assessment of papules and pustules can increase skin breakdown. Carefully assess skinfolds.
- Assess size, shape, location, warmth, and color of diaper rash; assess for maculopapular rash in the diaper area. Note areas of erythema, distribution of linear, circular, and generalized rash; assess for bleeding or weepy exudate.
- Assess if the rash comes and goes, if the rash is always present; assess for irritability and pain.

Diagnostics

- History and physical assessment.
- When *Candida albicans* is suspected, skin scraping is obtained and examined for microscopic examination with potassium hydroxide.

Nursing Interventions

- Instruct parents to change infant or child's diaper as soon as possible after urination and bowel movement and change diaper at least every 2 hours.
- Wash the area with soap and water, and pat dry.
- Instruct parents to use alcohol-free baby wipes.

Special Considerations

- **Prevention:** Keep clean and dry as often as possible.
- Application of water-impermeable barrier protectant, such as zinc oxide and protective powders.
- When *Candida albicans* is present, apply antifungal topical medications as prescribed.

FUNGAL INFECTION: ORAL CANDIDIASIS (THRUSH)

Description

- Yeast infection located in the mouth
  - Acute conditions can occur with newborns.
  - Children who are immunocompromised or who use corticosteroid inhalers.

Assessment

Characterized by white patches in the oral mucosa that are not easily removed. Removal can cause bleeding.

Diagnostics

- Physical examination, clinical appearance
- Microscopic examination and skin scraping

Nursing Interventions

- Prevention, teach sterilization for bottle nipples and pacifiers.
- Instruct good hand hygiene to decrease transmission of fungal infection.
- May need to treat breastfeeding mothers; apply nystatin to nipples.

Special Considerations

- Instruct parents of children who have asthma and have frequent inhaler use to rinse mouth out well after use of inhaler.
- Teach parents proper administration of oral nystatin. Proper application after feeding in mouth and on tongue.

FUNGAL INFECTION: TINEA INFECTIONS

Description and Assessment

- Tinea refers to all fungal infections.
  - Tinea Pedis (athletes' foot)
    - Areas of erythema on the foot and between toes.
    - Fissures may occur between the toes.
    - May be weepy.

- Itchy and painful.
- Occurs most frequently in adolescents.
- Common spread in locker rooms, public showers, and swimming pools.

- Tinea Corporis (ringworm involving trunk, extremities, and groin)
  - **Characteristic lesions:** Ring-shaped (annular)
  - Superficial dermatophyte featuring annular borders with peripheral red, raised scaling; center of ring can be clear (healing) or include vesicles
  - Person to person transmission and/or animal to person transmission, commonly seen in wrestlers

- Tinea Capitis (ringworm involving scalp)
  - Common in school-aged children, includes scaling scalp and associated hair loss
  - Spreads in circular pattern, may be caused by person-to-person transmission or animal to person transmission

- Tinea Cruris (jock itch)
  - Inflammation in the folds of the groin
  - Itching with sweating and exercising on warm days
  - Rare in preadolescent children

Diagnostics

Physical assessment

Nursing Interventions

- May require oral and topical antifungal medication treatment.
- Apply antifungal powder, creams, shampoo, and lotions to affected areas as prescribed.
- Clean contaminated objects, hairbrushes, combs, towels, and bedding sheets.
- Instruct family members to not share objects such as hairbrushes, combs, towels, and bedding sheets.
- Shower after exercise and softly pat affected area dry.
- Eliminate conditions such as heat and perspiration.
- Use clean light "breathable" fabric, such as cotton socks, avoidance of occlusive clothes, and underwear.

Special Considerations

- Assess for coexisting bacterial infections with break in skin.
- Instruct family to carefully assess for resistant healing.

INSECT STINGS AND SPIDER BITES

Description

- Common in children and generally not problematic.
- Exceptions include stings and bites that are caused by parasites, venomous spider bites, or those that carry communicable diseases such as mosquitos and ticks.

Assessment

- Mosquitoes and fleas
  - Red papules and edema, itching, pruritic wheals, and bullae after repeat exposure.
  - Rare systemic reactions include generalized urticaria, angioedema, wheezing, nausea, vomiting, manifestations of anaphylaxis.

- Bed bugs
  - Localized inflammation, pruritic papules in clusters, new lesions commonly assessed in the morning
- Bees, wasps
  - Localized reaction, including localized inflammation, which includes erythema, edema, mild localized pain
  - Systemic reactions
    - **Cutaneous:** Urticaria, flushing, angioedema, hives, and pruritus
    - **Gastrointestinal:** Abdominal pain, nausea, vomiting, and diarrhea
    - **Respiratory:** Hoarseness of voice, dysphagia, throat tightening, wheezing, and cough
    - **Circulatory:** Hypotension, tachycardia, dizziness, and change in the level of consciousness
- Spiders (black widow and brown recluse)
  - Black widow localized reaction
    - Onset 1 to 3 hours; peak 3 to 12 hours; diminish within 72 hours
    - Stinging sensation, erythema, edema, petechiae, and two fang marks
  - Black widow systemic reaction
    - Muscle cramping at injury site
    - Muscle rigidity of chest and abdomen
    - Malaise, diaphoresis, restlessness, nausea, vomiting, insomnia, hypertension, cardiac dysthymias, oliguria
  - Brown recluse localized reaction
    - Onset within 2 hours; peak 1 to 2 days
    - Pain, depressed blue macule with halo of inflammation at the site of bite
    - Hemorrhagic blister, with necrotic center
  - Brown recluse systemic reaction
    - Fever, chills, nausea, vomiting, and hemolysis

Diagnostics

- Physical assessment
- Comprehensive history

Nursing Interventions

- Supportive therapies, cool compresses, apply ice to the site, clean wounds with soap and water, application of antihistamines, topical corticosteroids as prescribed.
- Oral corticosteroids as prescribed for severe allergic reactions.
- Opioids may be prescribed for severe pain with spider bites, antivenom administered IV for severe reactions. Excision and skin grafting for severe cases of necrosis with brown recluse spider bites.

Special Considerations

- Prevention strategies, teaching children to avoid bees and wasps and to remain calm when present and slowly walk away.
- Instruct use of insect repellants, reapply once washed off, instruct parents/caregivers to wash all diethyltoluamide (DEET) products off of children when returning indoors.
- Antibiotics for secondary infections.

Discharge Planning; Patient and Family Education

- Instruct caregiver/parental use of nonperfumed hygiene products such as shampoo, powder, soap, or lotions.

- Avoid dressing children in brightly colored clothes while outside, encourage light-colored clothes, smooth textured clothes, wearing long sleeves and pants while outside.
- Avoid eating sweetened food and beverages while outside; pour beverages in clear cups and avoid drinking from a can.

PEDICULOSIS (LICE)

Description

- Most common in children 3 to 14 years old.
- Uncommon in African American children due to characteristics of hair shaft.
- Transmission of parasitic louse infestation by direct hair to hair contact or indirect contact through the sharing of hairbrushes, hats, towels, and bedding. Occur only on human-to-human contact.
- Lice do not jump or fly; need blood source on scalp for meal.

Assessment

- Intense pruritus and dandruff that sticks to hair.
- Inspect hair for nits behind the ears and near the scalp.
- Inspect hair for wingless insects the size of a sesame seed.
- Assess for secondary symptoms, such as inflammation, pustules, and bacterial infection.

Diagnostics

Based upon physical assessment

Nursing Interventions

- Treatment includes antiparasitic/pediculicide shampoo, including pyrethrins and enzymatic lice egg remover, according to medication label instructions.
- Use permethrin shampoo first; apply to dry hair and scalp, leave in hair for 10 minutes and rinse with cool water, towel dry, remove nits with fine tooth comb. Repeat in 7 to 10 days.
- Use of permethrin cream rinse, shampoos, and conditioners only after shampoo product use first. Cream rinse can be applied after shampooing leave in hair for 10 minutes, rinse, towel dry, remove nits with fine tooth comb. Repeat in 7 to 10 days.
- Instruct strict adherence to product instructions and time specified time, due to nature of risk of harms related to pesticide usage with children.
- Keep product out of eyes, mouth, and mucous membranes.
- Teach child to avoid sharing hats, hair combs, clothing.
- Teach proper care of cleaning fine tooth combs and tweezers with isopropyl alcohol.
- Ensure proper removal of all nits from hair shaft, requires manually removing and pulling down from hair shaft with fine tooth comb, fingernails, tweezers. Inform parents that process of removal is time consuming and repeat removal. Parents should be instructed to assess hair every 2 to 3 days to remove additional nits.
- Encourage transparency on parental notification of those whom the child has had contact within schools and day cares.

Special Considerations

- Daily laundering of bedding and clothing with detergent and hot water. Do not hang dry clothes; dry clothes in hot dryer.
- Instructions for parents/caregivers to store all nonessential bedding, clothing in tightly sealed plastic bags for 2 to 3 weeks.
- Provide emotional support.
- Encourage caregivers to send child to school; do not need to stay home until no nits are found.

Discharge Planning; Patient and Family Education

- Prevention of reinfection.
- Potential of lice resistance to selected products; seek alternative pediculicide treatment when needed.

PRESSURE ULCERS

Description

- Rare in children
- Increased risk for hospitalized and medically fragile children
- Typically occur in sacrum, scapula, occiput, and ears in children

Assessment

- Identify patients at risk, with professional skin risk assessment score evaluations.
- Assess for reddened areas over bony prominence.
- Assess for incontinence and increased moisture to skin.
- Palpate for intact skin and areas that become "boggy."
- Assess nutritional intake.

Diagnostics

Use Braden Q Scale.

Nursing Interventions

- Frequent repositioning, frequent turning at least every 2 hours.
- Use of pillows, rolls, and positioning support devices.
- Reduction of sheer or friction injury, reduction moisture management.
- Use disposable underpads, with frequent cleaning and changing of soiled clothes and under-garments.
- Nutrition consult and management.

Special Considerations

Frequent skin and pressure ulcer risk management assessments scales are recommended for children at risk.

Discharge Planning; Patient and Family Education

- Educate caregivers about condition and interventions; important for children who are immobile; child in wheelchair can experience pressure ulcers.
- Provide resources; may need home care/wound care.
- Encourage adequate nutrition.

SCABIES

Description

- Caused by the microscopic *Sarcoptes scabiei* mite; causes intense pruritus, especially at bedtime.
- Human to human transmission, highly contagious through direct contact and indirect contact. Indirect contact includes sheets, towels, clothing.
- Frequent transmission in same household—treat household; increased transmission in crowded living conditions.
- Pregnant female mites burrow into the epidermis and lays eggs. The eggs hatch in 3 to 4 days and proceed to skin surface, leaving linear threadlike burrows.

Assessment

- Assess skin for rash, burrows, papules, and pustules.
- Assess common locations of lesions, which include axillae, palms, wrists, elbows, inner thighs, and waist. In children less than 2 years old, assess insteps of feet, back of head, neck, face, palms, and soles of feet.
- Appearances similar to ectopic dermatitis.
- Assess secondary infections from scratching and irritation.

Diagnostics

- Physical examination for burrows
- Microscopic examination/skin scrapings
- Assessment of moving mites, fecal debris, eggs, and nits

Nursing Interventions

- Prior to treatment, ensure a warm soap and water bath; ensure skin is cool and dry before treatment.
- Instruct treatment of scabicide as ordered by clinician.
  - Ensure proper use of prescribed scabicide over entire body, except face.
- Instruct the importance of keeping medication on skin for 8 to 48 hours (the recommended time on label); reapply on hands after handwashing.
- Keep socks on hands and feet and carefully avoid ingestion of scabicide with children who suck fingers, thumb, and hands.
- Ensure and instruct use of treatment for all household family members.
- Oral use of antiparasitic product Ivermectin may be prescribed for children greater than 15 kg as a second-line therapy when other treatment interventions are unsuccessful.

Special Considerations

- Daily laundering of bedding and clothing with detergent and hot water. Do not hang dry clothes, dry clothes in hot dryer.
- Instructions for parents to store all nonessential bedding, clothing, toys in tightly sealed plastic bags for 2 to 3 weeks.
- Provide emotional support.

Discharge Planning; Patient and Family Education

- Prevention of reoccurrence.
- Instruct risk of secondary infections.

STEVENS–JOHNSON SYNDROME (ERYTHEMA MULTIFORME MAJOR)/TOXIC EPIDERMAL NECROLYSIS

Description—Features

- A transient hypersensitivity reaction affecting the skin and mucous membranes; appearance of rash, eruptions; the term "multiforme" refers to the many forms/shapes/appearances of the rash; toxic epidermal necrolysis used to be considered a separate condition but now it is referred to as the most severe form of the condition, which is composed of a disease spectrum.
  - Dermatologic emergency as it can be life-threatening; etiology unknown; but increased risk associated with sulfonamides and antibiotics; most common infectious organisms (entero- and/or adenoviruses, *Mycoplasma pneumonia*); and possibly food reactions.
  - Skin tissue dies and detaches.
  - Can progress to other body systems.

Assessment

- Obtain history about prodromal symptoms of previous illness: high fever, flu-like symptoms.
- Within 1 to 3 days after start of illness, assess for burning, itching, fever, sore throat, headache, and fatigue.
- Assess for painful oral lesions; ulcers may appear on mouth, lips, conjunctiva, and genital areas.
- Assess for rash, ring pattern, or bulls-eye pattern; characterized by widespread erythema rash throughout the body and then followed by macule formation, blistering, and epidermal detachment from the dermis, sloughing and progressive erosion of skin and mucous membranes (multimorphology rash—"multiforme").

Diagnostics

- Comprehensive history related to use of medications that increase patient risk and physical assessment; chest x-ray to rule out infectious organism discussed previously
- Cytology studies; CBC
- May need skin biopsy

Nursing Interventions

- Immediately discontinue medications and/or food, if cause.

PEDIATRIC PEARLS

- If *Mycoplasma pneumonia* is determined to be the cause of erythema multiforme major, be sure to administer the medication to treat infection/organism; do not stop it.

- Refer to dermatology; interprofessional team will determine severity and plan of care for hospitalization in ICU, burn unit, or dermatology unit.
- Provide standard treatment used for burns.
- Monitor hydration status and hemodynamic stability; administer IV fluids; encourage oral hydration.
- Aseptic technique with all care/wound care; prevent sepsis and monitor for secondary infections.
- Administer pain medication.
- Administer antihistamine for pruritus.
- Refer to an ophthalmologist if eyes involved to prevent permanent damage; may need to perform saline rinses, apply lubrication/artificial tears/antibiotic drops.
- Monitor for mouth ulcers; frequent mouth care, decrease pain using oral anesthetics or mouth rinses/wash.
- Monitor nutritional status.

Special Considerations

Thermoregulation—maintaining normal temperature

Discharge Planning; Patient and Family Education

- Offer supportive emotional care and emphasize that condition does resolve on its own within days—weeks; offer psychological support and referrals as needed.
- Educate caregiver on condition, wound care, pain management, and supportive care such as with mouth care; instruct to call clinician if secondary infections noted.
- Encourage oral hydration and educate on the importance of adequate nutrition.

WOUNDS

Description of Injuries

- Three phases of overlapping wound healing phases:
  - 1. **Inflammatory phase:** Lasting 3 to 5 days
    - Characterized by acute inflammatory response
  - 2. **Proliferative Phase:** Lasting 4 days to 2 weeks
    - Characterized by natural debridement and removal of necrotic tissue
    - Reconstruction and epithelialization, through restoration of *structural* integrity
  - 3. **Remodeling (maturation):** Lasting months to 2 years
    - Characterized by remodeling and restoration of *functional* integrity through regeneration and maturation of cells

Assessment

- Healing by intention
  - Primary intention
    - Wounds that heal with minimal tissue loss.
    - Wound edges are connected, closed, and healing with minimal epithelization.
  - Secondary intention
    - Wounds that are open, large, and craterlike, which heal from the bottom up and heals slowly. Wounds that heal via secondary intention are at increased risk for infection and scarring from replacement of connective tissue
  - Complications of healing
    - Infection, poor perfusion, ulceration, dehiscence, keloids, adhesions, chronic inflammation
    - Dysfunctional wound repair associated with poor nutrition, hypoxemia, hypovolemia, hemorrhage, chronic conditions, and corticosteroid use

Diagnostics

- Main diagnostic techniques are inspection of individual lesion; patient and family history.
- **Dermatoscopy:** Examination of skin with the use of a lighted instrument with magnification.
- **Biopsy:** Most common diagnostic test for evaluating skin lesion.
- Stains and cultures to assess and determine fungal, viral, bacterial infections.

Nursing Interventions

- Comprehensive history and physical assessment.
- Accurate documentation of wound location, size, shape, color, and assessment findings, such as drainage, redness, cellulitis, loss of function, and deformity.
  - Monitor healing process.
- Wound care as ordered; may include gently washing injury site with warm antibacterial soap and water, high pressure wound irrigation with normal saline or lactated ringers solution to all open wounds, or cool/warm compresses to affected areas (depending on type and clinician orders); may need topical antibiotic ointment to prevent further infection or skin barrier ointments.

- Careful review of immunization record, ensuring current tetanus shot records or need for required tetanus booster shot depending on cause of wound, such as an animal bite.
  - Administer pain medication as needed.
- Provide emotional support.

Special Considerations

- Refer to "Pressure Ulcer" section in this chapter.

Discharge Planning; Patient and Family Education

- Educate child and caregivers on wound care.
- Provide resources for wound care supplies.
- Refer to wound care specialist and home care as needed.

BIBLIOGRAPHY

American Burn Association. (2018). *Advanced burn life support course: Provider manual 2018 update*. American Burn Association.

Braun, C., & Anderson, C. (2017). *Applied pathophysiology: A conceptual approach to the mechanisms of disease* (3rd ed.). Wolters Kluwer.

Genetic and Rare Diseases Information Center (GARD). (2018, October). *Stevens-Johnson syndrome/toxic epidermal necrolysis*. U.S. Department of Health and Human Services, National Institute of Health. https://rarediseases.info.nih.gov/diseases/7700/stevens-johnson-syndrometoxic-epidermal-necrolysis

Hockenberry, M., Wilson, D., & Rodgers, C. (2017). *Wong's essentials of pediatric nursing* (10th ed.). Evolve Elsevier.

Meadows, O. (2019). *Pediatric nursing made incredibly easy* (3rd ed.). Wolters Kluwer.

Ricci, S., Kyle, T., & Carmen, S. (2021). *Maternity and pediatric nursing* (4th ed.). Wolters Kluwer.

KNOWLEDGE CHECK

1. Which layer of the skin helps to regulate temperature and blood pressure?

   A. Epidermis
   B. Dermis
   C. Subcutaneous
   D. Hypodermis

2. A nurse is caring for an infant, diagnosed with contact dermatitis to the diaper area. Which action should the nurse include in the plan of care?

   A. Avoid using name brand absorbent diapers
   B. Change the diaper immediately after urination and bowel movement
   C. Administer antifungal medication
   D. Remove all crusted lesions with sterile gloves

3. What is the most common cause of cellulitis?

   A. Lymphangitis
   B. *Pseudomonas* folliculitis
   C. *Staphylococcus aureus*
   D. *Minutissimum* bacteria

4. A nurse is caring for a child in the emergency department 3 days after being scratched by the family cat. The nurse suspects localized cellulitis after assessing which of the following findings?

   A. Warmth, redness, and pain
   B. Swelling, fever, and redness
   C. Fever and elevated white blood cell count
   D. Positive blood cultures and lymph node enlargement

5. A 5-year-old patient is diagnosed with severe impetigo. The nurse is informed during report that the child has papules, erosion, and honey-colored crust formation on the right ear. How should the nurse most accurately describe the papule?

   A. Circumscribed, elevated lesion that is filled with purulent fluid, and is less than 1 cm in size.
   B. Circumscribed, elevated, plateau like, solid lesion that is greater than 1 cm in size.
   C. Raised circumscribed lesions that is intact and filled with clear liquid fluid that is 1 cm or less in size.
   D. Circumscribed, elevated solid lesion that is accentuated with oblique lighting, and is 1 cm or less in size.

6. A 3-month-old infant is being breast fed. The primary care clinician notices white patches in the oral mucosa. What is the priority nursing education for the mother?

   A. Instruct hand hygiene with only alcohol-based products
   B. Rinse all pacifiers and bottles with warm water
   C. Instruct use of oral nystatin and application of nystatin to nipples
   D. Instruct family members to not share towels and bedding sheets

KNOWLEDGE CHECK

1. **Correct Answer: B) Dermis.** The dermis is richly supplied by arteriovenous circulation and capillaries that connect the arteries and veins that assist in oxygenation, temperature regulation, and blood pressure. The arterial capillary blood supply provides oxygenation, nutrients to cells, regulating blood flow through dilation and constriction. Blood vessels that dilate allow for heat evaporation, and blood vessels that constrict allow for the preservation of heat in response to environmental temperatures.

2. **Correct Answer: B) Change the diaper immediately after urination and bowel movement.** Nursing management of contact dermatitis located in the diaper area includes removal of irritant, urine, and stool as soon as possible. Urine and bowel movements increase risk for irritation, redness of skin, and skin breakdown caused by increased pH and ammonia. The use of absorbent diapers is recommended. Antifungal medications are prescribed for fungal infections and crusted lesions occur with impetigo.

3. **Correct Answer: C) *Staphylococcus aureus*.** The most common cause of cellulitis is *Streptococcus* bacteria or *Staphylococcus aureus* bacteria. Cellulitis is caused by bacteria entering the skin, releasing bacterial toxins that cause inflammation of the subcutaneous tissue.

4. **Correct Answer: A) Warmth, redness, and pain.** Acute localized cellulitis is characterized by swelling, warmth, redness, and pain. Systemic manifestations of cellulitis include fever, chills, lymph node enlargement. Bacterial infections caused by cellulitis include positive blood cultures and elevated white blood cell count.

5. **Correct Answer: D) Circumscribed, elevated solid lesion that is accentuated with oblique lighting, and is 1 cm or less in size.** Pustules are circumscribed, elevated lesions, filled with purulent fluid filled lesions, that are less than 1 cm in size. Macular lesions are flat, color changes occur in circumscribed areas and are up to 1 cm in size. Vesicular rashes are raised circumscribed lesions with intact filled clear fluid, up to 1cm in size. Plaque lesions are circumscribed, elevated, plateau like, solid lesions, that are greater than 1 cm in size.

6. **Correct Answer: C) Instruct use of oral nystatin and application of nystatin to nipples.** Mothers who are breastfeeding will need to treat the baby and self with nystatin as ordered; additionally, good hand and body hygiene that utilizes soap, water, and friction is required to decrease the transmission of the fungal infection. Pacifiers and bottles must be properly sterilized. Separating towels and bedding is not required for oral candidiasis.

7. A patient is discharged from outpatient surgery after sustaining an open leg wound during an automobile accident. Postoperatively, the wound edges are sutured closed. The nurse determines that this type of wound healing is identified as:

    A. Primary intention
    B. Inflammatory phase
    C. Secondary intention
    D. Remodeling phase

8. A child is diagnosed with moderate acne. What is the best description of this type of acne?

    A. Nodular and cystic in nature, commonly found on face, chest, and back
    B. Numerous inflammatory papules, comedones, found on face, chest, and back
    C. Inflamed papules, pustules, and comedones, with mild symptoms
    D. Noninflammatory lesions found on face and back

9. A nurse is caring for a child with a deep partial thickness burn. The child reports severe pain. What is the nurse's best action?

    A. Administer IV morphine sulfate
    B. Administer meperidine intramuscular (IM) route
    C. Keep the child close to the nurses' station to continuously evaluate
    D. Speak to the social worker for a psychiatric evaluation

10. A child is admitted to the emergency department after a house fire and is assessed to have greater than 40% TBSA of burns. The child has difficulty swallowing and speaks with a hoarse sound in their throat. What is the nurse's priority of care?

    A. Maintain strict aseptic technique with all wound care
    B. Assess airway, provide supplemental oxygen, and secure the airway
    C. Administer hypotonic saline solution immediately
    D. Obtain BMP to assess electrolyte levels

KNOWLEDGE CHECK

7. **Correct Answer: A) Primary intention.** Wounds that heal by primary intention include surgical wounds, wounds that heal with minimal tissue loss, and wound edges are connected, closed, and healing with minimal epithelization. The inflammatory phase of wound healing is characterized by acute inflammatory response; wounds that heal by secondary intention are open large and craterlike, and they heal slowly from the bottom up; remodeling is characterized by restoration of functional integrity after the regeneration during the last phase of wound healing.

8. **Correct Answer: C) Inflamed papules, pustules, and comedones, with mild symptoms.** Inflamed papules, pustules, and comedones that are associated with mild symptoms include the correct elements of moderate acne. Severe acne is described as nodular and cystic in nature, commonly found on face, chest, and back. Moderately severe acne is associated with numerous inflammatory papules, comedones, commonly found on face, chest, and back. Mild acne is noninflammatory.

9. **Correct Answer: A) Administer IV morphine sulfate.** Burn pain is associated with severe levels of pain due to the association of nerve damage and exposure of nerve endings after severe heat associated with dermatologic damage, associated with traumatic burn injury. Pharmacologic treatment is necessary to adequately treat the pain associated with burns. All opioids should be administered via the IV route to avoid delayed absorption of medication associated with IM injections. The IM injection route is contraindicated. Close observation of the child will not adequately address the child's pain needs, nor will providing social service interventions to initiate a psychological evaluation to properly manage the child's report of pain.

10. **Correct Answer: B) Assess airway, provide supplemental oxygen, and secure the airway.** Difficulty swallowing, difficulty speaking with associated assessment of speech attempts that are "hoarse" are associated with acute upper airway inflammation and risk for airway obstruction. Maintaining strict aseptic technique with all wound care is an essential component of burn care; however, airway is the current priority in this case scenario. Patients with burns are treated with isotonic fluid resuscitation, not hypotonic solutions. Obtaining essential lab studies is important in the care of patients with burns; however, the immediate management of the patient's airway takes priority in the analysis.

CHAPTER 14

Infectious Diseases and Immunizations

Jessica L. Peck and Mary Koslap-Petraco

INTRODUCTION

An important component to infectious diseases is the chain of infection. Chain of infection is a term used to illustrate the circle of links needed for transmission of infectious diseases in humans. This chapter will explore those common communicable diseases that can affect children.

- Although great advances have been made in public health, communicable disease is the leading cause of illness in infants and children.
- The role of the nurse is to promote prevention through immunization and hygiene measures such as handwashing, to prevent the spread of disease, to offer symptomatic comfort care, and to identify early signs of potential complications.

FEVER OF UNKNOWN ORIGIN

Description

- Fever is the body's response to assist the immune system in destroying foreign antigens.
- Temperature >101°F (38°C) on several occasions for >3 weeks and failure to reach a diagnosis after 1 week of intense evaluation and testing.

Assessment

- Assess for immunization status, family pets, and past medical history.
- Assess hydration status.
- Assess for general state of contentment or discontentment with activity versus lethargy.

Diagnostics

Work-up may be limited or extensive depending on length and severity of symptoms. Studies may include complete blood count (CBC); inflammatory markers (erythrocyte sedimentation rate [ESR], C-reactive protein [CRP]); blood culture; urinalysis; tuberculosis (TB) skin test; chest x-ray; head CT; and echocardiogram.

Nursing Interventions

Support adequate hydration and nutrition, as fever accelerates fluid losses.

PEDIATRIC PEARLS

Fever Reduction Measures	
Antipyretics	Ibuprofen, acetaminophen Give 1 hour prior to implementing cooling measures to lower set point
Environmental Cooling Measures	Apply cool, moist compresses to the skin; remove extra layers of clothing; cover with a light sheet or blanket only; encourage hydration efforts
Not Recommended	Aspirin is not recommended because of association between use in children with influenza or varicella with Reye's syndrome; avoid ice or fans that cause compensatory shivering; sponging or tepid baths are ineffective and uncomfortable and should be avoided
When to Seek Care for Fever or Alert Clinician	<2 months of age, T > 105°F, lethargic or sick-looking, rash, trouble breathing, inconsolable, fever > 24 hours with no other symptoms, pain with urination

Special Considerations

- Digital thermometers are quickest and most accurate.
  - Rectal is the most accurate method for <3 years but not always the best choice depending on development and diagnosis. For rectal temps, insert approximately ½ to 1 inch into the anal opening with a lubricated tip.
  - Oral is best for kids 4 to 5 years. For oral temperatures, wait 20 to 30 minutes after eating or drinking and place it under the tongue.
  - Axillary is not accurate but acceptable as a first screen if no other options.
  - Less preferable are temporal artery thermometers measure heat waves on the forehead in infants >3 months.
  - Tympanic thermometers measure heat waves from the eardrum in infants >6 months.
  - Plastic strip, pacifier, glass mercury, and smartphone temperature app thermometers are not recommended.

Discharge Planning; Patient and Family Education

Fever is one of the most common reasons for parental anxiety; reassurance and education should be given on when to seek care.

INFECTIOUS DISEASES THAT ARE NOT VACCINE-PREVENTABLE

Table 14.1 lists the infectious diseases for which there is no vaccine.

TABLE 14.1: Infectious Diseases That Are Not Vaccine-Preventable

Bacterial illnesses	Group A beta-hemolytic *Streptococci* Group B beta-hemolytic *Streptococci*
Parasitic illnesses	*Cryptosporidium* *Giardia* Parasitic worms
Vector-borne illness	Lyme disease Zika
Viral illnesses	Coxsackie virus Erythema infectiosum Roseola infantum Infectious mononucleosis

GROUP A BETA-HEMOLYTIC *STREPTOCOCCI* AND GROUP B *STREPTOCOCCUS*

Description

- Group A beta-hemolytic *Streptococci* (GABHS) is a form of pharyngitis more commonly known as strep throat.
  - Untreated, it causes risk for rheumatic fever, an inflammatory illness affecting the heart, joints, and central nervous system.
- Group B *Streptococcus* (GBS) is a naturally occurring bacterium many people carry asymptomatically in the gastrointestinal (GI) and genitourinary (GU) tracts but can be harmful to neonates. It can cause neonatal pneumonia, sepsis, and meningitis.

Assessment

- **GABHS**
  - Assess for fever, tender/swollen anterior cervical lymph nodes, and exudate or inflammation of the tonsils.
  - Small children may complain of abdominal pain.
- **GBS**
  - Assess for risk factors of early-onset disease including preterm birth, rupture of membranes >18 hours, maternal fever, previous maternal history of GBS.
  - Early-onset symptoms manifest in the first 24 hours, with late-onset between 1 week and 3 months.

Diagnostics

- **GABHS**
  - 80% to 90% of pharyngitis cases are viral, but because of potential long-term sequelae, GABHS is commonly screened with a rapid test using a throat swab, with a follow-up confirmatory culture recommended for negative rapid screens.
- **GBS**
  - Pregnant women are generally screened with a vaginal and/or rectal swab at 36 to 38 weeks of pregnancy, with prophylactic antibiotic treatment for women who screen GBS+.

Nursing Interventions

- **GABHS**
  - Provide symptomatic care including rest, cool fluids, warm saltwater gargles, and antipyretics.
  - Provide a new toothbrush after 24 hours of antibiotics; discard the old toothbrush.
  - Provide liquids, such as water, Pedialyte®, apple juice, or popsicles.
    - Give small amounts of liquid often.
  - Provide soft foods that are easy to swallow, such as applesauce, mashed potatoes, hot cereal, or eggs.
  - To soothe a sore throat offer:
    - For children over age 1, warm fluids such as chicken broth or apple juice.
    - For children over age 4, throat or cough lozenges or throat sprays.
      - Do not use throat sprays that contain benzocaine, as this could cause a drug reaction.

- For children over age 6 who are able to gargle without swallowing, a mixture of ½ teaspoon of table salt in 8 ounces of warm water. Swish and gargle the mixture 2 to 3 times a day for the next few days.
  - Avoid swallowing the salt water; have them spit it out.
- Completion of a prescribed 7- to 14-day course of antibiotics is essential.
- **GBS**
  - Treatment is in the neonatal intensive care because of high morbidity and mortality.

Special Considerations

- GABHS can also cause acute otitis media and pneumonia, skin and soft-tissue infections, sepsis, and meningitis.
- Invasive forms of GABHS can cause necrotizing fasciitis.

Discharge Planning; Patient and Family Education

- **GABHS:** Emphasize completion of all prescribed antibiotics.
- **GBS:** Families need holistic support during hospitalization and long-term care. Late-onset GBS = 5% mortality. 50% of survivors develop permanent neurologic damage.

METHICILLIN-RESISTANT *STAPHYLOCOCCUS AUREUS*

Description

- Methicillin-resistant *Staphylococcus aureus* (MRSA) is a bacterial infection commonly occurring in the skin. Previously seen primarily in nursing homes, the rise of community-acquired infections in children is steep.
- MRSA is staph that can't be killed with common staph antibiotics, such as cephalexin.
- MRSA is usually limited to the skin.
  - It can be life-threatening if it spreads to the lungs, the bloodstream, or other organs.

Assessment

- Assess for a bump (papule) that is painful, red, leaking fluid, or swollen.
- Assess for bumps under the skin that are swollen or firm, skin around the sore that is warm or hot.
- Rash or fluid-filled blisters (vesicles).
- Bump that gets bigger quickly or doesn't heal.
- Painful sore along with a fever, chills, headache, sleepiness, dizziness, or fainting.
- Assess for signs of spreading or worsening infection.

Diagnostics

- A skin swab, to check for MRSA.
- Cultures of samples of blood, spit, or fluid from a sore to check for MRSA.
- X-ray of the lungs, to see if the lungs may be infected.
- Echocardiogram of the heart, to see if the heart may be infected.
- CT scan or MRI, to see if any other tissue, bones, or joints are infected.
- The infected site can be cultured for confirmation of MRSA with antibiotic sensitivities.

Nursing Interventions

- Emphasis is on preventing spread of infection and complications.
- Handwashing is mandatory for patient care and ordered isolation precautions should be strictly adhered to.

- Family members should not share washcloths or towels.
- Clothing should be changed daily.
- Disposable razors should be discarded after each use.

Special Considerations

- Some strains are resistant to all oral antibiotics and require hospitalization or home care for intravenous (IV) antibiotic therapy. Systemic infections or localized abscesses can occur.
- Some children (especially those with atopic dermatitis or eczema) can be colonized with MRSA under fingernails and in nares. Daily use of topical antibiotics may be prescribed.

Discharge Planning; Patient and Family Education

Emphasize hygiene practices noted previously. Some specialists recommend a chlorine bath twice weekly with one tsp of chlorine per gallon of water.

MYCOBACTERIUM TUBERCULOSIS

Description

Globally, TB is the leading cause of death from a single infectious disease agent, and about ¼ of cases in the United States are children > 14 years. Risk factors include HIV infection, malnutrition, and exposure to unpasteurized milk. Children are usually infected by a household contact. Primary lesions extend and cause progressive tissue destruction.

Assessment

- Assess for high-risk exposures—children with weakened immune systems.
- Assess for a child with close contacts of a person with infectious TB disease.
- Assess children from families who have immigrated from areas of the world with high rates of TB.
- Assess for groups with high rates of TB transmission, such as homeless youth, injection drug users, and persons with HIV infection.
- **Assess for symptoms:** fever, fatigue, anorexia, weight loss, persistent cough, chest pain or tightness, hemoptysis (rare), respiratory distress.

Diagnostics

- The tuberculin skin test administers a dose of purified protein derivative intradermally on the forearm.
- Tuberculin skin testing (TST) is considered safe in children and is preferred over TB blood tests for children less than 5 years of age.
  - Skin reactions are assessed within 48 to 72 hours.
  - The size of the induration is measured, not the erythema.
  - ≥5 mm induration is positive if:
    - Immunocompromised (including HIV infection)
    - Contact to an active TB case
    - Radiographic or clinical evidence of active TB disease
  - ≥10 mm induration is positive if:
    - Child younger than 4 years old
    - Medical conditions (lymphoma, Hodgkin disease, diabetes mellitus, chronic renal failure, or malnutrition)

- Child or parent from high-prevalence countries
- Frequent exposure to high-risk adults (HIV infected, users of illicit drugs, homeless)
  - ≥15 mm induration if positive if:
    - Child ≥ 4 years of age without risk factors
  - TST is not recommended for children, but screening for risk factors facilitates targeted testing.

Nursing Interventions

- For active TB, hospitalization with airborne precautions and a negative pressure room is required, along with the use of an N-95 or N-100 mask for all patient contacts.
- Sputum specimens may need to be collected after aerosolized normal saline for 10 to 15 minutes followed by CPT and suctioning or lavage of the nasopharynx.
- Asymptomatic children may be able to go to school and be in the community.

Special Considerations

Most children recover from a primary TB infection, but younger and immunocompromised children are at risk for disseminated disease.

Discharge Planning; Patient and Family Education

- Emphasize adherence to long-term pharmacotherapy, which can last 6 to 12 months.
- Emphasize the importance of preventive care and immunizations.

PARASITIC ILLNESS (*SALMONELLA, GIARDIA LAMBLIA, ENTEROBIASIS*)

Description

- ***Salmonella:*** Bacteria passed from person-to-person, undercooked meats and poultry, and pets. Diarrhea may persist 2 to 3 weeks while shedding virus 5 weeks to 1 year.
- ***Giardia lamblia:*** Protozoan passed from person-to-person or in contaminated water. Nonmotile stage can last for months on surfaces, making day-care centers at high risk.
- **Enterobiasis:** Commonly known as pinworm infection, infection begins with inhalation or ingestion of *Enterobius vermicularis* eggs which migrate through the intestine and hatch on the rectal mucosa.

Assessment

- ***Salmonella:***
  - Assess for nausea, vomiting, bloody diarrhea, fever.
    - May lead to meningitis or sepsis
- ***Giardia lamblia:***
  - Assess for diarrhea, vomiting, anorexia; malodorous, pale, watery, greasy stools.
- **Enterobiasis:** Often nocturnal rectal itching is the only symptom.

Diagnostics

- ***Salmonella:*** Stool cultures, stool leukocytes and occult blood, CBC
- ***Giardia lamblia:*** Stool specimens for trophozoites or cysts
- **Enterobiasis:** Worms visualized at the anus, microscopic examination with tape test

Nursing Interventions

- **Salmonella:** Watch for early signs of meningitis or sepsis, deteriorating status.
- **Giardia lamblia:** Carefully monitor hydration status, contact the local health department for reportable illness; may resolve without treatment or require pharmacotherapy.
- **Enterobiasis:** Morning baths, clip nails, avoid scratching and nail-biting, hand hygiene.

Special Considerations

- **Salmonella:** Antibiotics are only considered for infants <3 months, or those with preexisting immunosuppressive illness or prescribed therapies.
- **Giardia lamblia:** Complications can cause malabsorption, anorexia, weight loss, and FTT.
- **Enterobiasis:** Recurrence is common, but subsequent infections are treated the same.

Discharge Planning; Patient and Family Education

- **Salmonella:** Nausea, vomiting, bloody diarrhea, fever. May lead to meningitis or sepsis.
- **Giardia lamblia:** Avoid swimming until 2 weeks after symptoms resolve.
- **Enterobiasis:** Ensure prescribed medication is taken; 1 dose at diagnosis with a repeat dose in 2 weeks. Educate family members and school setting about transmission.

VECTOR-BORNE ILLNESS (LYME DISEASE AND ZIKA)

Description

- Lyme disease is the most common tick-borne disorder in the United States, with most cases reported in the Northeast.
  - It occurs in three stages: (a) tick bite followed in 3 to 31 days by *erythema migrans* at the bite site; (b) systemic neurologic, cardiac, and musculoskeletal involvement; (3) late-stage chronic musculoskeletal pain and arthritis with possible deafness and encephalopathy.
- Zika is a mosquito-borne flavivirus identified in Brazil in 2015. For most adults, the virus is self-limiting but can have devastating neonatal impacts including microcephaly, intrauterine growth restriction, subcortical brain calcifications.

Assessment

- Assess for exposure to ticks, and manifestation of symptoms listed in stages.
  - Ring-shaped rash that looks like a bull's-eye. It may be pink in the center and have a darker red ring around it. The rash does not occur in every case of Lyme.
  - **Several days or weeks after a bite from an infected tick:** Headache, stiff neck, aches and pains in muscles and joints, low fever and chills, tiredness, loss of appetite, swollen glands.
  - **Weeks to months after the bite:** Nervous system symptoms, such as inflammation of the nervous system (meningitis) and weakness and paralysis of the facial muscles (Bell palsy); heart problems, such as inflammation and heart block; inflammation of the eyes.
  - **Months to a few years after a bite:** Inflammation of the joints (arthritis), nervous system symptoms such as numbness in the arms and legs, tingling and pain, and trouble with speech, memory, and concentration.
- Assess for fever, headache, arthralgia, and maculopapular rash.
  - Screen for risk of exposure or travel for pregnant women in areas with high rates of Zika transmission.

Diagnostics

- Lyme disease is best diagnosed by early rash recognition and later, serologic testing.
- Diagnostic tests can detect Zika viral RNA in the first 14 days. A + antibody test may indicate past infection of another flavivirus like dengue. Fetal ultrasounds are indicated.

Nursing Interventions

- Prevention is most important. Avoid tick-infested areas, wear light-colored clothing to spot ticks easily, perform regular full body assessment for ticks, use insect repellent containing 30% or less diethyltoluamide (DEET) for children >2 years.
  - Apply sparingly and avoid the face. Wash treated skin with soap and water when indoors.

Special Considerations

Other vector-borne illnesses include malaria, yellow fever, chikungunya fever, West Nile virus, Japanese encephalitis, and Chagas. Most of these are preventable.

Discharge Planning; Patient and Family Education

Families will likely need long-term support to manage complex chronic illnesses.

VIRAL EXANTHEMS (TABLE 14.2)

Description

Viral exanthems are skin eruptions related to a viral infection. These are quite common in pediatrics, and most will resolve spontaneously with only supportive care.

TABLE 14.2: Viral Exanthems

Virus	Transmission	Incubation	Communicability	Rash description
Coxsackie virus	Respiratory droplets; Oral/Fecal	1–5 days Usually 2	At first symptoms until rash resolves	Macular, maculopapular, or vesicular rash on the hands, feet, and mouth
Erythema infectiosum (fifth disease or parvovirus)	Respiratory secretions and maternal/fetal transmission	4–20 days	1 week prior to rash eruption	"Slapped cheek syndrome" with lacy rash on extremities
Infectious mononucleosis	Direct contact	4–6 weeks	Unknown	Generalized maculopapular, quite common with ampicillin administration
Roseola infantum (human herpesvirus 6 and 7)	Respiratory droplets and saliva	5–15 days	Until 24–48 hours after fever resolution	Generalized maculopapular rash appears within 24 hours of resolution of fever

Assessment

- Assess hydration status, especially with febrile illnesses.
  - Coxsackie virus causes blisters in the mouth, which are painful and can cause decreased oral intake.

Diagnostics

Most of these exanthems are identified based on clinical presentation of specific rash characteristics. A rapid test with peripheral blood collection can detect mononucleosis.

Nursing Interventions

- No special care is needed for rash presentations other than general good hygiene.
- Children with mono may have splenomegaly and need activity restriction until resolved.

Special Considerations

If a child with erythema infectiosum has exposure to an expectant mother, they should be advised to consult their obstetric clinician. Rarely, fetal exposure (especially in the first trimester) in a nonimmune mother can result in fetal demise and miscarriage.

Discharge Planning; Patient and Family Education

- Emphasize adherence to long-term pharmacotherapy, which can last 6 to 12 months.
- Emphasize importance of preventive care and immunizations.

INTRODUCTION TO IMMUNITY AND IMMUNIZATIONS

- **Immunity** is the ability of the human body to tolerate the presence of material indigenous to the body and to eliminate foreign substances.
- The discriminatory ability to eliminate foreign substances is performed by a complex system of interacting cells called the *immune system*.
- The immune system develops a defense against **antigens**, which are substances that can stimulate the immune system. This defense is known as the *immune response*.
  - **Passive immunity** is protection by antibody or antitoxin produced by one animal or human and transferred to another. Passive immunity provides immediate protection against infection, but that protection is temporary.
  - **Active immunity** is protection produced by a person's own immune system. The immune system is stimulated by an antigen to produce antibody and cellular immunity. Unlike passive immunity, which is temporary, active immunity usually lasts for many years, often for a lifetime.
- The persistence of protection for many years after the infection is known as *immunologic memory*.
  - **Live attenuated vaccines** are derived from "wild" viruses or bacteria. These wild viruses or bacteria are attenuated (weakened) in a laboratory, usually by repeated culturing.
  - **Inactivated vaccines** are not live and cannot replicate.
  - A **polysaccharide vaccine** is a unique type of inactivated subunit vaccine composed of long chains of sugar molecules that make up the surface capsule of certain bacteria. These vaccines are not consistently immunogenic in children younger than 2 years of age, probably because of immaturity of the immune system.
  - **Recombinant** vaccine antigens are produced by genetic engineering technology.

VIRAL DISEASES AND VACCINES FOR PREVENTION

BACTERIAL DISEASES VACCINES

Diphtheria Tetanus Pertussis containing vaccines (Inactive):
- Diphtheria-Tetanus-Pertussis (Acellular; DTaP)
- Tetanus-diphtheria-acellular pertussis (Tdap)
- Tetanus-diphtheria (Td)
- Tetanus toxoid (TT)

Vaccine Schedule DTaP

- Three-dose primary series at age 2, 4, and 6 months.
- Primary series interval of 4 to 8 weeks and minimum interval 4 weeks.
- Boosters at age 15 through 18 months and age 4 through 6 years.
- Minimum interval for dose 4 is 6 months from dose three, and minimum age is 12 months.
- If dose four is given on or after 4th birthday, the fifth dose is optional.
- DT is used in place of DTaP if child has a valid contraindication to pertussis vaccine.

Vaccine Schedule Diphtheria Toxoid-Containing Vaccine

Tdap
- One dose at age 11 through 18 for adolescents who have completed DTaP series
- Booster dose of Td or Tdap every 10 years for all persons
- One dose for every pregnancy preferably in third trimester

Td
- Three doses of tetanus- and diphtheria-containing vaccine (one dose should be Tdap) for adolescents and adults without previous history of primary series

Special Considerations (Nursing Interventions)

- Screening for contraindications/precautions prior to DTaP, Tdap, Td, DT, TT
- **Contraindications**
  - Severe allergic reaction to vaccine component or following a prior dose
  - Encephalopathy not attributable to another identifiable cause within 7 days after vaccination*
- **Precautions**
  - Moderate or severe acute illness
  - Progressive or unstable neurologic disorder*
  - Uncontrolled seizures*
  - Progressive encephalopathy*
  - Guillain–Barré syndrome (GBS) within 6 weeks after a previous dose of tetanus-toxoid containing vaccine**
  - History of Arthus-type hypersensitivity reactions after a previous dose of diphtheria toxoid- or tetanus toxoid-containing vaccine**

---

* DTaP and Tdap

Vaccine Schedule *Haemophilus influenzae* (PRP-T, PRP-OMP; Inactive; Table 14.3)

- Immunization Action Coalition has an excellent *Screening Checklist for Contraindications for Children and Teens*: www.immunize.org/catg.d/p4060.pdf
- Parent/caregiver must be provided with Vaccine Information Statement for specific vaccines administered according to federal regulations: www.immunize.org/vis/

TABLE 14.3: Vaccine Schedule *Haemophilus influenzae* (PRP-T, PRP-OMP; Inactive)

Vaccine type	Vaccine trade name	2 months	4 months	6 months	12–15 months
PRP-T	ActHIB	Dose 1	Dose 2	Dose 3	Booster
	Pentacel	Dose 1	Dose 2	Dose 3	Booster*
	Hibrix	Dose 1	Dose 2	Dose 3	Booster+
PRP-OMP	PedvaxHIB	Dose 1	Dose 2	--	Booster
	Vaxelis	Dose 1	Dose 2	Dose 3~	Not indicated

Note: *The recommended age for dose 4 of DTaP-IPV/Hib (Pentacel) is age 15 through 18 months, but it can be administered as early as 12 months, provided at least 6 months have elapsed since dose 3.
+The recommended age for dose 4 of Hib (PRP-T; Hiberix) is age 15 months, but to facilitate timely booster vaccination, it may be administered as early as age 12 months.
~The recommended minimum age for dose 3 of DTaP-IPV-Hib-HepB (Vaxelis) is 24 weeks, the minimum age for completion of the hepatitis B vaccine series.

MENINGOCOCCAL VACCINES

Vaccine Schedule Meningitis B (MenB-FHbp, MenB-4C)

- **FHbp (Trumenba)**
  - 0, 1, and 6 months—if second dose of Trumenba is administered at an interval of 6 months or more, a third dose is not needed.
- **MenB-4C (Bexsero)**
  - 0 and 1 month or longer

Special Considerations (Nursing Interventions)

- Screening for contraindications/precautions prior to meningitis B vaccine.
- Both meningitis B vaccines can be used for persons 10 years of age or older who are at increased risk of serogroup B meningococcal disease.
- Preferred age is 16 to 18 years of age.
- FHbp and MenB-4C are NOT interchangeable. Must use same vaccine for all doses in series including boosters.

** DTaP , DT , Tdap , Td

Precautions

Latex sensitivity for MenB-4C

Vaccine Schedule Meningococcal (MenACWY-D, MenACWY-CRM; Inactive)

- One dose at age 11 or 12 years.
- Booster dose at age 16 years.
- Healthy persons who receive first dose at or after age 16 years do not need a booster dose unless they become at increased risk for meningococcal disease.

PNEUMOCOCCAL VACCINES (INACTIVE)

Vaccine Schedule Pneumococcal Conjugate (PPSV23)

Children 24 months of age and older with chronic lung disease, heart disease, diabetes, cerebrospinal fluid leak, cochlear implant, functional or anatomic asplenia, including sickle cell disease, or immunocompromising conditions should receive PPSV23 at least 2 months after final dose of PCV13. A second dose of PPSV23 is indicated 5 years after the last dose as long as child remains in high-risk group.

Vaccine Schedule Pneumococcal Polysaccharide (PCV13)

- Three-dose primary series at age 2, 4, and 6 months.
- Booster at age 12 through 15 months.
- Minimum age for dose one is 6 weeks.
- Minimum interval for doses before age 1 year is 4 weeks and age 1 year or older is 8 weeks.
  - Unvaccinated children 7 months or older require fewer doses.

Special Considerations (Nursing Intervention)

- Screening for contraindications/precautions prior to each vaccine administered
- **Contraindications**
  - Severe allergic reaction to vaccine component or following prior dose
- **Precautions**
  - Moderate or severe acute illness

Discharge Planning; Patient and Family Education

- Prevention is of the utmost importance with adequate immunization.
- Review potential serious side effects such as temperature of 105 degrees F; child is very noticeably less active or responsive; crying uncontrollably for more than 3 hours; child's body is shaking, twitching, or jerking; and advise parent to seek medical treatment.
- Provide parent/caregiver with instructions for supportive care following vaccines such as cool compresses to swollen, red, hot injection site; encourage fluids; review clinician's instructions for antipyretics.
- Immunization Action Coalition has an excellent handout for parents, *After The Shots...*: www.immunize.org/catg.d/p4015.pdf

VIRAL DISEASES VACCINES

The Centers for Disease Control and Prevention (CDC), along with the American Academy of Pediatrics and other major medical groups, continues to recommend COVID-19 vaccination for people 5 years and older.

Vaccine Schedule Pfizer-BioNTech COVID-19 Vaccine (Inactive)

- Two shots, 21 days apart
- Minimum age is 5 years
- Indications for COVID-19 vaccination include*:
  - A 2-dose primary series to individuals 5 years of age and older
  - A third primary series dose to individuals 12 years of age and older who have been determined to have certain kinds of immunocompromise
  - A single booster dose to individuals 18 years of age and older who have completed a primary series with Pfizer-BioNTech COVID-19 vaccine or COMIRNATY®
  - A single booster dose to individuals 18 years of age and older who have completed primary vaccination with a different authorized COVID-19 vaccine

Special Considerations (Nursing Interventions)

- Screening for contraindications/precautions prior to Pfizer-BioNTech COVID-19 vaccine.
- Based on the latest evidence, myocarditis appears to be an extremely rare side effect.
- **Contraindications:**
  - Previous immunizations in past 14 days
  - Severe allergic reaction (anaphylaxis) to any ingredient in a messenger RNA (mRNA) COVID-19 vaccine (such as polyethylene glycol)
  - Severe allergic reaction (anaphylaxis) after getting the first dose of the vaccine
- **Precautions:**
  - Immediate allergic reaction to any other vaccine or injectable therapy (e.g., intramuscular, IV, or subcutaneous vaccines or therapies)

Discharge Planning; Patient and Family Education

- Review potential side effects pain, swelling, erythema at the injection site, localized axillary lymphadenopathy (on the same side as the vaccinated arm) and systemic (e.g., fever, fatigue, headache, chills, myalgia, arthralgia).
- Provide parent/caregiver with instructions for supportive care following vaccines such as cool compresses to swollen, red, hot injection site; encourage fluids; review clinician's instructions for antipyretics.

Immunization Schedule Hepatitis A Vaccine (Inactive)

- Two-dose series at age 12 and 18 months.
- Children who are not vaccinated by 2 years of age can be vaccinated at subsequent visits.

Immunization Schedule Hepatitis B Vaccine (Inactive)

- Three-dose series at 0, 1, and 6 months.
- All children and adolescents through age 18 years not previously vaccinated.

Inactivated Polio Vaccine Schedule (Inactive)

- Typically administered at age 2, 4, 6 through 18 months, and 4 through 6 years.
- Do not administer earlier than age 6 weeks.

---

* Subject to change as information becomes available and is released by the CDC.

Special Considerations (Nursing Interventions)

Screen for contraindications and precautions for inactivated polio vaccine (IPV).

Influenza Vaccine Schedule (Inactivated Influenza3 [IIV3], Inactivated Influneza4 [IIV4], and Live Attenuated Influenza Vaccine [LAIV])

- One dose each influenza season for persons age 9 years or older
- One or two doses each influenza season for children age 6 months through 8 years
- One dose if two or more doses are documented prior to July 1
- Two doses administered at least 4 weeks apart if two or more doses are not documented prior to July 1

Special Considerations (Nursing Interventions)

- **Precautions to IIV3, IIV4, LAIV**
  - Moderate or severe acute illness
  - History of GBS within 6 weeks of receipt of influenza vaccine
- **Precautions to LAIV**
  - Receiving aspirin or salicylate-containing medications
  - Age 2 to 4 years with history of asthma or wheezing
  - Immunocompromised due to any cause (including medications and HIV infection)
  - Anatomic or functional asplenia
  - Close contacts or caregivers of severely immunosuppressed persons who require a protected environment
  - Pregnancy
  - Cochlear implant
  - Cerebrospinal fluid-oropharyngeal communication
  - Children less than age 2 years
  - Received influenza antiviral medications oseltamivir or zanamivir within the previous 48 hours, peramivir within the previous 5 days, or baloxavir within the previous 17 days

Human Papilloma (9vHPV) Vaccine Schedule (Inactive)

- Can be started at age 9 years but usual recommendation is age 11 to 12 years
- Catch-up vaccination recommended for all persons not adequately vaccinated through age 26 years
- Before 15 years: a two-dose series with an interval between 6 and 12 months after the initial vaccination
- After age 15: a three-dose series with the second dose given at 1 to 2 months after initial vaccination and then again 6 months following the second vaccination

Special Considerations (Nursing Interventions)

- **Contraindications**
  - Severe allergic reaction to vaccine component or following a prior dose.
  - History of immediate hypersensitivity to yeast.
  - To prevent fainting-related injuries, people receiving HPV vaccines should sit or lie down during vaccination, then patients should be observed for 15 minutes after immunization.
- **Precautions**
  - Moderate or severe acute illness

Measles–Mumps–Rubella Vaccine Schedule (Live Attenuated)

- Two-dose series at age 12 through 15 months and at age 4 through 6 years.
- MMRV (Measles–Mumps–Rubella–Varicella) preferred for dose two and dose one at age 48 months or older.
- Minimum interval from dose one to two is 4 weeks for MMR and 3 months for MMRV (although a 4-week interval is valid). Minimum age is 12 months.

Special Considerations (Nursing Interventions)

- Screen for contraindications and precautions.
- **Contraindications:**
  - Severe allergic reaction to vaccine component or following a prior dose
  - Severe immunocompromise
  - Systemic high-dose corticosteroid therapy for 14 days or more
  - HIV infection, regardless of immunocompetence status*
  - Family history of congenital or heredity immunodeficiency in first-degree relatives
  - Receipt of antibody-containing blood products (wait 3–11 months to vaccinate)
  - Pregnancy
- **Precautions:**
  - Moderate or severe acute illness
  - Alpha-gal allergy (consult with physician)
  - History of thrombocytopenic purpura or thrombocytopenia
  - Need for TST or interferon-gamma release assay testing
  - Simultaneous use of aspirin or aspirin-containing products*
  - Personal or family history of seizures of any etiology*
  - Receipt of specific antiviral drugs 24 hours before vaccination*

Rotavirus (RV1, RV5) ROTARIX®, ROTATEQ® Schedules (Live Attenuated)

- Two-dose series for RV1 vaccine (at age 2 and 4 months)
- Three-dose series for RV5 vaccine (at age 2, 4, and 6 months)
- For both rotavirus vaccines
  - May be started as early as 6 weeks of age.
  - Maximum age for first dose is 14 weeks 6 days.
  - Minimum interval between doses is 4 weeks.
  - Maximum age for any dose is 8 months 0 days.

Special Considerations (Nursing Interventions)

- Screen for contraindications and precautions for all vaccines administered.
- **Contraindications:**
  - Severe allergic reaction to vaccine component or following a prior dose
  - Severe latex allergy for RV1 only so use RV5 instead
  - History of intussusception
  - Severe Combined Immunodeficiency (SCID)
- **Precautions:**
  - Moderate or acute illness including gastroenteritis (defer until well)
  - Altered immunocompetence (SCID is a contraindication)

---

* MMRV only

Varicella (VAR) Vaccine Schedule (Live Attenuated)

- Two-dose series at age 12 through 15 months and age 4 through 6 years
- Minimum interval for dose one to two is:
  - 3 months for children between the ages of 12 months to 12 years (although a 4-week interval is valid)
  - Weeks for persons age 13 years and older (VAR only)

Special Considerations (Nursing Interventions)

- **Contraindications**
  - Severe allergic reaction to vaccine component or following a prior dose of any vaccine administered
  - **Contraindicated for MMRV; contraindicated for VAR depending on CD4 count
- **Precautions**
  - Moderate or severe acute illness
  - Alpha-gal allergy (consult with physician)
  - Need for TB testing
  - Receipt of specific antiviral drugs 24 hours before vaccination
  - Simultaneous use of aspirin or aspirin-containing products
  - Personal or family history of seizures of any etiology*

Discharge Planning; Patient and Family Education

- Review potential serious side effects such as temperature of 105 degrees F; child is very noticeably less active or responsive; crying uncontrollably for more than 3 hours; child's body is shaking, twitching, or jerking; and advise parent to seek medical treatment especially for pertussis containing vaccines.
- Review potential side effects for MMR and VAR vaccines such as rash, fever, and temporary joint pain in adolescents which can occur 3 to 30 days after vaccines.
- Provide parent/caregiver with instructions for supportive care following vaccines such as cool compresses to swollen, red, hot injection site; encourage fluids; review clinician's instructions for antipyretics.
- Immunization Action Coalition has excellent handout for parents *After The Shots...*: www.immunize.org/catg.d/p4015.pdf

BIBLIOGRAPHY

Centers for Disease Control and Prevention. (2021, April 27). *Interim clinical considerations for use of COVID-19 vaccines currently authorized in the United States.* https://www.cdc.gov/vaccines/covid-19/info-by-product/clinical-considerations.html#Contraindications

Garzon Maaks, D. L., Barber Starr, N., Brady, M. A., Gaylord, N. M., Driessnack, M., & Duderstadt, K. (Eds.). *Burns' pediatric primary care* (7th ed.). Elsevier.

Hamborsky, J., Kroger, A., & Wolfe, S. (Eds.). (2020, June). *Epidemiology and prevention of vaccine-preventable diseases.* Centers for Disease Control and Prevention.

Hockenberry, M., Wilson, D., & Rodgers, C. C. (Eds.). (2017). *Wong's essentials of pediatric nursing* (10th ed.). Elsevier.

Immunization Action Coalition: https://www.immunize.org/

Kroger, A., Bahta, L., Hunter, P., & General Best Practice Guidelines for Immunization. (2020, November). *Best practices guidance of the advisory committee on immunization practices (ACIP).* Centers for Disease Control and Prevention.

New Jersey Medical School National Tuberculosis Center: http://globaltb.njms.rutgers.edu/downloads/products/wallchart.pdf

KNOWLEDGE CHECK

1. A nurse is caring for a child who has been diagnosed with *Giardia lamblia*. Which assessment finding is the nurse most likely to find?

   A. Rectal itching
   B. Bloody stools
   C. Pale, greasy stools
   D. Nuchal rigidity

2. A nurse is assessing an infant's temperature with a digital rectal thermometer and documents a finding of 102.8°F, rectally. What is an appropriate action to take at this time?

   A. Request an order to administer an oral dose of baby aspirin
   B. Recheck rectal temperature with a glass mercury thermometer
   C. Apply ice compresses to the baby's axilla, face, and neck
   D. Assess the infant's hydration and nutrition status

3. A nurse is caring for a school-aged child with newly diagnosed pharyngitis caused by group A beta-hemolytic *Streptococci*. Which statement by the parents indicates the need for further teaching?

   A. "My daughter will need to take medication for the rest of her life."
   B. "Saltwater gargles may help to ease the pain she has in her throat."
   C. "We should give her ibuprofen or acetaminophen for fever or discomfort."
   D. "We will be sure that our child completes the entire course of antibiotics."

4. A nurse is caring for an adolescent with active TB. The clinician orders contact precautions in a regular room. How should the nurse respond?

   A. "This patient has active TB and should be on airborne precautions in a negative pressure room."
   B. "I will need to get fit tested for an N-95 mask before I can provide care in this room for this patient."
   C. "I need to have a tuberculin skin test with a negative result in 72 hours before I can care for this patient."
   D. "This patient will need to have no visitors until antibiotics have been administered for at least 48 hours."

5. A nurse is explaining passive immunity to a parent. Which of the following can be used as an example for the parent?

   A. MMR vaccine
   B. Varicella vaccine
   C. Hepatitis B immunoglobulin
   D. Tetanus diphtheria vaccine

6. A nurse is explaining how vaccines work to a parent. Which term should be used to describe the mechanism of immunization?

   A. Active immunity
   B. Passive immunity
   C. Incubation
   D. Adjuvant

KNOWLEDGE CHECK

1. **Correct Answer: C) Pale, greasy stools.** *Giardia* is often associated with pale, greasy stools. Rectal itching is a classic hallmark sign of enterobiasis (pinworm infection). Bloody stools are frequently associated with a GI disorder called Meckel's diverticulum. Nuchal rigidity is associated with meningitis, which can occur as a complication of *Salmonella*.

2. **Correct Answer: D) Assess the infant's hydration and nutrition status.** Hydration assessment is critical in a febrile infant as fever accelerates fluid losses. It may be appropriate in this scenario to also give a dose of acetaminophen or ibuprofen, depending on the age of the child and presence of a clinician order. Aspirin is contraindicated in children because of the association of certain viral febrile illnesses with Reye's syndrome. Glass mercury thermometers are no longer recommended because of the dangers of breakage and chemical spillage. Ice compresses are contraindicated, as they can cause compensatory shivering and increase the patient's temperature.

3. **Correct Answer: A) "My daughter will need to take medication for the rest of her life."** Some children who develop rheumatic fever following a strep throat infection may require lifelong medication, but most cases of group A beta-hemolytic *Streptococci* pharyngitis will resolve easily with a 7- to 14-day course of antibiotics. Saltwater gargles can provide pain relief. Antipyretics are indicated for fever and will also provide pain relief. Completing the course of prescribed antibiotics is essential to help prevent rheumatic fever.

4. **Correct Answer: A) "This patient has active TB and should be on airborne precautions in a negative pressure room."** Active TB is highly contagious and requires airborne precautions and a negative pressure room. The nurse should wear an N-95 or N-100 mask but must do so in a negative pressure room. It is too soon for the nurse to get a tuberculin skin test; before exposure has occurred, the test is not indicated. Visitors may be restricted but is not dependent on antibiotic therapy.

5. **Correct Answer: C) Hepatitis B immunoglobulin.** Hepatitis B immunoglobulin (HBIG) is a purified solution of human immunoglobulin that has high titers of antibody to hepatitis B surface antigen (anti-HBs). It is derived from plasma donated by individuals immune to hepatitis B viral infection. HBIG is widely administered to confer passive prophylactic immunity against the hepatitis B virus because of the ability of anti-HBs to neutralize hepatitis B virions. MMR vaccine and varicella vaccine are live virus vaccines and invoke the immune system to make antibodies. Tetanus diphtheria vaccine is a killed virus vaccine that also invokes the immune system to make antibodies. MMR, varicella, and tetanus diphtheria vaccines all inspire an active immunity in the individual.

6. **Correct Answer: A) Active immunity.** Active immunity is protection produced by a person's own immune system. The immune system is stimulated by an antigen to produce antibody and cellular immunity. Unlike passive immunity, which is temporary, active immunity usually lasts for many years, often for a lifetime. Passive immunity is protection by antibody or antitoxin produced by one animal or human and transferred to another. Passive immunity provides immediate protection against infection, but that protection is temporary. Incubation is the development of an infectious disease from the entrance of the pathogen to the appearance of clinical symptoms. An adjuvant is a substance which enhances the body's immune response to an antigen. It is used in vaccines to make the vaccine more effective.

7. A nurse is doing patient teaching for the parent of a 2-month-old child who is to receive Diphtheria-Tetanus-Acellular Pertussis vaccine for the first time. Which statement indicates the parent needs further teaching?

    A. "I heard that vaccine is better than the one that was given some years ago."
    B. "I can put cool cloths on my baby's legs if they are red and sore after the vaccine."
    C. "I need to make sure my baby drinks enough after the vaccine."
    D. "I heard that vaccine causes autism."

8. A nurse is screening a 2-month-old for contraindications and precautions prior to immunizations and the parent tells the nurse that the baby had an anaphylactic reaction to latex. Which is the appropriate action to take?

    A. Advise the clinician that the office does not have any vaccines that are safe to give this baby
    B. Give the baby rotavirus 5 (RV5) vaccine
    C. Tell the parent that all vaccines that are appropriate for age are safe to give this baby
    D. Give the baby rotavirus 1 (RV1) vaccine

9. A nurse is assessing the HPV immunizations for a 16-year-old and notes that a dose of HPV vaccine was administered at age 12 years. What is the appropriate action to take?

    A. Give a dose of HPV vaccine
    B. Give nothing
    C. Give a dose of HPV vaccine today and make an appointment for another dose in 2 months
    D. Make an appointment for another dose of HPV vaccine in 6 months

10. A nurse receives a call from a parent whose 12-month-old has a fine rash on the entire body. The nurse asks more questions and notes that the child received Varicella and MMR vaccines 7 days ago. The child is mildly fussy but is eating and drinking as usual. What should the nurse do?

    A. Advise the parent to force fluids and call the office if child is not getting better or is getting worse
    B. Advise the parent to stay home because the child probably has a mild case of chickenpox
    C. Advise the parent to stay home because child probably has a mild case of measles
    D. Advise the parent that rash was probably a side effect of MMR vaccine and to call back if child gets worse or does not get better

KNOWLEDGE CHECK

7. **Correct Answer: D) "I heard that vaccine causes autism."** There is no evidence that DTaP vaccine or any other vaccine causes autism. This misinformation has been circulating especially on social media for years. Nurses can respond to parents' concerns in a positive nonjudgmental manner with empathy and offer the parent reliable scientific information to increase the comfort of the parent in accepting vaccines. Acellular pertussis vaccines were introduced because they have a lower incidence of causing high fevers which can lead to febrile seizures, and irritability. Encephalopathy was a very rare event with the previous whole cell DTaP vaccine, and it is even more rare with the acellular vaccine. Putting cool cloths on warm, red sites of vaccination and encouraging fluids are recommended comfort measures following immunizations.

8. **Correct Answer: B) Give the baby rotavirus 5 (RV5) vaccine.** It is important to screen for latex allergy prior to immunization since some packaging contains latex, notably included is the rotavirus vaccine. The Rotarix (RV1) dispenser contains latex and the RotaTeq (RV5) vaccine does not. Prefilled syringes have latex stoppers and protective tips, so nurses need to be aware of this so that other presentations such as vials are selected for any child with a latex allergy. All vaccines have alternatives that do not contain latex so children can receive all vaccines appropriate for their age and medical condition. CDC has updated information on latex in packaging: www.cdc.gov/vaccines/pubs/pinkbook/downloads/appendices/B/latex-table.pdf

9. **Correct Answer: A) Give a dose of HPV vaccine.** The total number of HPV doses an adolescent receives depends on when the first dose was given. If the first dose was given before the 15th birthday only one more dose is indicated at least 6 months after the first dose. If the first dose is administered on or after the 15th birthday then the adolescent needs a second dose 4 weeks after the first and a third dose 6 months after the first dose.

10. **Correct Answer: D) Advise the parent that rash was probably a side effect of MMR vaccine and to call back if child gets worse or does not get better.** An expected side effect of both MMR and VAR vaccines is a rash most likely occurring 7 to 10 days following administration of the vaccines. Therefore, the parent should be advised of this side effect, and only call back if the child's health does not improve. Post vaccine teaching for all vaccines includes encouraging fluids, but forcing fluids is not advised at this time. MMR and VAR vaccines do not cause the diseases they are intended to prevent; however, they may cause side effects which mimic the diseases which indicate a robust immune response to the vaccines.

CHAPTER 15

Immunology and Allergies
Maureen Fitzgerald

INTRODUCTION
Children with alterations in their immune system function or dysfunction are at high risk for infection. The main priority of nursing intervention is to prevent infection in the child.

- *Immunity:* A condition to resist disease
  - **Humoral immunity (antibody protection):** Immunoglobulins (antibodies) are main part of humoral immune response which are formed from B cells; secrete antibodies to attack the antigen and eliminate infectious source.
    - **Immunoglobulins (Ig):** IgA, IgD, IgE, IgG (crosses the placenta), and IgM
  - **Cellular immunity (cell-mediated immune response):** T cells, cytokines attack foreign cells, not antibodies.
- *Immunodeficiency:* Failure of the immune system to produce an appropriate immune response due to absence or insufficiency of a substance or process

ALLERGIES (HYPERSENSITIVITIES)

Description
- A condition where the body has an immunologic response to a foreign substance resulting in an adverse reaction
- **Types**
  - *Eczema (atopic dermatitis)*
    - Altered function in skin barrier in flexor surfaces (e.g., elbows, popliteal area), with an immune response in elevated IgE levels; acute or chronic (Figure 15.1)
    - Family history
    - At risk for asthma development
  - *Food allergies*
    - Immune-mediated response by IgE to an ingested food
    - 90% of food allergens from six main foods or food groups: cow's milk, soy, eggs, peanuts, tree nuts (all nuts in hard shells), and wheat
  - *Latex allergies*
    - Immune-mediated response by IgE to a latex exposure
    - **Latex:** A product made from rubber; latex gloves commonly used in healthcare settings

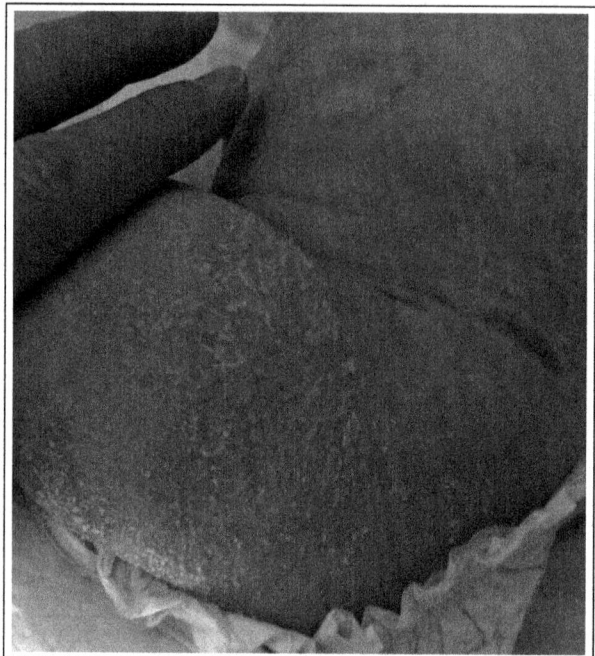

FIGURE 15.1: Atopic dermatitis (eczema) on the abdomen and thigh of an infant
Source: Courtesy of GZ, https://commons.wikimedia.org/wiki/File:Atopic_dermatitis_child_3.jpg

Assessment

- Obtain history for suspected allergens such as latex, foreign substances, and food consumption, depending on the type of hypersensitivity.
- Assess for duration and amount of exposure to the allergen.
- Assess for environmental factors.
- Assess for signs and symptoms of allergies such as eye or mouth and throat itching; coughing; skin changes/lesions such as erythema, pruritis, rash/hives, lichenification, facial swelling; rhinorrhea; sneezing; abdominal pain and bloating; nausea; vomiting; diarrhea; colic; and severe symptoms include wheezing, shortness of breath, swelling of tongue, uvula, pharynx, or upper airway, respiratory distress, hypotension.

Diagnostics

- Elimination diet
- **Oral food challenge:** Child consumes the possible food allergen over a one-hour time period, in a clinician's office or hospital setting
- Skin test for allergy testing

Nursing Interventions

- Document all allergies including foods and latex.
- Educate families on avoiding the identified allergen, foreign or food substance; if food allergy, remove food allergen from diet.
- Observe for risk of malnutrition if many food allergens.
- **For eczema:** Assess for secondary skin infections due to pruritis; rehydrate skin with daily lukewarm baths using mild soap and applying cream emollients.
- Administer antibiotics as ordered for secondary skin infections.
- Administer steroids as ordered to reduce inflammation.
- Administer antihistamines and epinephrine, as necessary. See Pediatric Skill 15.1.

HUMAN IMMUNODEFICIENCY VIRUS INFECTION (A SECONDARY IMMUNODEFICIENCY)

PEDIATRIC SKILL 15.1: ADMINISTRATION OF EPINEPHRINE

1. Hold the EpiPen® or EpiPen Jr® with a fist, ensuring that the colored end with needle tip is facing down; remove the safety release at the top with the opposite hand.
2. Position arm holding EpiPen® down near upper, outer thigh. Swing fist out and then swing fist in to stab the outer thigh at a 90° angle (you will hear a click), holding position of needle in thigh for at least 3 to 10 seconds.
3. After removing the EpiPen® from thigh, massage the injected area for another 10 seconds.
4. Get medical attention immediately. If symptoms continue or recur, then another injection may be necessary.
5. Discard EpiPen® in safety container (you can show a healthcare clinician and have them discard it safely).

Special Considerations

- Understand the difference between a true food allergy and a food intolerance; intolerance occurs with an adverse physiologic response but not an immune-mediated response.
- Educate child and family on secondary infection prevention by decreasing pruritis during bedtime with the use of hand coverings such as mittens; keep fingernails trimmed short.

Discharge Planning; Patient and Family Education

- Teach the child and family what signs and symptoms may occur with allergic reactions.
- Instruct the child and family to always bring an EpiPen® with them; develop a written emergency plan and share with school and day care; wear a medical ID bracelet to indicate allergies.
- Avoid the allergen such as latex items, especially latex gloves; if a food allergen, educate on the importance of reading food labels; discuss a referral to a registered dietician and allergist.
- Educate child and family about eczema exacerbations with temperature extremes and sweating; recommend the use of a humidifier.

PEDIATRIC PEARLS

- Breastfeeding for a minimum of 6 months is a preventative measure in hypersensitivity reactions.

HUMAN IMMUNODEFICIENCY VIRUS INFECTION (A SECONDARY IMMUNODEFICIENCY) AND ACQUIRED IMMUNE DEFICIENCY SYNDROME

Description

- *HIV:* A virus that attacks cells that help the body fight infection, making a person more vulnerable to other infections and diseases, primarily T-lymphocytes called the CD4 T cells.
- *AIDS:* The late stage of HIV infection that occurs when the body's immune system is badly damaged because of the virus.
  - The person with HIV demonstrates a CD4 cell (also called "T cell") count **below 200 μL of blood** and so progresses to the AIDS diagnosis.
  - They develop one or more opportunistic infections regardless of their CD4 count.
- It is spread by contact with certain bodily fluids of a person with HIV; may occur through:
  - **Maternal transmission:** Occurring through utero or perinatal transmission from an HIV+ mother; HIV virus is transmitted through breast milk

- Contact with infected blood or blood products
- During unprotected sex (sex without a condom or HIV medicine to prevent or treat HIV) or through sharing injection drug equipment
  - Medication to prevent transmission includes pre-exposure prophylaxis (**PrEP**; Truvada) which helps to keep the virus undetectable and prevents transmission to high-risk individuals (can be taken by non-HIV infected individuals to prevent transmission as well).
  - World Health Organization (WHO) guidelines recommend PrEP for high-risk HIV+ pregnant women. PrEP is started in pregnancy and lactation for women who are HIV+ (in combination therapy with antiretroviral therapy [ART]) and high-risk negative pregnant patients.
  - ART controls the replication of HIV in the body.

Assessment

- Obtain history for frequent and severe occurrences of common childhood bacterial infections (e.g., otitis media, sinusitis, pharyngitis, and pneumonia).
- Obtain history for reoccurrences of fungal infections (e.g., candidiasis or thrush not responding to standard antifungal therapy, histoplasmosis, and cryptococcosis).
- Obtain history for recurrent or unusually severe viral infections, such as recurrent or disseminated herpes simplex or zoster infection or cytomegalovirus (CMV) retinitis.
- Assess for growth failure and presenting failure to thrive (FTT); note if wasting syndrome is present (progressive involuntary weight loss of >10% of baseline body weight in the setting of chronic infection and/or chronic diarrhea).
- Assess for developmental delay; such delays, particularly impairment in the development of expressive language, may indicate HIV encephalopathy.
  - Assess for behavioral issues (in older children), such as loss of concentration and memory, may also indicate HIV encephalopathy.
  - Assess for persistent generalized lymphadenopathy, fatigue, fever, diarrhea, and/or night sweats.
  - Assess for recurrent opportunistic infections (e.g., *Pneumocystis jiroveci* [formerly *carinii*]) pneumonia CMV infections, chronic and recurrent mucosal and esophageal candidiasis, herpes zoster, nontuberculous mycobacteria (principally mycobacterium avium-intracellulaire complex [MAC]), cryptosporidium enteritis, and mucocutaneous herpes simplex virus infections. HIV-infected children also have an increased incidence of common childhood infections such as otitis media, sinusitis, viral respiratory infections, bacterial pneumonia, bacteremia, and meningitis.

Diagnostics

- Because of the persistence of the maternal HIV antibody, infants younger than 18 months require virologic assays that directly detect HIV in order to diagnose HIV infection.
  - In infants, virologic assays include HIV DNA polymerase chain reaction (PCR) and HIV RNA assays. For known HIV-exposed infants, test three times within 6 months of age.
  - In older children and adults, an enzyme-linked immunosorbent assay (ELISA) to detect HIV antibody, followed by a confirmatory Western blot (which has increased specificity), should be used to diagnose HIV infection.
  - Rapid HIV tests provide results in minutes, simplify and expand the availability of HIV testing. Their sensitivity is as high as 100%, but they must be followed with confirmatory Western blotting or immunofluorescence antibody testing, as with conventional HIV antibody tests.
  - Ratio of $CD4^+$ to $CD8^+$ counts is persistently inverted.

Nursing Interventions

- Assist the child with developing coping mechanisms regarding the emotional burden of serious illness and body image (common with wasting or other opportunistic infections such as Kaposi sarcoma [KS], *Pneumocystis jiroveci*, or molluscum lesions).
- Administer prescribed medications such as ART.
- **Implement standard precautions:** Hand hygiene; use of personal protective equipment such as gloves for handling body secretions, mask, goggles and gowns when risk of splashing is present; sharp safety safe injection practices; clean and disinfected environmental surfaces.
- Use normal saline or bicarbonate mouthwash for daily oral rinsing.
- Provide a diet high in nutritional value, high protein, high calorie, cook meats thoroughly, and wash all produce. Avoid:
  - Raw eggs or foods that contain raw eggs (e.g., homemade cookie dough)
  - Raw or undercooked poultry, meat, and seafood
  - Unpasteurized milk or dairy products and fruit juices
- Ensure adequate enteral or parental fluid intake during episodes of diarrhea. HIV-infected children benefit from both high dose vitamin A supplementation and the addition of zinc to oral rehydration therapy for the treatment of diarrhea.
- Inspect the skin and mucous membranes frequently. Provide skin care.

Special Considerations

Educate on risk reduction and prevention.

Discharge Planning; Patient and Family Education

- Educate patient and family on the importance of medication adherence.
- Educate on the importance of safer sex practices (adolescents).
  - Emphasize that abstinence is the most effective way to prevent transmission.
- Educate the patient and family regarding signs of impending infection and the importance of seeking immediate medical attention.
- Avoid crowded areas and people with known infections.
- Ensure child gets properly vaccinated.
- Tell the child and parents that the child should not donate blood, blood products, organs, tissue, eggs, sperm, or breast milk.
- Provide referral to infectious disease specialist as needed.

HYPOGAMMAGLOBULINEMIA (A PRIMARY IMMUNODEFICIENCY)

Description

Disorder where the child has low serum immunoglobulin or does not form antibodies appropriately; physiologic hypogammaglobulinemia may occur as maternal antibodies wear off.

Assessment

- Assess for history of recurrent respiratory, gastrointestinal, or genitourinary infections, family history of primary immunodeficiency.
- Palpate for enlarged lymph nodes.
- Determine if treated in the past with antibiotics for two months or longer.

Diagnostics

Rapid diagnosis to avoid risk of recurrent infections; laboratory tests (CBC with differential, serum immunoglobulin levels); genetic testing

Nursing Interventions

Monthly administration of intravenous immunoglobulin (IVIG; Pediatric Skill 15.2)

PEDIATRIC SKILL 15.2: INTRAVENOUS IMMUNOGLOBULIN ADMINISTRATION

- Exogenous IgG antibodies—a plasma product.
- **Indications:** Primary immune deficiencies, HIV infection, myasthenia gravis.
- **Assessment:** Assess for infections since last infusion.
- **Nursing Implications:** Do not shake the medication; do not mix with other intravenous (IV) medications/fluids; do not give intramuscular (IM) or subcutaneous (SQ); may need to premedicate with antipyretic or antihistamine; monitor vital signs and observe for signs of adverse reactions and anaphylaxis; oxygen, epinephrine, antihistamine, and IV steroids should be at bedside.

Discharge Planning; Patient and Family Education

- Educate families about infection prevention (hand hygiene).
- Discuss referral to immunologist.

PEDIATRIC PEARLS

- Assess for FTT due to congenital hypogammaglobulinemia.

SEVERE COMBINED IMMUNODEFICIENCY (A PRIMARY IMMUNODEFICIENCY)

Description

- Severe Combined Immunodeficiency (SCID) is an inherited disorder that typically presents in infancy and results in profound immune deficiency where the individual is unable to fight off even mild infections. It is considered to be the most serious primary immunodeficiency disorder and is potentially fatal.
  - SCID is caused by genetic defects that result in the **deficiency** or **absence** of both T-lymphocyte and B-lymphocyte functioning.
    - Natural killer (NK) cells develop separately from T and B cells and can provide a degree of protection in individuals with T and B cell dysfunction. Assessing for the presence of NK cells helps determine the severity and prognosis of the SCID.
  - Most commonly identified type is linked to a problem in a gene on the X chromosome, affecting only males. Since starting newborn screening for SCID, recessive forms of the disease that can affect boys and girls have been identified with increased frequency.
  - Other forms of SCID are caused by a deficiency of the enzyme adenosine deaminase (ADA) and a variety of other genetic defects. ADA is an enzyme found in lymphocytes responsible for removing certain toxins produced by their metabolism.

Assessment

- Obtain **family history** for presence of SCID.
- Assess for extreme susceptibility to infection within the first few months after birth.
  - Usually appears around six months of age (because of protection by maternal immunoglobulin G [IgG]) with opportunistic infections caused by bacteria, viruses, fungi, and protozoa.

- Infections by rare microorganisms.
- Assess for septicemia and bacteremia.
- Assess for FTT, diarrhea.
- Assess for frequent use of antimicrobials without noticeable improvement.

Diagnostics

- Quantitative serum measurement of immunoglobulins, Ig levels are usually low or absent, but IgG may be normal because of transplacental maternal IgG.
- A lymphocyte function test shows severely diminished or absent T-cell number and function.
- Absolute lymphocyte count is less than 3,000 cells/mm^3, with T cells making up less than 20% of total lymphocytes.
- Noted lymphopenia.
- Currently, many states have added SCID to their newborn screening panel.

Nursing Interventions

- Provide for strict protective isolation (germ-free environment), standard precautions.
- Administer IV infusion of immunoglobulins; check serum IgA levels, as ordered, before administering IVIG to prevent possible life-threatening allergic reaction.
- Institute possible parenteral or enteral nutrition supplementation.
  - Caution with breastfeeding as some infections can be passed through breast milk.
- Antibiotic, antiviral, or antifungal agents to treat infections.
- Minimize invasive procedures, provide skin care, and promote rest.
- Refrain from administering live vaccines.
- Prepare the child and family for bone marrow or stem cell transplantation, as appropriate.
- Collaborate with a genetic counselor to obtain genetic testing if the family consents.

Discharge Planning; Patient and Family Education

- Family teaching regarding proper technique for strict protective isolation.
- Family teaching regarding signs and symptoms of infection and the need to promptly notify a clinician if any occur.
- Inform family that IVIG may be given every three to four weeks but that the exact schedule is adjusted to maintain adequate levels (adverse effects may include headache and aseptic meningitis).
- Inform family of the need to avoid live-virus vaccines for the child and siblings living in the same household.
- Avoid all sick contacts; isolation from crowded facilities.

PEDIATRIC PEARLS

- If transfusion is prescribed, only administer blood that has been **irradiated** to destroy white blood cells.

BIBLIOGRAPHY

Healthy Children by American Academy of Pediatrics: https://www.healthychildren.org/English/healthy-living/nutrition/Pages/Common-Food-Allergies.aspx

Huq, M., Bhatnagar, N. K., & Hostoffer, R. W. (2020). Hypogammaglobulinemia. In *StatPearls* [Online]. StatPearls Publishing. https://www.ncbi.nlm.nih.gov/books/NBK563134/

Justiz Vaillant, A. A., & Mohseni, M. (2020). Severe combined immunodeficiency. In *StatPearls* [Online]. StatPearls Publishing. https://www.ncbi.nlm.nih.gov/books/NBK539762/

Meridian Medical Technologies. (2020). *EpiPen® and EpiPen Jr®*. https://dailymed.nlm.nih.gov/dailymed/fda/fdaDrugXsl.cfm?type=display&setid=7560c201-9246-487c-a13b-6295db04274a#section-15

Ricci, S. S., Kyle, T., & Carman, S. (2021). *Maternity and pediatric nursing* (4th ed.). Wolters Kluwer.

Rivera, D. (2020). *Pediatric HIV infection.* https://emedicine.medscape.com/article/965086-overview

Silbert-Flagg, J., & Sloand, E. D. (Eds.). (2017). *Pediatric nurse practitioner certification: Review guide* (6th ed.). Jones & Bartlett Learning, LLC.

Wolters Kluwer Clinical Drug Information. (2020). *Lexi-comp online.* http://online.lexi.com/lco/action/doc/retrieve/docid/pdh_f/129550

KNOWLEDGE CHECK

1. A pediatric nurse is caring for a 3-month-old infant with atopic dermatitis (eczema). Which intervention would the nurse recommend to the caregiver?

   A. Maintain a dry, warm environment
   B. Keep the fingernails trimmed short
   C. Bathe infant with a harsh soap that dries the skin
   D. Avoid baths and moisturizing lotions

2. Which is the priority nursing assessment when administering IV immunoglobin to a child with hypogammaglobulinemia?

   A. Observe for signs of adverse reactions and anaphylaxis
   B. Monitor urine output
   C. Assess for pain
   D. Evaluate family's understanding of treatment

3. A pediatric nurse is teaching a health promotion class to parents about hypersensitivity reactions. Which factor should be included in the teaching plan?

   A. Formula feeding helps reduce the risk of allergies
   B. Keep the food allergen in the diet to decrease exacerbations
   C. Discourage use of humidifiers
   D. Encourage breastfeeding for at least six months

4. A caregiver has received discharge instructions about using an EpiPen®. Which response by the caregiver would indicate that further education is needed?

   A. "Multiple doses can be given with the same syringe."
   B. "I will push the EpiPen® firmly into my child's upper, outer thigh at a 90° angle."
   C. "I will hold the EpiPen® firmly in the injection site for at least 3 to 10 seconds."
   D. "I will call for medical help right away after giving the EpiPen® to my child."

5. A pediatric nurse is caring for a 4-year-old child who has been diagnosed with AIDS. Which precaution measures should be taken?

   A. Standard precautions
   B. Droplet precautions
   C. Airborne precautions
   D. Enteric precautions

6. The nurse is providing discharge instructions with a parent who has a child positive for HIV. Which of the following information would be important for the nurse to include?

   A. Separate plates and utensils during mealtimes
   B. Avoid the annual influenza vaccination
   C. Avoid large crowds and people with known infections
   D. Administer aspirin for pain control

KNOWLEDGE CHECK

1. **Correct Answer: B) Keep the fingernails trimmed short.** Educate child and family on secondary infection prevention with eczema by decreasing pruritus during bedtime with the use of hand coverings such as mittens; keep fingernails trimmed short. Educate child and family about eczema exacerbations with temperature extremes and sweating. A use of a humidifier is recommended. It is important to rehydrate skin with daily lukewarm baths using mild soap, then apply cream emollients after bath.

2. **Correct Answer: A) Observe for signs of adverse reactions and anaphylaxis.** The priority nursing assessment when administering IVIG is to monitor vital signs and observe for signs of adverse reactions and anaphylaxis. Although it is important to monitor the urine output, assess for pain, and to evaluate the family's understanding of the treatment, the most immediate priority must be focused on adverse reactions to the IVIG.

3. **Correct Answer: D) Encourage breastfeeding for at least six months.** Breastfeeding for a minimum of six months, not formula feeding, is a preventative measure in hypersensitivity reactions. It is important to avoid known food allergens, eliminating them from one's diet. Use of humidifiers is recommended, especially during winter months.

4. **Correct Answer: A) "Multiple doses can be given with the same syringe."** Each EpiPen® or EpiPen Jr® (epinephrine injection, USP) Auto-Injector (or their authorized generics) contains a single dose of epinephrine. When a child is having an allergic emergency, instruct caregivers to immediately give their child epinephrine by using the EpiPen®. Instructions for administration of EpiPen® include: position arm holding EpiPen® down near upper, outer thigh; swing fist out and then swing fist in to stab the outer thigh at a 90° angle (you will hear a click), holding position of needle in thigh for at least 3 to 10 seconds; get medical attention immediately; if symptoms continue or recur, then another injection may be necessary.

5. **Correct Answer: A) Standard precautions.** Standard precautions combine the major features of universal precautions (UP) and body substance isolation (BSI) and are based on the principle that all blood, body fluids, secretions, excretions except sweat, nonintact skin, and mucous membranes may contain transmissible infectious agents. Standard precautions include a group of infection prevention practices that apply to all patients, regardless of suspected or confirmed infection status, in any setting in which healthcare is delivered. The Centers for Disease Control and Prevention have established three new elements to standard precautions, which include: respiratory hygiene/cough etiquette, safe injection practices, and use of masks for insertion of catheters or injection of material into spinal or epidural spaces via lumbar puncture procedures (e.g., myelogram, spinal, or epidural anesthesia). Droplet precautions are intended to prevent transmission of pathogens spread through close respiratory or mucous membrane contact with respiratory secretions. Airborne precautions prevent transmission of infectious agents that remain infectious over long distances when suspended in the air (e.g., rubeola virus [measles], varicella virus [chickenpox]). Enteric precautions are taken to prevent infections that are transmitted primarily by direct or indirect contact with fecal material.

6. **Correct Answer: C) Avoid large crowds and people with known infections.** Educate the child and family on prevention of infection, which may include obtaining a yearly vaccination, avoiding crowded areas and individuals known to have an infection to protect the child from any opportunistic infection. It is not necessary to separate dishes or eating utensils. Dishes used by a person infected with HIV do not require special methods of cleaning. Acetaminophen, non-steroidal anti-inflammatory drugs (NSAIDs), or opioids should be administered to a child who has pain; however, aspirin should not be given due to the possible development of Rye Syndrome.

7. A child with HIV has developed *Pneumocystis jiroveci* pneumonia. What does the nurse conclude from this new diagnosis?

    A. CD4 count is likely above 200 μL of blood
    B. Viral load is likely low
    C. Ratio of $CD4^+$ to $CD8^+$ counts are rising
    D. Child has progressed onto AIDS

8. The nurse is teaching an adolescent about HIV/AIDS transmission. Which statement made by the adolescent would require further teaching?

    A. "You can contract HIV/AIDS through casual kissing."
    B. "Sharing needles can contribute to HIV/AIDS infection."
    C. "Infants can get infected while in utero, during birth, after birth, and during breastfeeding."
    D. "Condoms and barrier methods can help to reduce the chance of HIV/AIDS transmission."

9. The most important reason for a pediatric clinician to prescribe a combination of antiretroviral medications to a child with HIV is to delay:

    A. Appetite suppression
    B. Progression to AIDS
    C. Medication resistance
    D. Onset of pain response

10. Which clinical manifestation in the child diagnosed with SCID should the pediatric nurse expect to find?

    A. Fatigue
    B. Presence of stress fractures
    C. Susceptibility to infection
    D. Prolonged bleeding

7. **Correct Answer: D) Child has progressed onto AIDS.** *Pneumocystis jiroveci* pneumonia remains the most common AIDS-indicator disease among HIV-infected children, accounting for 33% of AIDS cases overall. The presence of the opportunistic infection indicates that the child with HIV infection has progressed to AIDS. This occurs when at least one complicating illness develops or when there is a significant decline in the body's ability to defend itself from infection. CD4 counts would most likely be below 200 μL of blood, not above, and viral loads are expected to be elevated. HIV-negative clients generally have a greater number of CD4 cells than they have of CD8 cells. In HIV individuals, a declining $CD4^+/CD8^+$ ratio has been found to be a prognostic marker of HIV disease progression.

8. **Correct Answer: A) "You can contract HIV/AIDS through casual kissing."** HIV is transmitted via blood, semen, vaginal secretions, and breast milk. Vertical transmission can occur during the birthing process. There is no evidence that casual contact such as kissing will result in viral spreading.

9. **Correct Answer: B) Progression to AIDS.** Effective ART is the most important intervention in terms of improving longevity and preventing opportunistic infections in patients with HIV infection. Therapy should involve combinations of antiretroviral medications, which will hopefully prevent the progression of the HIV infection to AIDS. Although some HIV medicines may reduce the appetite and may alter the taste of food, it is not an indication for ART. Similarly, ART is not prescribed to delay resistance to medications nor delay the onset of a pain response.

10. **Correct Answer: C) Susceptibility to infection.** SCID is characterized by an absence of cell-mediated immunity, which would present with manifestations of infection. Fatigue may indicate a deficiency in the erythrocytes, whereas prolonged bleeding may indicate an issue with platelets or clotting factor. Presence of stress fractures may be seen with alterations in calcium levels or bone matrix, and leukemia disorders.

CHAPTER 16

Behavioral and Psychosocial Conditions

Stephen DiDonato and David Jack

INTRODUCTION

Mental/behavioral health is an important component of holistic health and wellness. Many behavioral disorders may manifest themselves along a continuum of individual symptoms and functioning. Promotion of healthy coping, stress reduction, early intervention, and self-awareness may mitigate some of the negative effects of these diseases/disorders.

ANXIETY DISORDERS

Description

Anxiety disorders are psychiatric disorders that present in a variety of forms and individual diagnoses, but the overarching theme is a sense of extreme fear or worry, which results in changes in the child's behaviors, sleep, mood, and/or eating.

- **Types**
  - **Generalized Anxiety Disorder**
    - Excessive worry and anxiety.
    - Individual finds it difficult to control the worry.
    - Individual may become restless, get easily fatigued, become irritable, have muscle tension, have sleep disturbances, have difficulty concentrating.
  - **Separation Anxiety Disorder**
    - Recurrent excessive distress when anticipating or experiencing separation from home or from major attachment figures
    - Persistent and excessive worry about losing a major attachment figure (e.g., death) or that something will happen to this figure (e.g., illness, injury)
    - Persistent reluctance to leave home and engage in school or other outside of the home activities because of the fear of separation
  - **Selective Mutism**
    - Consistent failure to speak in specific social situations where there is an expectation for speaking (e.g., school) despite speaking in other situations
  - **Specific Phobias**
    - Marked fear or anxiety about a specific object or situation (e.g., animals, heights, storms, needles, invasive medical procedures, elevators)

- **Social Anxiety Disorder**
  - Marked fear about one or more social situations in which the individual is exposed to possible scrutiny by others.
  - Individual fears they will act in a way where their anxiety symptoms are negatively evaluated by others.
- **Panic Disorder**
  - Recurrent or unexpected panic attacks (an abrupt surge of intense fear or intense discomfort that causes symptoms such as palpitations, sweating, trembling, chest pain, feeling of choking, fear of losing control, derealization; Figure 16.1)
- **Agoraphobia**
  - Marked fear about situations such as public transportation, being in open spaces, being in enclosed areas, standing in a crowded line, being outside of the home.
  - Individual fears the listed situations because they feel they cannot escape the situation or help may not be available if needed.

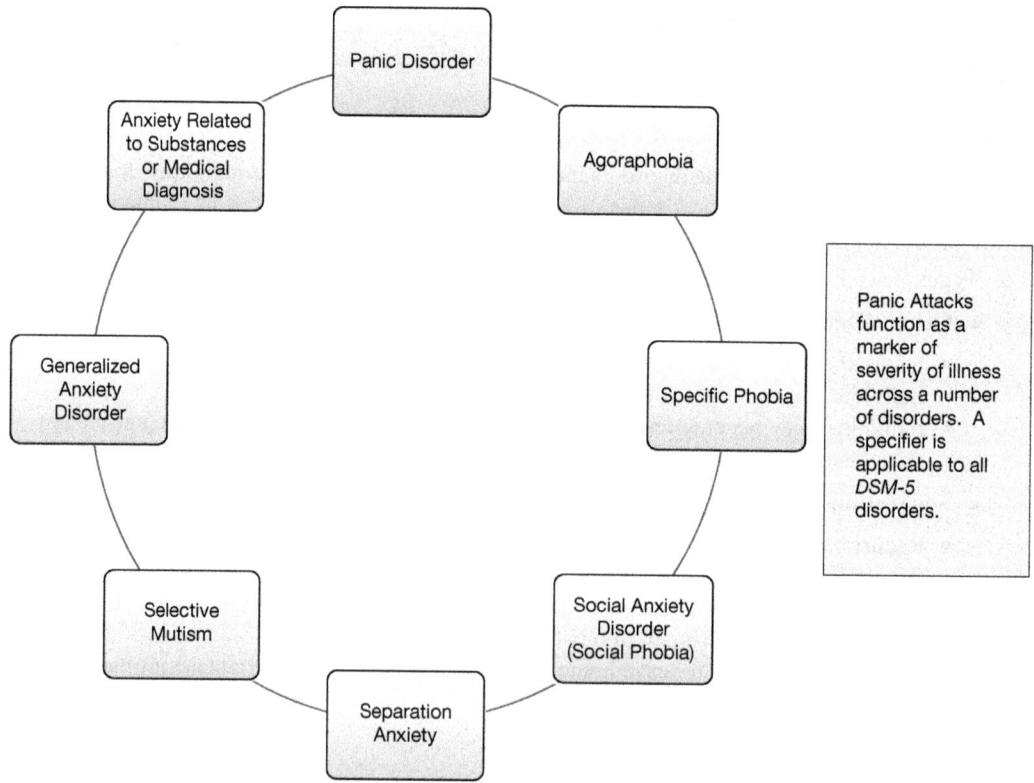

FIGURE 16.1: Categories of anxiety disorders from the *Diagnostic and Statistical Manual of Mental Disorders,* 5th Edition

Source: Adapted from American Psychiatric Association. (2013). *Diagnostic and statistical manual of mental disorders* (5th ed.). https://doi.org/10.1176/appi.books.9780890425596; Reprinted from Singleton, J. K. (2014). *Primary care: An interprofessional perspective* (2nd ed.). Springer Publishing Company.

Assessment

- Assess physiologic symptoms such as trembling and/or twitching, shortness of breath, tachycardia and tachypnea, elevated blood pressure, and sweating.
- Assess for reactions to a perceived threat that cause internal feelings of apprehension, dread, or uneasiness.
- Assess for worries, fears, and distress that are seen across life domains (home, school, and social) that child and/or parent report as disruptive.
- Assess patient for history of muscle aches and spasms; inability to relax; apprehension; fear; difficulty concentrating, eating, and sleeping; inability to control worrying; fatigue; irritability.

Diagnostics

- **Generalized Anxiety Disorder–7 (GAD–7):** Online self-report measure on generalized anxiety disorder
- **Screen for Child Anxiety Related Disorders (SCARED):** A child self-report and parent-report screening for multiple anxiety disorder in children

Nursing Interventions

- Set a calm and safe space for both the child and family.
- Administer medications as directed with education for caregivers around timing of day for administration, as per prescription.
- Help identify anxiety triggers and measures to alleviate them, such as distraction and deep breathing; assist with relaxation measures.
- Provide emotional support through active listening and developing an attuned relationship; emotional support is about the relationship and does not need to involve verbalization of feelings until the patient is ready.
- Institute suicide precautions or a no-harm contract if the patient exhibits suicidal ideation.
- Allow child to verbalize their feelings.

Special Considerations

- Initial symptoms of anxiety disorders present in adolescence.
- Exposure to childhood adversity may increase a child's or adolescent's sense of loss or control and lack of predictability in their lives, at times manifesting as symptoms that look like anxiety symptoms. For some children and adolescents, the exposure to adversity caused these symptoms and for others who had underlying anxiety, the exposure to adversity has exacerbated these symptoms.
- Showing symptoms of anxiety is typical during any life transition (e.g., puberty, change of schools, home stressors, applying to college).

Discharge Planning; Patient and Family Education

- Educate family on psychiatric medications, if applicable, including timeline for therapeutic effectiveness.
- Educate caregivers on realistic and clear expectations.
- Ensure caregivers have necessary information for behavioral health follow-up.
- Support caregivers with documentation for school, if necessary, and educate on communicating child's needs with school.
- Provide caregivers and child/adolescent with age-appropriate resources on coping skills (movement, progressive muscle relaxation, deep breathing, exercise).
- Support caregivers and child to praise their child/self for efforts to cope with fears and worry.

ATTENTION DEFICIT HYPERACTIVITY DISORDER

Description

Attention deficit hyperactivity disorder (ADHD) is a neurodevelopmental disorder characterized by persistent and pervasive patterns of inattentiveness and/or hyperactivity and impulsivity, with several symptoms present before the age of 12. ADHD is more likely to be diagnosed in boys and more than half of the children diagnosed with ADHD have at least one co-occurring disorder.

- **Types of Symptoms:** ADHD manifestations that are symptoms are predominantly inattentiveness, predominantly hyperactive and impulsive, or combined inattentiveness and hyperactive and impulsive.
  - **Inattentive Symptoms**
    - Fails to pay close attention to details or makes careless mistakes
    - Has difficulty sustaining attention
    - Often does not follow through on instructions and fails to complete tasks (e.g., schoolwork, chores)
    - Is often easily distracted by extraneous stimuli
    - Often avoids or dislikes activities that require sustained attention (e.g., school, completing reports)
    - Often does not seem to listen when spoken to directly
  - **Hyperactive or Impulsive Symptoms**
    - Often fidgets with or taps hands or feet, squirms in seat
    - Often talks excessively, blurts out answers, or interrupts others
    - Is often "on the go" acting as if "driven by a motor"
    - Often leaves seat in situations when remaining in seat is expected
    - Often unable to engage in quiet activities

Assessment

- **Assess for duration:** Symptoms must be present for at least 6 months.
- **Assess for pervasiveness:** Symptoms must be present across at least two domains of the child's life.
- Assess for inability to sustain attention, lack of eye contact, constant movement, or fidgeting.

Diagnostics

- **Children 6 to 12 years old:** National Institute for Children's Health Quality (NICHQ) Vanderbilt Assessment Scale, which provides a parent and teacher report measure
- Behavior rating scales (parent report, child/adolescent self-report, or teacher report) or utilize the criterion within the *Diagnostic and Statistical Manual of Mental Disorders*, Fifth Edition (*DSM-5*)

Nursing Interventions

- Maintain a safe environment for the child and others.
- Implement positive reinforcement and behavioral checklists for task completion.
- Obtain the child's attention before giving instructions, breaking down tasks into short steps with clear expectations of task completion.
- Implement a consistent, structured routine.
- Implement modeling behaviors to demonstrate acceptable behaviors.
  - Set clear limits on unacceptable behaviors and be consistent in your approach to redirect or correct unacceptable behaviors.

- Focus on child's and family's strengths, assist with developing effective coping mechanisms.
- Set a calm, firm, and respectful approach for both the child and family.
- Administer medications as directed.
  - Psychostimulants are often used to increase focus and attention.
    - Short acting medication is effective for 4 hours.
    - Long-acting medication is effective for 8 to 12 hours; do not chew long-acting tablets.
    - Assess for complications such as sleep disturbances and anorexia.

Special Considerations

ADHD prevalence rates are higher in children who have been exposed to potentially traumatic events.

Discharge Planning; Patient and Family Education

- Educate caregivers on realistic and clear expectations.
- Ensure caregivers have necessary information for behavioral health follow-up.
- Educate family on psychiatric medications, if applicable, including timeline for therapeutic effectiveness.
- Provide resources on sleep hygiene (e.g., showering at night to calm, no technology within 30 minutes of bedtime).
- Support caregivers with documentation for school, if necessary.
- Empower caregivers to set realistic expectations for their own parenting and celebrate the strengths that ADHD brings (e.g., critical thinking, creativity).
- Referral to a qualified behavioral healthcare professional (psychologist, psychiatrist, professional counselor, clinical social worker).

AUTISM SPECTRUM DISORDER

Description

Autism spectrum disorder (ASD) is a developmental disorder that affects social interaction and communication and other behavior. Symptoms of ASD must be present in early developmental period. The disorder is four times more likely to occur in boys than girls. Autism can be diagnosed at any age, but it is typically referred to as a "developmental disorder" because symptoms generally appear in the first 2 years of life.

- Types of Symptoms
  - **Deficits in Social Communication and Social Interaction**
    - Deficits in social-emotional reciprocity (e.g., abnormal social approach, failure to engage in back-and-forth conversation, failure to initiate or respond to social interactions)
    - Deficits in nonverbal communication behaviors (e.g., abnormalities in eye contact and body language, deficits in understanding and use of gestures, lack of facial expression)
  - **Restricted and Repetitive Behaviors, Interests, or Activities**
    - Stereotyped or repetitive motor movements
    - Inflexible adherence to routines
    - Hyper- or hyporeactivity to sensory input

Assessment

- Assess for attainment or regression of developmental milestones (e.g., caregiver concerns).
- Assess for pervasive and persistent impairments in capacity to communicate and interact with others.

AUTISM SPECTRUM DISORDER

- Assess for lack of cuddling, attachment, or show of affection to caretaker.
- Assess for family history of autism.
- Assess for ability to adapt to changes in routine.
- Assess for savant behaviors where child excels in certain areas (e.g., art, puzzles, math, memory).
- Assess for lack of imaginative play.

Diagnostics

While diagnosis typically occurs during pediatrician well-visits or other visits, understanding a child's health history (e.g., parental concerns, family history) and current physical findings (e.g., decreased infant play, delayed smile response, repetitive play, not comforted by caregivers, cognitive delays) will expedite diagnosis process.

Nursing Interventions (see Pediatric Skill 16.1)

- Refer child for early intervention programs.
- Refer child as needed for physical, occupational, speech, and language therapy.
- Implement behavioral modification strategies and set realistic goals.
- Use of positive reinforcement.
- Promote increased social awareness.
- Promote verbal communication.
- Implement consistent behavioral expectations.
- Decrease environmental stimuli when appropriate.
- Minimize handling of the child to prevent upsetting the child.
- Provide comfort/coping aids (e.g., weighted vest, a swing).
- Recognize signs of sensory overload and implement, assist with calming and self-regulating strategies.
- Introduce child into new situations slowly, maintain consistency and structure of home routines.
- Administer medications as directed.
- Encourage a healthy diet.

Special Considerations

- ASD may manifest similar to intellectual impairments, language impairments, and other co-occurring mental health and neurodevelopmental conditions calling for an understanding of differential diagnosis.
- White children are more likely to be diagnosed than children from minority populations; we should consider a social justice lens to barriers of non-White children being screened for ASD.

Discharge Planning; Patient and Family Education

- Ensure caregivers have necessary information for developmental specialist (developmental pediatrician, neuropsychologist, speech–language pathologist) follow-ups.
- Support with education on behavioral techniques and positive reinforcement.
- Ensure caregivers understand the treatment regimen and next steps in care.
- Identify and plan for assisted daily living skill needs (e.g., hygiene).

PEDIATRIC SKILL 16.1: USE THERAPEUTIC COMMUNICATION

- Communication is the basis of a therapeutic relationship and is designed to assist with therapeutic goals.
  - A therapeutic relationship between the child's nurse and the child and family is defined as purposeful, respectful, based on caring with recognition of the unique qualities of the child and family, and one that is guided by professional boundaries.
  - In developing a trusting nurse–child–family relationship, key characteristics must include empathy, honesty, caring, respect, and genuineness in a supportive, nonjudgmental approach.
  - Nurses must establish and maintain dynamic, reciprocal, therapeutic relationships, not only with the child but also with their family.
- Communication techniques:
  - Numerous strategies exist that nurses can access to develop their knowledge and skills in effective relationship building. For example, communication skills such as active listening, paraphrasing, summarizing, reflecting, using silence, and questioning are fundamental to the development of rapport and empathic therapeutic relationships.
  - Recognize that cultural variations may exist (e.g., eye contact, touch, and close proximity).
  - Play is the universal language of children.
    - **Bibliotherapy:** Using books in a therapeutic and supportive process.
    - "What if" questions encourage the child to explore situations and to consider choices and problem-solving options.
    - **Drawing:** Includes spontaneous drawing and directed drawing.
- Family-centered care is a key concept in children's nursing, suggesting that children and families should consent and be actively involved in care decisions resulting in an agreed understanding between all stakeholders.

DEPRESSION

Description

- Depression is a mood disorder. Incidence of depression increases as child ages. Girls are twice as likely as boys to experience depression.
  - **Types of Symptoms**
    - Persistent sad, anxious, or "empty mood"
    - Loss of pleasure in activities
    - Anhedonia
    - Insomnia or hypersomnia
    - Change in appetite or weight
    - Psychomotor retardation or agitation
    - Low energy
    - Poor concentration
    - Thoughts of worthlessness or guilt
    - Somatic complaints

- **Disruptive Mood Dysregulation Disorder**
  - New diagnosis to characterize severe recurrent temper outbursts where the mood is irritable or angry throughout the day on most days, must be diagnosed between 6 and 18 years of age

Assessment

- Assess for family history.
- Assess for the use of illicit or prescription drugs and alcohol use.
- Assess for changes in psychological stressors (e.g., peer relationships, school, recent events).
- Assess for somatic complaints (e.g., fatigue, headaches, stomach aches).
- Assess for suicidal thoughts and ideations.
- Assess for patient's social support network.

Diagnostics

- Patient Health Questionnaire–9 (adolescents)
- Beck Depression Inventory (all ages)
- Children's Depression Inventory (7 to 17 years old)

Nursing Interventions

- Encourage patient to express emotions; allow for time to build rapport.
- Provide a structured routine.
- Help with appropriate hygiene and sleep routine (sleep hygiene interventions).
- Offer positive reinforcement consistently, specifically for small progress.
- Institute suicide precautions, as needed.
- Administer medication as directed.
- Encourage strength-based and empathetic dialogue from caregivers to child.

Special Considerations

- Approximately 10% of children/adolescents in medical settings experience depression.
- The American Psychological Association recommends against the use of clomipramine, imipramine, mirtazapine, paroxetine, and venlafaxine in adolescents because of the potential for increased suicide risk in youth taking these drugs.

Discharge Planning; Patient and Family Education

- Educate patient and caregivers on medication regime, including that many medications for depression take 2 to 6 weeks to reach therapeutic efficacy.
- Educate on the importance of follow-up mental healthcare.
- Educate on warning signs of suicidal thoughts and ideations.

EATING DISORDERS

Description

- Eating disorders are psychological disorders that refer to conditions related to abnormal eating behaviors and habits. The two primary types of eating disorders are anorexia nervosa and bulimia nervosa. Anorexia nervosa affects about one in every 100 adolescents, while underreported in males, females are ten to 20 times more likely to experience anorexia nervosa. Bulimia occurs in about one out of every four females, most likely between 13 and 18 years old.

- **Types of Eating Disorders**
  - **Anorexia Nervosa**
    - Low body weight (less than 85 percent of normal weight for height and age)
    - Disturbance in body weight, size, or shape (body image)
    - Intense fear of gaining weight or becoming fat, even if though underweight
    - *Two types*
      - **Restricting:** The primary means for weight loss is severe limiting of food intake.
      - **Binge Eating and Purging:** Periods of food intake are followed by compensations efforts (e.g., vomiting, use of laxatives or diuretics, excessive exercise).
  - **Bulimia Nervosa**
    - Binge eating followed by periods of shame, guilt, humiliation, depression, self-deprivation.
    - Self-induced vomiting, excessive exercise, use of diuretics or laxatives, or fasting to compensate for binge eating.
    - Patterns of eating show negative impacts on physiologic functioning.
    - *Two types*
      - **Purging:** Binge followed by self-induced vomiting, use of laxative/diuretics
      - **Nonpurging:** Binge followed by sharp restriction of food or excessive exercise

Assessment

- **General**
  - Assess for family history.
  - Assess for changes in social and family interactions, and academic performance.
  - Assess for symptoms of depression.
- **Anorexia**
  - Measure height, weight, and anthropometric measurements.
    - Assess for weight loss, specifically 15% loss.
  - Assess for fears and perceptions around body image and being "*fat.*"
  - Assess for delayed puberty, irregular menses, amenorrhea (absence of at least three consecutive menstrual cycles).
  - Assess for diet pills, laxatives, diuretics, and excessive enema usage.
  - Assess for excessive exercise and dieting.
  - Assess for dry skin, hypercarotenemia, lanugo body hair, atrophy of the breasts, swelling of the parotid and submandibular gland, peripheral edema, thinning hair.
  - Assess malnutrition, electrolyte disturbances, noting potassium level.
    - Cardiac arrhythmias can occur, especially long Q-T syndrome.
- **Bulimia**
  - Assess for issues with impulse control.
  - Assess for exaggerated feelings of guilt and shame.
  - Assess for dental issues such as enamel erosion.
  - Assess for abrasions, small lacerations, and calluses on the back of the hand overlying the knuckles.
  - Assess for metabolic alkalosis from vomiting.

EATING DISORDERS

Diagnostics

- Serum complete blood count (CBC) may show a decreased white blood cell count especially if malnutrition is present.
- Serum electrolytes may show abnormalities.
- Serum pH is typically increased but may be decreased if laxatives are used for purging.
- In girls, levels of luteinizing hormone (LH) and follicle-stimulating hormone (FSH) are decreased.
- Urine analysis may show diluted urine.
- Electrocardiography may show nonspecific S-T segment, T-wave changes, and prolonged PR interval; ventricular arrhythmias may be seen.

Nursing Interventions

- **General**
  - Correct fluid and electrolyte imbalance.
  - Support in restructuring perspectives of self and the world around them through group, family, and individual counseling.
  - Engage with interdisciplinary team to promote sustainable care plan.
    - Meal training, behavioral modification
  - Weight, height, body mass index, and muscle mass.
  - Collect urine specimen.
- **Anorexia**
  - Support with weight gain, should increase 0.2 to 1.5 kg per week.
  - Gradual reintroduction of food to prevent re-feeding syndrome (may require enteral feedings); work with adolescent to plan a well-balanced meal with appropriate calorie intake.
  - Negotiate food intake of a balanced diet and normal eating pattern with patient, food intake during initial period may vary and should increase over time.
  - Observe individual during eating and for 1 hour after.
  - Limit physical activity and calorie expenditure.
- **Bulimia**
  - Provide a pleasant and relaxing environment for eating, nonjudgmental.
  - Establish a food contract, how much and what food will be eaten at each meal.
  - Observe individual during eating and for 1 hour after.

Special Considerations

- Inpatient treatment is the most effective treatment for eating disorders in adolescents.
- Comorbid with depression often and history of childhood abuse is prevalent in patients.
- Monitor for 1 hour after food intake to ensure against self-induced vomiting, restrict bathroom use for this hour.

Discharge Planning; Patient and Family Education

- Provide psychoeducation on nutrition; role of foods, appropriate food intake, and choices.
- Provide psychoeducation on the effects of restrictive eating, purging, and binge eating.
- Ensure patent and caregivers understand the prognosis and treatment plan, as well as required follow-up care and warning signs that require medical attention.

INTENTIONAL SELF-INJURY

Description
Intentional self-injury, also referred to as deliberate self-harm, is a behavioral act that one engages in to purposively injure themselves physically, without the intent to commit suicide. Self-injury can include cutting, scratching, burning, drug overdose, poisoning, biting, pinching, pulling out hair, piercing skin with sharp objects, picking at existing wounds, jumping from high places (e.g., buildings or bridges), carving words or symbols into skin, among other acts an individual may take.

Assessment
- Assess for physical signs (scars, fresh cuts, burns, scratches, or bruises).
- Assess for behavioral signs (rubbing an area excessively to create a burn, wearing long sleeves or long pants, even in hot weather, difficulties with interpersonal relationships).
- Assess for mood and psychological signs (persistent questions about personal identity, emotional instability, impulsiveness, or unpredictability, saying that they feel helpless, hopeless, or worthless).
- Assess for sharp objects in hand or on person.
- Assess for depressive mood.
- Assess for changes in family, school, or social relationships/situations.

Diagnostics
Conduct a suicide assessment.

Nursing Interventions
- Remove any objects that patient can use to self-harm.
- Provide care to wounds and injuries.
- Use nonjudgmental language; stigma prevents individuals who self-harm from asking for help.
- Teach calm down and distraction activities (e.g., texting supportive people, mindfulness).
- Support patient to name their feelings and why they are self-harming.

Special Considerations
- Self-harm has been shown to occur between 10% and 40% in children/adolescents diagnosed with intellectual disabilities.
- LGBTQIA+ youth seriously contemplate suicide at almost three times the rate of heterosexual youth.
- Children and adolescents who engage in self-harm have been shown to also engage in other high-risk behaviors (unprotected sexual activity, substance use).

Discharge Planning; Patient and Family Education
- Educate patient and caregiver on local and national self-injury and suicide prevention resources (e.g., textlines, hotlines, online resources).
- Educate caregivers on warning signs.
- Educate patient and caregivers on follow-up behavioral healthcare.
- Educate patient and caregivers on longer-term risk factors of self-injury.

LEARNING DISABILITIES

Description

- Learning disabilities are due to genetic or neurobiological factors that impact a child's cognitive processes that are related to learning. Children will have difficulties learning and using academic skills. The academic skill deficit is substantially and quantifiably below those expected for the individual's chronological age and cause significant interference in academic performance or daily living activities.
  - **Types of Learning Disorders**
    - **Dyscalcia:** Affects individual's ability to understand numbers and learn math.
    - **Dysgraphia:** Affects individual's handwriting ability and fine motor skills.
    - **Dyslexia:** Affects reading and related language-based processing skills.
    - **Nonverbal Learning Disorder:** Has trouble interpreting nonverbal cues like facial expressions or body language and may have poor coordination.
    - **Oral/Written Language Disorder and Specific Reading Comprehension Deficit:** Learning disabilities that affect an individual's understanding of what they read or of spoken language. The ability to express oneself with oral language may also be impacted.

Assessment

- Assess the patient's communication skills and their preferred method of communicating.
- Assess the person with a learning disability's knowledge of hospitals and address any potential fears.
- Assess patient's preferred communication style.
- Assess for family history of learning disabilities or concerns.
- Assess for performance in social, academic, and developmental performance.

Diagnostics

- Referral to educational and/or psychological testing, typically consisting of intelligence (IQ) test and a standardized achievement (reading, writing, arithmetic) test
- Neurologic medical testing
- Referral to speech–language pathologist for a language assessment and to assess for child's ability to organize speech and thoughts

Nursing Interventions

- Make direct eye contact prior to verbal communication with patient.
- Allow caregiver to support in communication as they may have better understanding of communication preferences.
- Allow for extra time for patient to process information and communicate.
- Dependent upon learning disability type, be creative and interactive in communication (e.g., if patient has Nonverbal Learning Disorder, use direct verbal communication and fewer gestures and facial expressions to communicate).

Special Considerations

ADHD, dyspraxia (causes problems with movement and coordination, language, and speech), and executive functioning are often comorbid with learning disorders.

Discharge Planning; Patient and Family Education

- Ensure caregivers and child understand diagnosis, prognosis, and follow-up needs with other professionals.
- Provide psychoeducation to parents focused on communication styles dependent on type of learning disability.
- Identify child and family supports.
- Provide psychoeducation for caregivers focused on communicating child needs with school.

NEONATAL ABSTINENCE SYNDROME

Description

- Neonatal abstinence syndrome (NAS), also referred to as neonatal opioid withdrawal syndrome, is defined by signs and symptoms of withdrawal that infants develop after in utero exposure to opioids such as oxycodone, illicit substances such as heroin, or drugs used for opioid therapy maintenance, such as methadone or buprenorphine.
  - NAS symptoms appear at 2 to 3 days of life, 24 hours for heroin use.

Assessment

- Obtain a prenatal history for intrauterine opioid drug exposure, or lack of prenatal care.
- Assess for the presence of a positive maternal toxicity screen.
- Assess for excessive sucking, high-pitched excessive crying.
- Assess for poor feeding, which may be vomiting or just not sucking well at all.
- Assess for diarrhea, skin excoriation.
- Assess for tremors or jitteriness and irritability to sound or light.
- Sleep–wake disturbances.
- Alterations in muscle tone (hyperactive primitive reflexes, hypertonia, myoclonic jerks, tremors, and possible seizures).
- Autonomic dysfunction (sneezing, sweating, nasal stuffiness, fever, mottling, yawning).
- Respiratory changes (tachypnea, nasal flaring).
- Temperature instability.

Diagnostics

- Toxicology screenings of newborn's blood, urine, umbilical cord, and meconium.
  - Meconium toxicology is more sensitive than a urine test and has a longer window for substance detection.
- Neonatal hair analysis can detect in utero exposure to opioids, benzodiazepines, methadone, cocaine, and alcohol for up to 3 months after exposure. Hair is not commonly used (because a 2–5 mg of hair is needed to test for drug usage and many babies do not have enough hair.
- **Umbilical cord:** Newest method for drug testing, can be collected at the time of birth (6 inches are required) and stored up to 7 days; provides drug exposure within the last two trimesters of pregnancy.
- **Neonatal abstinence scales:** Scoring systems (e.g., Finnegan Neonatal Abstinence Scoring System [FNAST], Lipsitz Scoring Tool, Neonatal Narcotic Withdrawal Index) help to diagnose and determine the severity of withdrawal symptoms.

NEONATAL ABSTINENCE SYNDROME

Nursing Interventions

- **Neonate**
  - Monitor withdrawal severity using a neonatal abstinence scoring method, used to initiate and adjust pharmacologic therapy and to wean the neonate from it.
    - Pharmacology treatment with methadone or buprenorphine
  - Positioning; holding; rocking (gentle, vertical); and swaddling to reduce motoric hyperactivity.
    - **Swaddle:** In a flexed position with hands midline against chest and legs loosely swaddled in lumbar flexion; to decrease sensory stimulation
    - **Handling:** Handle gently and close to the body to increase sense of security
    - Skin-to-skin care with the mother/kangaroo care
  - Minimize environmental and physical stimulation (low lighting and noise level); do not use TV or mobiles, only soft voice and gentle touch to awaken baby and engage in care.
    - Reduce stimulation when signs of distress appear.
  - Pacifiers for nonnutritive sucking.
  - Cluster care activities.
  - Initiate breastfeeding, although controversial, or formula feeding (small, frequent feedings) as tolerated.
    - May required high-calorie formulas
    - Possible enteral feeding, if sucking difficulties are present
- **Mother**
  - Assist the mother with attaching emotionally to her neonate.
  - Provide positive reinforcement and immediate feedback on all caretaking activities.
  - Explain the neonate's behavior and sensitivity to the environment and that this behavior is not a rejection of her as a mother.
  - Teach the mother to intervene early with her crying baby, as it is easier to settle a baby earlier than later.

Special Considerations

The American Academy of Pediatrics (AAP) recommends breastfeeding for neonates experiencing withdrawal as long as the mother is in a supervised drug treatment program and the mother is HIV- and hepatitis C-negative.

Discharge Planning; Patient and Family Education

- If the baby will go home with medication to control the symptoms of NAS, ensure the mother knows how to administer the medication as well as how to obtain the medication.
- Arrange for a social worker to consult with the family regarding needs at home and expectations.
- Teach parents/caregivers to assess for dehydration or jaundice, especially if the neonate's intake is inadequate.

PEDIATRIC PEARLS

- Use the **WITHDRAWAL** acronym to familiarize yourself with NAS symptoms:
  - **W**akefulness; **I**rritability; **T**emperature variation (tachycardia, tremors); **H**yperactivity (high-pitched cry, hypertonia); **D**iarrhea (diaphoresis, disorganized suck); **R**espiratory distress (rub marks, rhinorrhea); **A**pneic attacks (autonomic dysfunction); **W**eight loss; **A**lkalosis (respiratory), **L**acrimation

OBSESSIVE-COMPULSIVE DISORDER

Description

- Obsessive-compulsive disorder (OCD) is a psychiatric condition characterized by recurrent obsessions (e.g., recurrent and persistent thoughts, urges, or images) and compulsions (e.g., repetitive behaviors or mental acts). The obsessions and/or compulsions serve as defense mechanism for the child against perceived threat. While the onset of OCD may occur at any point between preschool age through adulthood, onset is likely to occur between 8 and 12 (prepubescent onset more likely for boys) or in late teenage years (late teen onset more likely for girls). OCD occurs in boys and girls equally.
- **Pediatric Autoimmune Neuropsychiatric Disorder Associated with Streptococcus (PANDAS)/Pediatric Acute-Onset Neuropsychiatric Syndrome (PANS):** In rare cases, OCD seems to occur "overnight" with rapid changes in mood and severe anxiety. PANDAS and PANS are sub-types of pediatric OCD caused by an infection. When this occurs, the child's immune system gets confused and attacks the brain instead of the infection, causing severe symptoms of OCD seemingly all at once. The sudden appearance of symptoms is very different from general pediatric OCD, where symptoms appear more gradually.
- **Types of Symptoms**
  - **Obsessions**
    - Worrying about germs, getting sick, or dying
    - Preoccupation with body fluids or waste, dirt, germs/disease, chemicals, or sticky substances. Fear of becoming contaminated by and/or spreading perceived contaminants
    - Unwanted thoughts (e.g., violent images, forbidden thoughts or images about sex or taboo behaviors, worries about being gay)
    - Fear of losing control and doing something that is horrible or inconsistent with one's sense of self (e.g., stealing, harming others, harming self)
    - Concerns about evenness, symmetry, completeness, or doing something "just right" (e.g., reading or writing, arranging)
  - **Compulsions**
    - Excessive hand washing, showering, grooming, cleaning, or other efforts to decontaminate
    - Following rigid rules or ritualized behaviors to ensure safety (e.g., washing hands at 10 a.m. daily)
    - Excessive reassurance seeking (e.g., confessing, repeatedly asking questions)
    - Mental compulsions (e.g., rituals such as special sayings, prayers, mentally reviewing situations)
    - Repeating, counting, touching, ordering/arranging, do-overs, or undoing

Assessment

- Assess for obsessions and compulsions during daily activities, such as rituals, such as bedtime routines, morning routines.
- Assess for child's worry and concern related to daily activities.
- Assess for impairment in social and school functioning.
- Assess for skin irritation from behaviors like excessive hand washing.

Diagnostics

- A referral to a child psychologist or psychiatrist is best for children.
- Yale–Brown Obsessive-Compulsive Scale.
- Take a physical and mental health history that screens for obsessions and compulsions, and physical signs (e.g., skin irritation from excessive washing, hair loss from hair pulling). Explore patterns with caregivers and child to be able to inform mental health provider.

Nursing Interventions

- Be supportive, listen, and show empathy.
- Reassure child and parents that OCD is treatable and children can get better with support.
- Allow space and time for ritualistic behaviors to occur.
- Administer prescribed medication.
- Identify insights of child (and family) and promote behavioral change attempts and successes.
- Conduct suicide assessment and safety planning if necessary.

Special Considerations

While the obsessions and compulsions seem necessary for the patient typically, adult patients see these obsessions and compulsions as irrational, but children may lack this insight.

Discharge Planning; Patient and Family Education

- Ensure caregivers and child understand diagnosis, prognosis, follow-up needs with other professionals.
- Provide parents and child with at-home coping strategies (e.g., relaxation, stress relief, movement/exercise).
- Identify child and family supports.
- Provide psychoeducation for caregivers focused on communicating child needs with school.
- Provide psychoeducation and modeling with child to encourage communication with supports (e.g., peers and siblings).

OPPOSITIONAL DEFIANT DISORDER AND CONDUCT DISORDER

Description

- Oppositional defiant disorder (ODD) and conduct disorder (CD) are disruptive and impulse control behavioral disorders that often occur as a means for a child to gain control of their environment. ODD is often a means for the child to gain control over their own life, whereas CD is often a means for the child to gain control through controlling another person's life. Boys are more likely than girls to exhibit both ODD and CD.
  - **Differentiating ODD and CD**
    - **ODD**
      - Angry/irritable mood (e.g., often loses temper, often resentful, easily annoyed)
      - Argumentative/defiant behavior (e.g., argues with authority figures, deliberately annoys others, blames others for own mistakes)
      - Vindictiveness (spiteful or vindictive)

- **CD**
  - Child's behaviors violate the basic rights of others or major age-appropriate societal norms/rules are violated.
  - Aggression to people and animals (e.g., bullies, threatens, is physically cruel, forces someone into sexual activity).
  - Destruction of property (e.g., deliberate fire setting with intent for harm).
  - Deceitfulness or theft (e.g., shoplifting, lies to obtain goods or favors).
  - Serious violation of rules (e.g., runs away from home overnight, truant from school).

Assessment

- Assess for exposure to exposure to abuse, neglect, harsh punishment, household dysfunction (e.g., parental substance use), and other adversity.
- Assess for family history.
- Assess for disruptions in school (e.g., truancy, fighting/bullying, change in performance).
- **CD**: Assess for injuries from risk-taking behaviors.
- Assess for communication style (CD may seem more aggressive and attempt to gain control of room, whereas ODD may simply ignore opportunities to engage and listen for blaming of others for concerns).

Diagnostics

Diagnosis for both ODD and CD should be made by a qualified mental health professional through clinical interviewing and behavior or diagnostic measures.

Nursing Interventions

- Respond consistently to the patient's behaviors (consistency increases sense of control).
- Remain calm, convey unconditional acceptance, and provide a calm space.
- Establish trusting relationship with patient and caregivers.
- Provide clear boundaries and expectations.
- Assist patient in developing social skills (e.g., verbalizing emotions, greeting).
- Role-play situations to help child practice managing stress; improve confidence.
- **CD**: Be alert for potential violent outbursts toward staff and redirect outbursts.

Special Considerations

- Exposure to childhood trauma is highly likely in children diagnosed with ODD and CD.
- Some children with CD will present with limited prosocial emotions (e.g., lack of remorse/guilt, lack of empathy); this does not need to be present for a diagnosis of CD.
- ODD often comorbid with ADHD.

Discharge Planning; Patient and Family Education

- Ensure that patient, if appropriate, and caregivers understand medication plan, understand use of medication (if medication is for ODD or CD, or for a co-occurring disorder), and possible side effects.
- Ensure there is a mental health follow-up scheduled.
- Educate patient and caregivers on the diagnosis, treatment needs, and possible longer-term supports.
- Educate on community resources.
- Educate caregivers of the importance of consistent (at least daily) one-on-one time with child.

SUBSTANCE-RELATED DISORDER (ABUSE)

Description

- Substance-related disorders are psychological disorders related to the recurrent use of a substance that causes physical, mental, emotional, or social impairment and harm. Substance use-related disorders fall under various types: (a) Alcohol-Related, (b) Caffeine-Related, (c) Cannabis-Related, (d) Hallucinogen-Related, (e) Inhalant-Related, (f) Opioid-Related, (g) Sedative-, Hypnotic-, or Anxiolytic-Related, (h) Stimulant-Related, and (i) Tobacco-Related disorders.
  - **Categories:** Each type of substance use-related disorders fall under the following categories:
    - **Use Disorder:** Refers to a problematic pattern that leads to clinically significant impairment or distress
    - **Intoxication:** Use of the related substance that manifested in clinically significant impairment or distress shortly after use (NOTE: not related to a pattern)
    - **Withdrawal:** Physical symptoms related to the cessation or reduction in use of the related substance

Assessment

- Assess for behavioral or social problems (e.g., lack of sustained relationships).
- Assess for physical pain or chronic illness.
- Assess for mood swings.
- Assess for impairments in sleep routine.
- Assess for feigned illness or injury.
- Assess for uncooperative or violent behaviors.
- Assess for physical indications of substance use.
  - Needle marks
  - Constricted or dilated pupils
  - Inflammation or perforation of nasal mucosa or nasal septum
  - Increase in acne

Diagnostics

- Screening to Brief Intervention (S2BI)
- Brief Screener for Tobacco, Alcohol, and Other Drugs (BSTAD)
- National Institute on Alcohol Abuse and Alcoholism (NIAAA) Youth Alcohol Screen (Youth Guide)

Nursing Interventions

- Follow SBIRT (screening, brief intervention, and referral to treatment) for patient care.
- Maintain a nonjudgmental approach.
- Maintain a calm environment (e.g., minimize noise and external stimuli).
- Encourage gradual increase in self-care activities.
- Ensure well-balanced nutritional intake.
- Set clear limits with demanding behaviors.

Special Considerations

- Adolescents are at higher risk than any other age group to have health problems related to their substance use.

- More than 15% of individuals with mental health conditions have co-occurring substance-related conditions.

Discharge Planning; Patient and Family Education

- Ensure referral to psychological/mental health treatment is in place.
- Plan for relapse prevention.
- Educate on signs of withdrawal, if appropriate.
- Educate on resources, such as 12-step groups.
- Promote positive coping skills (e.g., self-care regimen).

SUICIDAL IDEATION

Description

- Suicidal ideation is an umbrella term that covers thoughts and urges related to suicide. Boys take their lives three to four times more than girls.
  - **Related terms**
    - Suicidal thoughts (thoughts of no longer wanting to be alive or killing oneself, thoughts of wanting to die)
    - Suicidal plan (an identified plan to kill oneself that includes steps that the individual identified to carry out the act)
    - Suicidal intent (desire to act on the suicidal thoughts)
    - Suicide attempt (an act that the individual engages in with the intent to die)

Assessment

- Assess for previous attempts.
- Assess for past self-injury.
- Assess for mood changes, depressive or anxious states.
- Assess for behavioral changes (academic performance, risk-taking behaviors, social relationships).
- Assess for changes in attitude or personality.
- Assess for substance use and other risky behaviors (unprotected sex).
- Assess for recent life changes and other stressors.

Diagnostics

- Conduct a suicide assessment.
  - Columbia Suicide Severity Rating Scale
  - IS PATH WARM (Ideation, Substance use, Purposefulness, Anger, Trapped, Hopelessness, Withdrawing, Anxiety, Recklessness, Mood changes)
  - Be direct! (Ask about thoughts to **die**, if the patient intends and wants to **kill** themselves, if the patient has a plan to **die**, if the patient has **access** to the means mentioned in plan)

Nursing Interventions

- Remove any objects and means the patient could use to harm or kill themselves.
- Be direct and open in communication.
- Use developmentally appropriate language, not clinical jargon.
- Teach regulation activities (progressive muscle relaxation, square breathing, mindfulness).
- Support patient to name their feelings and why they are feeling this way.
- Manage your own reactions, keep yourself calm.
- Model for family how to ask suicide risk questions.
- Validate caregivers' discomfort and stress.

Special Considerations

Suicide is the second leading cause of death among teenagers.

Discharge Planning; Patient and Family Education

- Educate patient and caregiver on local and national self-injury and suicide resources (textlines, hotlines, online resources).
- Educate caregivers on warning signs.
- Educate patient and caregivers on follow-up behavioral healthcare.
- Support caregivers in questions to ask, reassure that asking will not increase risk.

TOURETTE SYNDROME

Description

- Tourette Syndrome (TS) is a neurologic disorder that is characterized by sudden, repetitive, and unwanted movement or vocal sounds called tics. Children are typically diagnosed with TS between the ages of 5 and 10, and most before the age of 18. Most people experience their worst symptoms during their teenage years, but the symptoms typically decrease or plateau by late teens to early 20s. TS is more common in boys than girls. The frequency, type, location, and severity may vary, but symptoms will be present for more than 1 year. Children and adolescents can have either simple (sudden, brief, repetitive—limited muscle groups) or complex (coordinated patterns of multiple muscle groups).
- Types of tics
  - Motor tics
    - **Simple:** Eye movements, shoulder shrugging, facial grimacing, head or shoulder jerking
    - **Complex:** Might include facial grimacing with a shoulder shrug. May appear purposeful like a sniffle, hopping, jumping, bending, or touching objects
  - Vocal (phonics) tics
    - **Simple:** Throat clearing, barking, grunting
    - **Complex:** Repeating one's own words or phrases, repeating others' words or phrases, using obscene language, or swear words (coprolalia)

Assessment

- Assess for family history of TS or other tic disorders.
- Assess for decrease in social interactions and functioning.
- Assess for presence of motor and vocal (phonic) tics.
- Assess for increases in hyperactivity and distractibility.
- Assess for increases in aggressive behaviors.

Diagnostics

- Physical and mental health history taking, based on *DSM-5* criteria.
- Most children are diagnosed through referral to neuropsychiatric testing.

Nursing Interventions

- Assist with intervention therapy aimed at habit reversal training.
  - Assisting the child to recognize tic awareness, recognize the premonitory urge that proceeds the tic.
  - Assist child to engage in a voluntary physical behavior until the tic urge subsides (e.g., slow, rhythmic, diaphragmatic breathing).

- Develop a calm and safe environment that minimizes stimuli, including approaching the child/adolescent calmly and quietly in direct eyesight.
- Administer medications as directed.
- Evaluate the child's capacity to engage in daily living activities and provide psychoeducation to child and caregivers that focus on these skills.
- Encourage child and caregivers to express their fears and concerns related to symptoms and potential impacts on child and family.
- Reward positive behaviors and effort.

Special Considerations

Common co-occurring disorders: ADHD, OCD, learning disorders, ASD, and ODD.

Discharge Planning; Patient and Family Education

- Assess if caregivers, and child when developmentally appropriate, have a clear understanding of diagnosis, treatment, follow-up, and warning signs to be aware of; provide psychoeducation where appropriate.
- Ensure caregivers have necessary information for behavioral health and developmental follow-ups.
- Ensure caregivers can access (e.g., transportation, finances) follow-up appointments and medication, as needed.

BIBLIOGRAPHY

American Psychiatric Association. (2013). *Diagnostic and statistical manual of mental disorders* (5th ed.). https://doi.org/10.1176/appi.books.9780890425596

Hockenberry, M., Wilson, D., & Rodgers, C. (2017). *Wong's essentials of pediatric nursing* (10th ed.). Elsevier.

Lippincott Advisor for Education. (2021). https://www.wolterskluwer.com/en/solutions/lippincott-solutions

Meadows, O. (2019). *Pediatric nursing made incredibly easy* (3rd ed.). Wolters Kluwer.

National Institutes of Mental Health. (n.d.). *Health topics.* https://www.nimh.nih.gov/health/topics/index.shtml

National Institute of Neurological and Stroke Disorders. (2021). *Tourette syndrome fact sheet.* https://www.ninds.nih.gov/disorders/patient-caregiver-education/fact-sheets/tourette-syndrome-fact-sheet

Ricci, S., Kyle, T., & Carmen, S. (2021). *Maternity and pediatric nursing* (4th ed.). Wolters Kluwer; American Academy of Pediatrics. https://www.aap.org/en-us/Pages/Default.aspx

Roberts, J., Fenton, G., & Barnard, M. (2015). Developing effective therapeutic relationships with children, young people and their families. *Nursing Children and Young People, 27*(4), 30–5; quiz 36. https://doi.org/10.7748/ncyp.27.4.30.e566

Substance Abuse and Mental Health Services Administration. (2016). DSM-5 *changes: Implications for child serious emotional disturbance.* Substance Abuse and Mental Health Services Administration; *DSM-5* Child Mental Disorder Classification. https://www.ncbi.nlm.nih.gov/books/NBK519712/

Wachman, E. M., Schiff, D. M., & Silverstein, M. (2018). Neonatal abstinence syndrome: Advances in diagnosis and treatment. *JAMA, 319*(13), 1362–1374. https://doi.org/10.1001/jama.2018.2640

KNOWLEDGE CHECK

1. The pediatric nurse is aware that for a child to be diagnosed with ADHD, the provider assesses the

   A. Amount of time for a child to sit still in a busy classroom environment
   B. Intellectual functioning based on standardized testing
   C. Hobbies that the child engages in
   D. Behavioral functioning, both at home and at school

2. The best initial approach in communicating with a 6-year-old child who is autistic and non-speaking would be

   A. Nonverbally, through eye contact and simple gestures
   B. Nonverbally, by touching the child to get their attention
   C. Verbally, by giving full, detailed explanations
   D. Verbally, by using abstract language

3. A school-aged child is resistant to attending any social events unless a family member is present. This behavior is typical of which anxiety disorder?

   A. Depression
   B. OCD
   C. Agoraphobia
   D. Generalized anxiety disorder

4. The pediatric nurse is providing care to a child with a history of panic attacks. Which of the following interventions should be added to the plan of care?

   A. Encourage the child to face their fears
   B. Encourage the use of distraction techniques such as deep breathing during an attack
   C. Assist child and family in identifying anxiety triggers
   D. Establish a calm, safe space for the child and family

5. The nurse is discussing an adolescent's sexuality. Which of the following attitudes would be a blocker to communication?

   A. Accepting
   B. Nonjudgmental
   C. Straightforward
   D. Moralistic

6. The nurse is caring for an adolescent who is hospitalized in an eating disorder unit. The adolescent is observed during mealtimes and for 1 hour after eating. The best explanation for this intervention is to

   A. Develop a trusting relationship
   B. Maintain focus on the importance of nutrition
   C. Prevent purging behaviors
   D. Reinforce the behavioral contract

KNOWLEDGE CHECK

1. **Correct Answer: D) Behavioral functioning, both at home and at school.** According to the *DSM-5* criteria, several inattentive or hyperactive-impulsive symptoms need to be present before 12 years of age and are present in two or more settings, such as at home, school, or work; with friends or relatives; in other activities. There is clear evidence that the symptoms interfere with, or reduce the quality of, social, school, or work functioning and that the symptoms are not better explained by another mental disorder.

2. **Correct Answer: A) Nonverbally, through eye contact and simple gestures.** Gestures and eye contact can build a foundation for language. A common feature of autism and Asperger's is a lack of eye contact. It is important to encourage eye contact that promotes the child to read facial expressions. Children with autism may have sensory issues demonstrated by either over-responsiveness or under-responsiveness. Certain types of touch (light or deep) can feel extremely uncomfortable. Language also needs to be specific and simplified. Language that is concrete with tasks broken down into small steps is best for the child to comprehend. Refrain from using sarcasm and abstract language.

3. **Correct Answer: C) Agoraphobia.** Agoraphobia is a disorder characterized by avoidance of situations in which escape may not be possible or help may be unavailable. According to the patient presentation, the child is exhibiting a behavior typical of agoraphobia. Depression is a mood disorder characterized by persistent periods of sadness or "empty" mood or loss of pleasure in normal activities. OCD is a condition characterized by recurrent obsessions (e.g., recurrent and persistent thoughts, urges, or images) and compulsions (e.g., repetitive behaviors or mental acts). With generalized anxiety disorder, patients experience excessive worry and anxiety, which they find difficult to control and may affect their sleep or ability to concentrate.

4. **Correct Answer: B) Encourage the use of distraction techniques such as deep breathing during an attack.** Distraction techniques that promote relaxation are important. During an anxiety attack, the child may breathe at a faster rate, causing them to feel lightheaded, dizzy, or experience chest pain. Using slow, controlled deep breathing may reduce the physical symptoms of a panic attack and help the panic attack to pass more quickly. Panic attacks are usually in response to certain situations or objects. It is important to encourage them to face their fears carefully graded steps. For example, the child gets panicky in the car, gradually expose them by just sitting in car when parked. Identifying triggers and remaining in control with a calm approach to the child may help to resolve the panicky feelings.

5. **Correct Answer: D) Moralistic.** Blockers to communication are communication tactics that prevent the flow of ideas, possibly ending the discussion on the topic. Nurses who are judgmental, moralistic, and hold on to prejudices will not effectively keep communication flowing and the adolescent may find the nurse to not be trustworthy. Establishing a trusting therapeutic relationship that promotes open dialogue is important. Acceptance, being nonjudgmental and speaking clearly, plainly, and matter-of-factly will most likely facilitate the communication and establish a strong nurse–patient relationship.

6. **Correct Answer: C) Prevent purging behaviors.** Refeeding and normalizing eating behavior are main treatment aims for individuals admitted to inpatient eating disorder units. A structured environment where the adolescent is observed during mealtimes and 1 hour following is designed to prevent opportunities for the adolescent to engaging in purging behaviors. Restricted bathroom use for at least 1 hour after meals is a common intervention as well. Observing mealtimes does not seek to develop a trusting relationship, maintain focus on the importance of nutrition, nor reinforce the behavioral contract, although these are all important aspects of patient recovery.

7. Which of the following clinical manifestations would a nurse assess in an infant diagnosed with NAS?

    A. Tremors and restlessness
    B. Decreased muscle tone
    C. Coordinated suck and swallow reflex
    D. Constipation

8. The pediatric nurse is performing an assessment on a newly admitted adolescent girl diagnosed with anorexia nervosa. Which of the following assessment findings would be expected with this disorder?

    A. Height and weight in the 90% of the growth chart
    B. Irregular or absent menses
    C. Chronic pain in more than one site
    D. Hypertension and tachycardia

9. Which statement is true about the infant diagnosed with NAS?

    A. Methadone treatment by the mother will prevent withdrawal reaction in newborns
    B. Meconium sampling for fetal drug exposure is less accurate than neonatal urine sampling for looking at long-term usage
    C. Mothers of NAS infants do not want the pregnancy or the infant
    D. The most severe symptoms are observed in the infants of mothers who have taken large amounts of drugs over a long period

10. The pediatric nurse is teaching a couple how to use positive reinforcement techniques with their child. The nurse should make which of the following recommendations:

    A. Reward positive behaviors to promote their recurrence
    B. Control their child's behavior so there is no opportunity to misbehave
    C. Manipulate the child's environment to avoid negative interactions
    D. Use firmer discipline techniques until behavior is controlled

7. **Correct Answer: A) Tremors and restlessness.** Although the presentation of NAS can be variable, withdrawal symptoms most commonly seen in neonates are tremors, irritability, decreased sleep intervals, high-pitched cry, increased muscle tone, hyperactive reflexes, poor feeding, diarrhea, dehydration, poor weight gain, fever, mottling, and temperature instability. NAS neonates are more likely to display an abnormal, uncoordinated suck and swallow reflex.

8. **Correct Answer: B) Irregular or absent menses.** Physical signs of anorexia nervosa may include menstrual irregularities (amenorrhea). Anorexia nervosa is an eating disorder characterized by weight loss (or lack of appropriate weight gain in growing children); difficulties maintaining an appropriate body weight for height, age, and stature; and, in many individuals, distorted body image. It is characterized by a height and weight of less than 85% below average, according to the growth chart. Vital sign changes found in patients with anorexia nervosa include hypotension, bradycardia, and hypothermia. Chronic pain in more than one site is associated with somatoform pain disorder.

9. **Correct Answer: D) The most severe symptoms are observed in the infants of mothers who have taken large amounts of drugs over a long period.** Withdrawal symptoms are more severe for neonates whose mothers were chronic abusers. Additionally, symptoms are milder for premature infants. Since methadone is an opioid medication, infants exposed to it during pregnancy can experience signs of withdrawal after birth. Using methadone will help to get the pregnant mother away from using illicit drugs and onto a monitored regimen in conjunction with prenatal care, making both mother and infant safer throughout and following pregnancy. Withdrawal for pregnant women is especially dangerous because it causes the uterus to contract and may bring on miscarriage or premature birth. Meconium sampling is more accurate than urine, as it reflects drug use during the last two trimesters of pregnancy. The major disadvantage for urine toxicology is the short detection window; urine provides maternal drug use data only for a few days prior to delivery. Many mothers want their infant and desire to care for their infant; therefore, it is incorrect to assume mothers of NAS infants are any different.

10. **Correct Answer: A) Reward positive behaviors to promote their recurrence.** Positive reinforcement as a form of positive discipline founded upon the notion that children respond better to praise than they do to criticism or correction. By providing praiseful recognition, children are more likely to repeat behaviors (e.g., being kind to others, cleaning up their room) because they like the good feelings that come with positive attention. Controlling the child's behavior, manipulating the child's environment, and using firmer discipline techniques all do not ascribe to positive reinforcement strategies.

CHAPTER 17

Special Developmental Needs

Maryanne Halligan

INTRODUCTION

- Approximately 20% of children under the age of 18 have a special healthcare need.
- Diagnosis that incurs chronic developmental, physical, emotional, and behavioral condition that will require needs from the healthcare team that are beyond the type of care required by children.
- The children in this category will require multiple services from many different healthcare teams.
- The number of children living with the assistance of high-tech medical equipment and treatments is growing rapidly.
- Developmental concerns from infancy through adolescence occurs because of the illness and the physical and emotional delay experienced.
- Families experience increased stress because of the expectations and hope for the child have been altered. Life is also altered due to the physical needs of the child, technology, and frequent visits to and from healthcare clinicians.
- Some children may have an injury that requires long rehabilitation and technology to support their life.

FETAL ALCOHOL SYNDROME

Description

- This syndrome is associated with maternal alcohol consumption. There is no evidence on a safe time to drink or amount of alcohol consumed during pregnancy that would not affect the fetus or child long term.
- There is some evidence that suggests alcohol consumption in large quantities during the first trimester will contribute to facial dysmorphic features; also, the evidence suggests that alcohol use during the second and third trimesters may not contribute to facial features but will increase the incidence of adverse brain development causing a spectrum of disorders.
- Classic dysmorphic facial features include narrow forehead, small nose and midface, short palpebral fissures, deficient philtrum, and a long, thin upper lip (Figure 17.1). Intellectual disability (ID) is frequently associated as well.
- **Fetal Alcohol Spectrum Disorders (FASD):** Umbrella term associated with disorders and features caused by maternal alcohol consumption during pregnancy; fetal alcohol syndrome (FAS), the most severe classification within FASD, is considered the full-blown syndrome that includes every diagnostic feature of FASD.

314 FETAL ALCOHOL SYNDROME

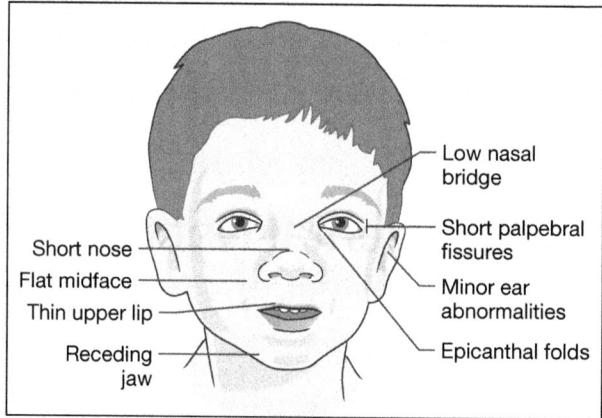

FIGURE 17.1: Typical facies noted with fetal alcohol syndrome. Note the thin upper lip and long philtrum

Source: Reprinted from Chiocca, E. M. (2021). *Advanced pediatric assessment* (3rd ed.). Springer Publishing Company.

Assessment

- Prenatal assessment for susceptibility to alcohol.
- Physical assessment at birth and in neonatal stages for dysmorphic features, growth deficiency and microcephaly.
- Assess developmental delay, cognitive and social abnormalities, and/or psychiatric conditions with a confirmed or a suspicion of maternal alcohol consumption.
- Assess sleep patterns in infancy and through childhood.
- Assess feeding and regurgitation during infancy.
- Assess for congenital heart defects, typically atrial septal defect (ASD) or ventricular septal defect (VSD).
- Assess the preschool-and school-aged child for hyperactivity and attention deficit.
- Assess for restless legs that may occur in infancy or in preschool-or school-aged children.

Diagnostics

- History of maternal alcohol use during pregnancy
- Clinical features
- Echocardiogram for congenital heart defect
- Four-digit diagnostic code (Table 17.1)

Nursing Interventions

- Height, weight, and head circumference should be followed through preschool age.
- These children may forget daily rules, especially those associated with activities of daily living (ADLs). Instruct families to reinforce rules daily.

TABLE 17.1: Four-Digit Diagnostic Code for Fetal Alcohol Syndrome

Growth deficiency	None 1, mild 2, moderate 3, significant 4
Facial dysmorphic features	None 1, mild 2, moderate 3, severe 4
CNS damage	None 1, mild 2, probable 3, definite 4
Prenatal alcohol consumption	None 1, unknown 2, probable 3, high risk 4

CNS, central nervous system.

Source: Adapted from Astley, S. J. (2004). *Diagnostic guide for fetal alcohol spectrum disorders: The 4-digit diagnostic code* (3rd ed.). FAS Diagnostic Prevention Network, University of Washington.

- Discuss regular bedtime routines to assist with insomnia. May recommend melatonin to assist with falling asleep.
- Provide supportive measures for the child to succeed in school.

Special Considerations

- Prevention is key: Educate child-bearing persons about not drinking during pregnancy or if planning a pregnancy. Discuss adverse effects on fetus and child.
- Children with this syndrome are subject to further family distress since the primary cause is due to a substance use disorder of the mother.
- Family treatment should be a primary goal. Assist mother in finding a treatment program. Children who are born with this syndrome may be placed in foster care until the mother has been treated for her substance use disorder.
- If a child exhibits the signs of FASD, the child may have already been exposed to substance use disorder in the home and social work should be involved to assure the safety of the child.

Discharge Planning; Patient and Family Education

- Educate the guardian of the potential signs and symptoms that may develop.
- Educate guardian that the child may have frequent spitting up and difficulty eating. Use specialized nipples and follow-up with pediatrician.
- Provide education regarding promoting sleep.

FRAGILE X SYNDROME

Description

- Most common inherited disorder that can cause ID and autism. The phenotype is caused by inactivation of the *FMR1* gene.
- The manifestations occur mostly in boys (mutation on X chromosome) and can be subtle until developmental milestones are delayed.
- Newborns with this disorder may appear completely normal. Signs and symptoms will relate to poor muscle tone, feeding problems, and chronic otitis media (OM).
- Physical manifestations may develop later in age. These include macrocephaly, tall forehead, elongated narrow face, large ears, and prominent jaw. Other manifestations include flat feet, droopy shoulders, related to muscle hypotonia, and macroorchidism (enlarged testes).
- Epilepsy can appear between 4 and 10 years of age. This occurs in about 20% of the children with FXS.
- Pathophysiologic changes in the brain include decreased size of the posterior cerebellar vermis and enlarged fourth ventricle.
- Although it is rare for females to have FXS, this can occur, and the physical features are similar to males. Ovarian insufficiency will occur in about 20% of the cases.

Assessment

- During infancy, identify any change in the child's growth and development.
- Assess motor development and feeding difficulties in infancy.
- Assess ability to walk and talk at the correct age.
- Assess physical attributes as the child becomes older if associated with developmental and physical delay.
- Assess for seizure activity that may be associated with sleeping.
- Assess for autism-like symptoms and behavioral disorders as the child progresses to school age.

Diagnostics

- Genetic blood test and/or prenatal testing
- MRI
- EEG if suspicious of seizures

Nursing Interventions

- Refer to genetic counselling especially if there are siblings involved.
- Assure that appropriate referrals are made to physical therapists, behavioral therapists, and occupational therapists.
- Refer to neurologist and cardiologist especially as the child grows into adulthood.
- Assure that ophthalmology and orthopedics are involved, especially if there is strabismus or flat feet identified.
- **Early intervention:** Speech and language therapist with experience working with FXS should be consulted.

Special Considerations

Families with a history of unexplained ID in boys should be considered for FXS.

Discharge Planning; Patient and Family Education

- Supportive care for the family.
- Assure the family has the supportive services for outpatient physical therapy, occupational therapy, and speech therapy.

HYPOXIC ISCHEMIC ENCEPHALOPATHY

Description

- This disorder is a major cause for neurologic disabilities in the term infant. Complications may include cerebral palsy and hearing/visual/speech/language impairments.
- There are numerous conditions that can occur that will interrupt cerebral blood flow. This will cause hypoxia and decrease glucose in the brain.
- Conditions that lead to hypoxic insult include placental abruption, umbilical cord compression, and uterine rupture. There are different phases of recovery once the brain is reperfused.
- Latent is the first hour to 6 hours, cell death occurs causing swelling and inflammation.
- Secondary phase includes seizures and mitochondrial death; this occurs over 6 to 12 hours.
- Tertiary phase occurs over the next 3 days to months after the injury. There will be late cell death and remodeling.

Assessment

- Assess Apgar scores, neurologic status, respiratory effort, tone.
- Assess infant through growth for seizure activity and neurologic function.
- Assess respiratory status as the infant grows. Implement respiratory support as required.
- Assess temperature.

Diagnostics

Clinical features

Nursing Interventions

- Infants may require ventilator support via a tracheostomy. Assess for signs of respiratory distress and suction as needed.

- Monitor for signs and symptoms of hypothermia. Temperature instability can be found throughout growth and development. Warmer beds should be utilized until the infant is able to maintain normal temperature 98.06°F (36.7°C) with bundling and blankets.
- Monitor nutritional status and ability to feed. Most infants have poor suck and swallow and will require a gastrostomy tube.
- Cooling procedures with a cooling blanket may be initiated 1 to 6 hours after birth and continue for 24 to 72 hours. Infants should be warmed slowly as per the hospital guidelines.

Special Considerations

- Infants who suffer from this disorder will have lifelong interaction with healthcare clinicians. Family support should be initiated and continued throughout the life of the child.
- Depending on the severity of the injury, and if cooling was successful, some families may face discussions with palliative care clinicians and receive support regarding quality-of-life questions and answers.

Discharge Planning; Patient and Family Education

- Determine discharge planning regarding technological support required in the home and home care nursing assistance.
- Discuss signs and symptoms of potential complications and what to do about them.
- Instruct the family on car seat safety as well as car seat use.
- Identify follow-up support for the family.
- Instruct the family on medication use and administration.
- Provide instructions for all special procedures, artificial airway care, suctioning, artificial feeding, and stimulation.
- Support infant–parent bonding and assess the parent's emotional status.

MITOCHONDRIAL DISORDERS

Description

- Mitochondria are essential to the cell's production of energy. Mitochondrial disease will interrupt that energy production and cause compromise to cellular function.
  - Organs most affected are brain and muscle because they rely on high energy to continue to function.
  - This can cause a variety of disorders in infants and children including intellectual and physical disabilities.
  - The prevalence of disorders from this is usually underestimated because of the variety of symptoms.
  - Mitochondrial disease onset can occur either in the neonate, which is usually more severe form with a high mortality rate, or in early childhood and can have varying degrees of severity.

Assessment

- Assess for hypotonia, nystagmus, neurologic impairment, and seizures, especially in the newborn period.
- Assess feeding difficulty, gastrointestinal (GI) dysmotility (constipation and vomiting).
- Assess for hepatomegaly, liver failure, and hypoglycemia.
- Assess for ataxia, muscle weakness, hearing loss.
- Assess for cardiac failure of unknown etiology.
- Assess for hematologic disorders such as pancytopenia or anemia.

Diagnostics

Muscle biopsy with genetic testing

Nursing Interventions

- Supportive care for families should be a priority when mitochondrial disorders occur.
- Multiple symptoms may occur throughout the child's life span, so it is important to work with families and assist with their navigation through the healthcare system.
- Some children will have frequent hospitalizations to receive high glucose intravenous (IV) therapy which will invigorate the mitochondria and may decrease symptoms.
- Provide assistance with ADLs as needed.
- Monitor for skin breakdown and if incontinent, keep skin dry.
- Positioning may be required for patients.
- Administer feeds and medications via G-tube if present. Identify issues with feeding and constipation.

Special Considerations

- Early intervention with social work and other services will assist the family with supportive measures for the home.
- Children with decreased motor ability and decreased developmental ability will need care and assistance constantly.
- Families can be directed through foundations and social security disability to assist with the financial needs of special equipment, such as wheelchairs, supplies for assisting with bathing, computers.

Discharge Planning; Patient and Family Education

- Discharge teaching will focus on the current needs of the child.
- If nursing care assistance is required, then families will be supported.
- Early intervention measures to help with socialization, physical, and occupational therapies may be instituted to optimize quality of life.
- Instruct families on the care of increased seizures and medication administration.
- Instruct families to monitor for changes in breathing, any fevers, since children with weakened muscles may be susceptible to pneumonias.
- Patients with feeding issues and failure to thrive may require a G-tube for feeding. Instruct families on how to care for the G-tube and administer feeding.

PREMATURE INFANT MEDICAL DISORDERS

Description

- Premature birth is a worldwide health issue, and in the United States one in eight births are delivered prematurely. Many of these neonates require technological intervention and spend time in the NICU.
- Children born very preterm, approximately 5% to 10%, may have significant neurologic deficits including motor, cognitive, behavioral, and sensory. After 30 weeks' gestation, most neonates develop without neurologic defects.
- Most prominent defect includes cerebral palsy (refer to Chapter 5) which is classified as a disorder that affects the child's ability to move.
- Mortality for neonates is also dependent on gestational age, with very preterm infants having the highest mortality.
- Preterm infants may suffer from lung disease because of the lack of lung development and poor surfactant production.
- Respiratory Distress Syndrome (RDS) occurs when the neonate has low surfactant production along with underdeveloped lungs.
- High oxygen delivery for the preterm infant will cause injury to the lung and will lead to chronic lung disease (bronchopulmonary dysplasia [BPD]). This contributes to lifelong complications in the respiratory system and may lead to frequent hospitalizations.

Assessment

- Assess preterm neonates for respiratory distress, cyanosis. If tracheostomy is present, suction as needed (Pediatric Skills 17.1 and 17.2).
- Assess temperature regulation. Hypothermia is noted to increase oxygen demand, mortality, apnea, and poor weight gain.
- Assess growth and nutrition. Monitor fluid status by assessing fontanels.
- Assess muscle tone and flexion.
- Assess for abnormal head circumference, movements, or poor neurologic response.
- Assess for heart murmurs.

PEDIATRIC SKILL 17.1: SUCTION OF A TRACHEOSTOMY TUBE

- Obtain suction catheter and kit.
- Perform personal protective equipment (PPE).
- Open suction kit with aseptic technique. Place sterile gloves on, and with dominant hand, take sterile suction catheter and wrap in hand to keep from contamination.
- Do not routinely use sterile saline for suctioning.
- Assure that the suction pressure is less than 10 cm Hg with nondominant hand. Connect the suction tubing with nondominant hand to the catheter and test the suction with thumb of dominant hand on Y port of catheter.
- Insert catheter down the tracheostomy tube without occluding Y port (without suctioning) to predetermined length. Gently apply intermittent suction as you withdraw the catheter for 5 to 10 seconds.
- Pause for oxygenation for at least 30 seconds and repeat as necessary.

PEDIATRIC SKILL 17.2: TRACHEOSTOMY SECUREMENT DEVICE CHANGE

- Position patient lying flat. Perform PPE and don clean gloves.
- A second person should assist to hold the tracheostomy in place as the ties or securement device is removed. The person holding the tracheostomy should do so with the thumb and pointer finger across the faceplate.
- Remove one side and assess the skin under the securement device, clean with soap and water. Place the clean ties on the empty side of the faceplate, repeat the same on the other side.
- Assure one finger depth between the ties and skin underneath.

Diagnostics

- Blood work that includes complete blood count (CBC), glucose, and blood gas
- Daily weights
- Head ultrasound
- Echocardiogram
- Electromyography (EMG)
- MRI

Nursing Interventions

- Administer oxygen as required by the newborn. Promote adequate respiratory effort and support breathing with mechanical devices.
- Maintain thermoregulation by using warming devices and radiation heat. May encourage kangaroo care with the mother or caregivers to assist with reducing hypothermia.
- Promote nutrition and fluid balance. Monitor intake and output carefully (Pediatric Skill 17.3).

TRISOMY 21 (DOWN SYNDROME)

- Measure daily weights.
- Monitor for feeding intolerance and encourage breastfeeding as tolerated.
- Monitor for signs and symptoms of infection. Use disposable equipment for the neonate.
- Encourage stimulation with parents, skin-to-skin contact, nutritive sucking.
- Cluster care to support rest when the newborn displays symptoms of overstimulation.
- Manage pain both in pharmacologic and nonpharmacologic fashion.
- Promote parent–infant bonding. Support the family and assist with coping.

Special Considerations

- Premature infants will have lifelong needs from the healthcare system.
- Provide ongoing support throughout the life span of the child to the family.
- Cognitive deficits may be difficult to identify in the infancy stage, so continued support and assessment for families is crucial.

Discharge Planning; Patient and Family Education

- Determine discharge planning regarding technological support required in the home.
- Discuss signs and symptoms of potential complications and what to do about them.
- Instruct the family on car seat safety as well as car seat use.
- Identify follow-up support for the family.
- Instruct the family on medication use and administration.
- Provide instructions for all special procedures, dressings, ostomy care, artificial airway care, suctioning, artificial feeding, and stimulation.
- Provide support for infant–parent bonding and assess the parent's emotional status.
- Assure appropriate equipment needs and home care plan as needed.
- Postoperative incision care for G-tube placement. Maintain the site and keep the area dry, clean, and maintained as described in Pediatric Skill 17.3.

PEDIATRIC SKILL 17.3 CARING FOR A GASTROSTOMY TUBE

- After the insertion of the tube, care for the insertion site using a cotton-tipped applicator soaked in sterile water. Do not raise the disk while sutures are present.
- When the site has healed, use a wet washcloth with soap to cleanse around the site.
- Pat the skin dry.
- Leave the site open to air unless there is drainage present. A gauze pad with slit may be used to capture drainage. Apply skin barrier or protectant to prevent skin breakdown.
- If patient has a Mic Key G-tube, once a week check the balloon by holding the tube in place with one hand (nondominant) and use the other hand to attach a nonslip syringe. Withdraw the fluid and then use sterile water to reinflate balloon.
- For feeding with a Mic Key G-tube attach the extension set and then attach the kangaroo bag to the feeding opening. Assure that the second port is completely closed. If administering medications flush with 3 mL to 10 mL of water to assure patency is maintained unless contraindicated.

TRISOMY 21 (DOWN SYNDROME)

Description

- A genetic disorder that is classified by an extra chromosome on the 21st chromosome caused by nondisjunction or translocation. This abnormality is the most common one associated with ID.

- Nearly one in 730 live births will result in Trisomy 21. The likelihood of having a child with this disorder will increase in relation to maternal age.
- There are common physical features that are part of this syndrome such as slanted eyes, flatter face, shorter neck, protruding tongue, poor muscle tone, shorter in height, small ears, Brushfield spots in eyes (white spots on iris), and small hands (may have simian crease) and feet.
- ID may vary as well with some children having an IQ that is low normal and most children are slow to speak.
- Congenital heart disease occurs in 50% of the children born with Trisomy 21.
- Hearing and vision problems occur in about 75% of the children and there is high incidence of thyroid disease.

Assessment

- Prenatal screening is performed routinely and will contribute to early diagnosis. Refer to genetic counselor.
- Risk factors for this include maternal age greater than 35, and poor prenatal care.
- Infants are usually diagnosed 1 to 2 days after birth due to the classic facial features associated with Trisomy 21. Some of these features include eyes that slant upward, small ears, small mouth that might make the tongue appear large, a short neck, and a small nose with a flattened bridge.
- Important assessments should focus on heart defects, hearing tests, thyroid disease, hematologic disorders, GI disorders, sucking or feeding problems, hypotonia, atlantoaxial instability, and delay reaching growth and development milestones.

Diagnostics

- Perform prenatal tests on the mother between 11 and 18 weeks of gestational age including alpha-fetoprotein in maternal blood. Ultrasound may demonstrate nuchal cord translucency.
- Tests that are performed after birth include a chromosomal analysis to confirm Trisomy 21.
- Echocardiogram to determine presence of congenital heart disease.
- Thyroid testing to determine if hypothyroidism is present.
- Ultrasound to determine any GI malformations or dysfunction.
- Hearing and vision screening to detect any abnormalities.
- Cervical x-ray to determine if atlantoaxial instability is present.

Nursing Interventions

- Support for families and children with this disorder is a key role of the nurse.
- Provide resources such as early intervention as early as possible to promote growth and development. Other support services will assist the family with coping and managing the frequent visits to the hospital or clinician's office.
- Promote nutrition, prevent complications, and recognize that children with Trisomy 21 will have slower growth development.

Discharge Planning; Patient and Family Education

- Provide emotional support to the family. Consider resources that will connect families with Trisomy 21.
- Hearing and vision tests should occur every 6 months.
- Performing hand hygiene will assist with decreasing infection.
- Monitor for signs and symptoms of respiratory viruses and/or ear infections.
- When performing a potentially hurtful procedure, prepare the child based on the developmental age, not the chronological age.

- Instruct families to report any changes in gait, weakness or tingling in the arms and legs, changes in bladder function, or stiffness in neck. This should be evaluated immediately with a cervical x-ray.
- Refer to interprofessional team (e.g., pediatric cardiologist, audiologist, ophthalmologist, occupational/physical/speech therapy).

PEDIATRIC PEARLS

CARE OF THE CHILD WITH SPECIAL DEVELOPMENTAL NEEDS

- Parents, siblings, grandparents, and all family members are a part of the care for any child with special developmental needs.
- Parents struggle with keeping the family unit as normal as possible. Frequent doctor visits, therapy sessions, physical needs of the child, and the emotional impact of loss play a significant role in how families cope with the chronic illness associated with children who have special developmental needs.
- It is important to identify support systems early and always have conversations about symptom management. There is a financial impact that may occur as well; social work can assist with care coordination.

BIBLIOGRAPHY

Back, S., & Miller, S. (2014). Brain injury in premature neonates: A primary cerebral dysmaturation disorder? *Annals of Neurology*, 75(4), 469–486. https://doi.org/10.1002/ana.24132

Boston Children's Hospital. (2021). *Feeding tube service*. https://www.childrenshospital.org/centers-and-services/programs/f-_-n/feeding-tube-service/patient-resources/three-column-page

Boston Children's Hospital. (2021). *Rhett syndrome/diagnosis and treatment*. https://www.childrenshospital.org/conditions-and-treatments/conditions/r/rett-syndrome/diagnosis-and-treatments

Bull, M. J., & Committee on Genetics. (2011). From the American academy of pediatrics: Clinical Report: Health supervision for children with Down syndrome. *Pediatrics*, 128(2), 393–406. http://pediatrics.aappublications.org/content/128/2/393.full

Centers for Disease Control and Prevention. (2020). *Facts about Down syndrome*. https://www.cdc.gov/ncbddd/birthdefects/downsyndrome.html

Centers for Disease Control and Prevention. (2021). *Fetal alcohol spectrum disorders*. https://www.cdc.gov/ncbddd/fasd/index.html

Douglas-Escobar, M., & Weiss, M. D. (2015). Hypoxic-Ischemic encephalopathy: A review for the clinician. *JAMA Pediatric*, 169(4), 397–403. https://doi.org/10.1001/jamapediatrics.2014.3269

Fernández Carvajal, I., & Aldridge, D. (2011). *Understanding fragile X syndrome a guide for families and professionals*. Jessica Kingsley Publishers.

Lissauer, T., & Anderson, M. (2016). *Neonatology at a glance* (3rd ed.). Wiley Blackwell.

March of Dimes. (n.d.). *Prematurity campaign*. http://www.marchofdimes.com/mission/prematurity-campaign.aspx

May, P., Tabachnick, B., Gossage, J., Kalberg, W., Marais, A., Robinson, L., Manning, M., Buckley, D., & Hoyme, H. (2011). Maternal risk factors predicting child physical characteristics and dysmorphology in fetal alcohol syndrome and partial fetal alcohol syndrome. *Drug and Alcohol Dependence*, 119(1), 18–27.

Popova, S., Lange, S., Probst, C., Gmel, G., & Rehm, J. (2017). Estimation of national, regional, and global prevalence of alcohol use during pregnancy and fetal alcohol syndrome: A systematic review and meta-analysis. *The lancet global health*, 5(3), e290–e299. https://doi.org/10.1016/S2214-109X(17)30021-9

Saneto, R. P. (2010). Disorders of mitochondrial metabolism. In S. Goldstein & C. R. Reynolds (Eds.), *Handbook of neurodevelopmental and genetic disorders in children* (2nd ed.; pp. 512–538). The Guilford Press.

Spohr, H., Noort, B., & Wolter, H. (2018). *Fetal alcohol syndrome: A lifelong challenge*. De Gruyter. https://doi.org/doi.org/10.1515/9783110436563

Taylor, C., Lynn, P., & Bartlett, J. L. (2012). *Lippincott course point for Taylor: Fundamentals of nursing*. (Course Point). https://coursepoint.vitalsource.com/#/books/9781975101336/

Thompson, C. E. (1999). *Raising a child with a neuromuscular disorder: A guide for parents, grandparents, friends, and professionals*. Oxford University Press.

Willemsen, R., & Kooy, F. (2017). *Fragile x syndrome: From genetics to targeted treatment*. Academic Press.

KNOWLEDGE CHECK

1. A 36-year-old mother arrives in the hospital in labor at 32 weeks. She states that she has had no prenatal care. The infant is born and appears to have a short neck, eyes that slant upward, and a small nose. The nurse suspects which developmental disorder?

   A. Trisomy 21
   B. FXS
   C. Mitochondrial disorder
   D. Premature infant disorder

2. An infant with the diagnosis of Trisomy 21 is admitted with a history of poor feeding, diaphoresis, fatigue, and increase respiratory rate. What diagnostic test is the priority?

   A. Chest x-ray
   B. Arterial blood gas test
   C. Echocardiogram
   D. Ultrasound of abdomen

3. A 10-year-old female with a primary diagnosis of Trisomy 21 is admitted for dysuria. She begins to complain about her legs falling asleep and feeling funny. What does the nurse anticipate as a priority for this patient?

   A. Obtain a cervical x-ray
   B. Obtain a chest x-ray
   C. Obtain a renal ultrasound
   D. Administer antibiotics for a urinary infection

4. The mother of a well-presenting 1-year-old female arrives to the clinic and states that her daughter is having difficulty falling asleep, is hyperactive, and complains of her legs "not sitting still." Upon assessment, the nurse notes a long, smooth philtrum and microcephaly. The nurse should have a high suspicion for which disorder?

   A. FAS
   B. Mitochondrial disorder
   C. Autism spectrum disorder
   D. FXS

5. A 6-month-old male who has a history of being diagnosed with FXS is admitted to the pediatric unit with difficulty breathing and OM. He is diagnosed with pneumonia. A possible contributing factor to the development of this infection is:

   A. Gastroesophageal reflux and microaspiration
   B. Immune disorder related to the diagnosis of Rhett syndrome
   C. An increase in seizure activity
   D. Presence of precious teeth development

6. A 3-month-old female with a history of hypoxic ischemic encephalopathy (HIE) and failure to thrive is admitted for G-tube insertion. Discharge instructions for the family include which of the following?

   A. Cleanse the area daily with an alcohol-based solution
   B. Cover the area with an occlusive dressing
   C. Check balloon of Mic Key button G-tube once a week
   D. Change Mic Key button G-tube once a month

KNOWLEDGE CHECK

1. **Correct Answer: A) Trisomy 21.** Infants born with Trisomy 21 often present with the following features: eyes that slant upward, small ears, small mouth that might make the tongue appear large, a short neck, and a small nose with a flattened bridge. The patient presentation does not align with FXS, mitochondrial disorder, nor premature infant disorder.

2. **Correct Answer: C) Echocardiogram.** Infants with Trisomy 21 have a high risk of congenital heart disorders, so an echocardiogram is the highest priority. The Echocardiogram would allow visualization of any cardiac defect anomaly that could be associated with this patient's history of Down syndrome (Trisomy 21). The most common heart disorder is atrioventricular (AV) canal defect, and the second most common is VSD, both of which would be revealed visually through an echocardiogram. Poor feeding, diaphoresis, fatigue, and an increase in respiratory rate are signs and symptoms of a cardiac defect or condition. Due to the patient presentation, a chest x-ray, arterial blood gas test, and ultrasound are not as important as an echocardiogram in determining the heart function and possible congenital anomalies.

3. **Correct Answer: A) Obtain a cervical x-ray.** Atlantoaxial instability, characterized by neck pain, paresthesia, bowel and bladder dysfunction, and gait disturbance, can occur in a child with Trisomy 21 and should be identified immediately. A cervical x-ray will be the only test to confirm this diagnosis.

4. **Correct Answer: D) FAS.** FAS is classically characterized by dysmorphic facial features, growth deficits, and central nervous system (CNS) conditions. According to the presentation, mitochondrial disorder, autism spectrum disorder, and FXS is not suspected.

5. **Correct Answer: A) Gastroesophageal reflux and microaspiration.** FXS is the most common inherited form of ID. Gastroesophageal reflux and swallowing difficulties are frequently seen in children with FXS, leading to microaspiration and lung and ear infections. Rett syndrome is a rare genetic neurologic disorder that occurs primarily in girls and more rarely in boys; the disorder is like FXS, but is distinct, so it would not be a contributing factor to the development of OM and pneumonia in a child with FXS. Although epilepsy can be associated with Fragile X disorder, it is unlikely that this would be the cause of the OM and pneumonia. The eruption of teeth, which usually begins around 6 months of age, should not be a factor in this presentation.

6. **Correct Answer: C) Check balloon of Mic Key button G-tube once a week.** It is important to ensure that the integrity of the balloon remains intact so that the button G-tube does not dislodge. Clean the area with soap and water, occlusive dressings should not be used, and changing the G-tube is not recommended.

7. An 8-month-old infant born prematurely with a history of a 7-week stay in the NICU is admitted to the hospital with respiratory distress. This is the third time since discharge from the NICU. What is the most likely rationale for the frequent hospitalization following the NICU discharge?
   A. Preterm infants are more susceptible to lung infections
   B. Preterm infants administered oxygen are more likely to acquire BPD
   C. Preterm infants tend to have a poor immunity
   D. Preterm infants may have neuromuscular deficits that impair respiratory effort

8. An infant is admitted with a tracheostomy for issues handling secretions after being born with a diagnosis of HIE. The infant currently has humidified oxygen at night. While being assessed, the patient begins to become cyanotic and appears to be drooling more. Which nursing intervention should be the first priority for this patient?
   A. Administer a nebulized treatment via the tracheostomy
   B. Perform suction via the tracheostomy using aseptic technique
   C. Provide 100% oxygen via tracheostomy and notify clinician
   D. Immediately change tracheostomy because the infant has a plugged tracheostomy

9. Mitochondrial disorders in infancy cause a high mortality rate. Which organ is most affected by mitochondrial disorders?
   A. Brain
   B. Lungs
   C. Heart
   D. Liver

10. Parents raising a child with special developmental needs face many challenges. A parent of a 7-year-old who suffers from a significant intellectual and developmental disability and is nonverbal states during a routine visit to the nurse, "I am so tired, I can't sleep, and I feel very overwhelmed with everything." The most appropriate response for the nurse is:
    A. "I hear you say that you are tired, I wonder if your sleep is being interrupted."
    B. "It must be hard some days, what kind of support do you have at home?"
    C. The nurse sits down, says nothing at first, and then says, "How can I help?"
    D. "I will talk to the doctor about prescribing something to help with your anxiety."

KNOWLEDGE CHECK

7. **Correct Answer: B) Preterm infants administered oxygen are more likely to acquire BPD.** Preterm infants administered oxygen is most likely to account for the frequent hospitalizations after NICU discharge because preterm infants generally require some oxygen support which may lead to a chronic lung condition known as BPD where there is airway damage, and tissue destruction (dysplasia). BPD can cause longer-term complications. Patients with BPD are often more at risk for respiratory infections, such as influenza (the flu), respiratory syncytial virus (RSV), and pneumonia. And when they get an infection, they tend to get sicker than most children do. Although it is likely that the rationale may be that preterm infants are more susceptible to lung infections, preterm infants tend to have a poor immunity, and preterm infants may have neuromuscular deficits that impair respiratory effort, the presentation points to BPD as a result of oxygen administration to the preterm infant.

8. **Correct Answer: B) Perform suction via the tracheostomy using aseptic technique.** Tracheostomies must be evaluated and suctioned as needed or at the minimum every 4 hours for children, especially those children with decreased neurologic status related to poor perfusion and hypoxemia at birth. Administering the nebulized treatment or providing 100% oxygen via the tracheostomy will not be effective until the airway obstruction (e.g., mucous, secretions) has been removed by tracheal suctioning. It is not likely that the tracheostomy is plugged, therefore it should not be immediately changed.

9. **Correct Answer: A) Brain.** The brain relies on high energy, especially as it develops during infancy and childhood. Mitochondria provide that energy; therefore, any disorders associated with this crucial energy source will affect how the brain functions.

10. **Correct Answer: C) The nurse sits down, says nothing at first, and then says, "How can I help?"** Although acknowledging and validating the parent's concerns can be considered therapeutic communication, silence can be a more effective way to elicit important information from parents feeling overwhelmed with caring for a child with a chronic illness that also has a significant developmental delay.

CHAPTER 18

Child Maltreatment and Neglect

Angela Karakachian and Maryanne Halligan

INTRODUCTION

- Defined as "a recent act or failure to act on the part of a parent or caretaker which results in death, serious physical or emotional harm, sexual abuse or exploitation; or an act or failure to act which presents an imminent risk of serious harm" (U.S. Department of Health and Human Services, 2020), child maltreatment is a universal concern.
- Child maltreatment covers a broad spectrum of abuse including physical abuse, sexual abuse, and neglect, and victims of child maltreatment suffer lifelong physiologic and psychological consequences (Cicchetti, 2016).
- In 2019, in the United States, Child Protective Services received over three million reports of child maltreatment suspicion, and over 600,000 of these reports were confirmed cases of child maltreatment (U.S. Department of Health and Human Services Children's Bureau, 2019).
- In 2019, it is estimated that over 1,800 children died as a consequence of child maltreatment (U.S. Department of Health and Human Services Children's Bureau, 2019).
- Almost 80% of victims of child abuse suffer from single type of maltreatment, and over 15% suffer from two or more types of maltreatment (U.S. Department of Health and Human Services Children's Bureau, 2019).

BACKGROUND

- According to U.S. Department of Health and Human Services (2019):
  - Over 77% of perpetrators are a parent of the victim.
  - Child neglect is the most single maltreatment accounting for over 60% of cases.
  - Child physical abuse accounts for 10% of cases of child maltreatment.
  - Children who are in their first year of life have the highest rate of victimization (25.7%) per 1,000 children.
  - Girls are at higher risk of being maltreated than boys (9.4% per 1,000 girls compared to 8.4% per 1,000 boys).
  - Native American or Alaska Native children have the highest rate of victimization at 14.8% per 1,000 children.
  - African American children have the second-highest rate of victimization at 13.7% per 1,000 children of the same ethnicity and race.

CONSEQUENCES OF CHILD MALTREATMENT

Victims of child maltreatment have lifelong emotional, physical, developmental consequences such as

- developmental delays in infancy;
- mood disorder, anxiety, and poor peer relationship in childhood;
- substance abuse in adolescence; and
- personality and psychiatry disorders including abusing own children in adulthood.

CHILD NEGLECT

Description

- Failure of a parent or the person legally responsible for the child to meet the child's educational, emotional, physical, and medical needs.
- Parent or legally responsible person may leave the child unattended or with an irresponsible person.
- Combination of factors such as poor stress-coping skills, families experiencing financial and environmental stresses, parent/caretakers with mental health disorders, unsupportive family circumstances, and parent/caretakers abusing drug and alcohol can lead to child neglect.
- There are four types of child neglect:
  - **Physical neglect:** Parent or responsible person fails to provide clothing, food, shelter, supervision, and/or protection from harm to the child.
  - **Emotional neglect:** Parent or responsible person fails to provide love, affection, or any kind of emotional support. The child may be rejected, ignored, and/or prevented from socializing with other children.
  - **Medical neglect:** Parent or responsible person may not obtain medical care when the child is sick, or delay treatment for physical injuries or mental well-being.
  - **Educational neglect:** Parent or responsible person may not enroll the child in school in a conventional setting or in their homes.

Assessment

- Assess the barriers affecting the parent/caregivers from providing adequate care to their child/children.
- Determine if the lack of care lead to seriously harming the child; if yes, a report must be submitted. If no, then it may not be necessary to report the case to child protective services.
- Assess for:
  - Growth failure, signs of malnutrition (e.g., abdominal distention, thin extremities)
  - Eating disorder
  - Poor hygiene
  - Dirty clothing or clothing that is not appropriate for weather (e.g., shorts in cold season, sweater during summer season)
  - Poor healthcare
  - Stealing food
  - Frequent injuries from lack of supervision
  - Sleep disorder
  - Enuresis
  - Absenteeism from school
  - Substance abuse

Diagnostics

To diagnose child neglect, systematic measures are necessary:

- **Measures for quality of parent/caretaking:**
  - **Polanksy's Childhood Level of Living Scale:** Helps the healthcare clinician measure the quality of physical and cognitive/emotional care in young children.
  - **Child Well-Being Scale:** Helps the healthcare clinician measure the dimension of care related to social, physical, and psychological needs of children. The child performance, the availability of parent/caretakers, and household adequacy are measured.
  - **HOME Inventory:** Helps the clinician measure the quality and the safety of the child's home environment. This tool also measures parent/caretakers' interaction with the child to provide intellectual stimulation.
  - **CLEAN Checklist:** Helps the clinician to determine if the item is clean or dirty.
  - **Home Accident Prevention Inventory:** Checks the safety hazards of the house (e.g., fire hazards, risk of poison, risk of suffocation, and presence of firearms).

- **Observational measures:**
  - CARE-Index that assesses parent–child behavior such as facial and vocal expressions; body position and contact; signs of affection (eye contact, physical holding, positive verbal message from the parent to the child)

- **Measures for risk assessment with the use of the** Neglect Scale (contains nine items to predict the likelihood of child neglect):
  - Previous reports of neglect
  - Out-of-home placement
  - History of neglect for the caretaker as a child
  - History of alcohol and drug abuse (caretaker)
  - Single parent or caretaker
  - Age of the parent or caretaker
  - Number of children at home
  - Caretaker's social relationship
  - Willingness of caretaker to change behavior

Nursing Interventions

- Determine if the child is safe.
- Determine if parents or caretakers have the resources to care for their child.
- Assume that parent/caretakers of a neglected child want to improve their behavior.
- Support parent/caretakers and help them recall their experiences as a child.
- Encourage parent/caretakers to express feelings about their own parents which may help them avoid the repeated cycle.
- Provide parent/caretakers with the resources (e.g., job training and placement, food, housing, recreational activities, medical care) they need.
- Check the child's height and weight and compare them to the normal values for age and based on the child's family background.
- Assess for signs of malnutrition (e.g., lack of smile and lack of stranger anxiety in infancy, lethargy, thin extremities, and irritability in childhood).
- Determine if the child is extremely compliant or has demanding behaviors.
- Check for delayed emotional and physical development.
- Check for signs of depression.
- Assess if the child has a history of delayed medical or dental care.
- Provide the child with therapeutic activities to stimulate and enrich the child's growth and development.

Special Considerations

- Primary prevention:
  - Educate new parents on normal growth and development, anticipatory guidance, and routine healthcare needs of a child.
  - Teach parent/caretakers about the damage of neglect on children.
  - Plan home visits to identify neglect, intervene, and report the cases as early as possible.
- If the child is hospitalized, treat as any other sick child, not as a victim; promote the child's development, play interest, and physical needs.
- Monitor signs of distress on the child (e.g., depression, changes in sleeping patterns, refusal to eat, refusal to go to school).
- Refer parent/caretakers to appropriate social services.

Discharge Planning; Patient and Family Education

- Discharge planning starts as soon as the legal authorities decide on the appropriate placement for the child (e.g., home, temporary foster home, or permanent termination of the rights of parent/caretakers).
- Discuss with parent/caretakers about guidelines on caring for a child.
- Help parent/caretakers to strengthen their social support (encourage them to be involved in activities in the community and in other supportive organizations).

FACTITIOUS DISORDER IMPOSED ON ANOTHER/MUNCHAUSEN BY PROXY

Description

- Initially named in 1977 by Roy Meadow based on cases of poisoning children that occurred and caused the children to seek repetitive medical treatment
- Also classified as medical child abuse and fabricated or induced illness
- Active and unintended contribution of doctors to harm a child based on the fictitious report from the parent/caretaker (usually mothers)
- A pattern of behavior that a caregiver does to create a physical or psychological illness that requires attention from medical professionals

Assessment

- Patients can present with a variety of symptoms or potential disorders.
- It is important that identifying the type of abuse whether it be actual physical harm that the caregiver caused or if there is history that has been fabricated to encourage harm to the child with invasive medical procedures.
- Perpetrators are usually mothers who appear to be caring, concerned, and unselfish in nature.
- Investigation into the perpetrator will usually elicit a history of psychiatric disorders that may or may not have been clear.
- Most cases are not identified initially, and it can take months to years to confirm a case.
- Caregivers will continue the abuse even when in the hospital, by continuing to exaggerate or fabricate symptoms. This process leads to more invasive medical treatments and/or procedures.
- Risk assessment is difficult because the pediatric clinician assumes the caregiver is telling the truth. It is important to search for other historians who are involved with the child but may see a different picture.

- Patients who may have been identified as at risk would benefit from closer observation of how the parent/caretaker and child interact.

Nursing Interventions

- Consider the history of the illness and compare to what is presented. The illness does not match up to the subjective findings on exam.
- Suspicion of diagnosis when the signs and symptoms from the patient only occur when the caregiver is present.
- Parent/caretaker who does not show appropriately relief regarding improvement of the child or no clinical diagnosis is found.
- May observe no improvement of the illness with normal treatment.
- Stop current medications and observe and document findings.
- Perform food challenges preferably with the parent/caretaker out of the room.
- Involve social work and child protection once suspicion is confirmed.

Special Considerations

- Terminology has changed over the years to assist with clarification of the disorder and for the parents/caretakers own psychiatric disability.
- Pediatric Condition Falsification is a condition that the parent/caretaker falsifies psychological or physical illness. The child is then treated by health professions in both invasive and noninvasive means to determine the extent of illness.
- The person who fabricates the information has a psychiatric disorder that is classified as Factitious Disorder by Proxy. This person usually has deep psychological and past psychiatric history, usually the mother.
- When a patient is admitted with symptoms of malnutrition, introduce food and nutrition slowly to avoid refeeding syndrome.
- It is difficult to identify and treat this specific disorder because the person who is the perpetrator also appears concerned and anxious regarding the illness of the child.
- Other siblings may also suffer from different or similar symptoms and should raise suspicions for healthcare workers.

Discharge Planning; Patient and Family Education

Child protection teams and social work should evaluate the home to determine when the child and potentially siblings should return to the caregiver.

PHYSICAL INJURY

Description

- The National Child Maltreatment report (2021) identified that 17.5% of the maltreatment was identified as physical abuse. Physical abuse is identified is the second most common maltreatment type identified.
- Physical injury is defined as a nonaccidental injury that either caused demonstrable harm to a child or could have caused harm to the child. There is a strong correlation between corporal punishment and physical abuse in children.
- Some of the most common forms of physical injury are soft tissue damage. These are easily identified as bruises that may have various stages of healing.
- Children under the age of 4 years old account for 79% of nonaccidental trauma injuries.
- Fifty percent of fractures that are diagnosed in children under the age of 1 year have occurred because of nonaccidental trauma.

Assessment

- The physical assessment of an injury includes discussion surrounding how the injury occurred. The healthcare clinician should determine if it is plausible that the injury occurred unintentionally.
- When interviewing the parent/caretaker and patient about how the injury occurred the healthcare worker should be alert for inconsistencies in the story, especially, how it relates to the injury that is being treated and the child's developmental age (e.g., leg bruises if not walking/cruising). If there is a high suspicion that nonaccidental trauma occurred, the patient and parent/caretaker should be interviewed separately by a trained clinician (Figure 18.1).
- As a mandatory reporter for suspected child abuse, when an injury does not match the description of how it was obtained, social work and child protective services should be notified to investigate the nature of the injury.
- When performing the physical assessment, the most common areas found to be affected are the face, head, neck, back, trunk, buttocks, and thighs. Soft tissue injury can include welts and bruises and there may be irregular patterns that look like the shape of an object used to cause the injury.
- Observe the degree of healing found on bruises on the skin or radiographic imaging if there is a fracture. There is a high suspicion for physical abuse if the healing has occurred in different time frames. Table 18.1 demonstrates a timetable of healing based on radiographic changes in children's fractures.
- Burn injuries can occur in many different patterns and on many different areas of the body. One common area from tub or water submersion is the genitalia and buttocks and legs (Figure 18.2). Toddlers that are toilet training are susceptible to suffering from this injury. Burns that appear circular in fashion and are found on the soles of the feet, palms, or buttocks can be attributed to cigarettes (Figure 18.3). Other burn injuries may have patterns that could be caused by an iron or grill.

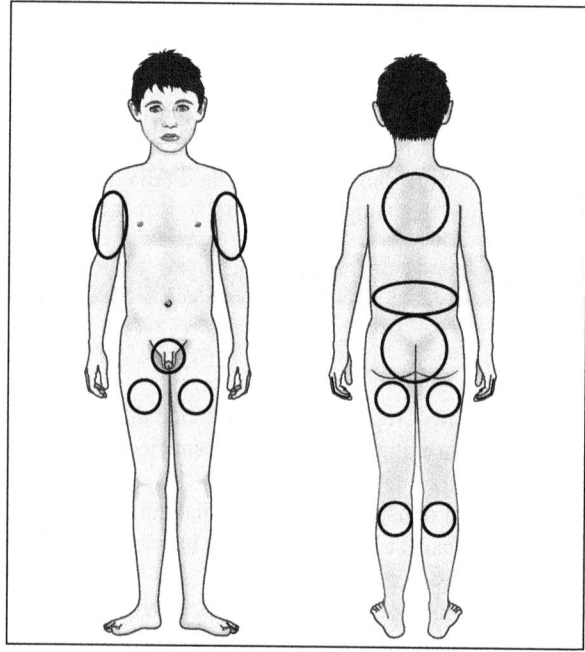

FIGURE 18.1: Injury sites on a child's body that raise suspicion for abuse

Source: Reprinted from Chiocca, E. M. (2021). *Advanced pediatric assessment* (3rd ed.). Springer Publishing Company.

PHYSICAL INJURY

TABLE 18.1: Timetable of Radiographic Changes in Children's Fractures

Category	Early	Peak	Late
Resolution of soft tissues	2–5 days	4–10 days	10–21 days
Periosteal new bone	4–10 days	10–14 days	14–21 days
Loss of fracture line definition		10–14 days	14–21 days
Soft callus		10–14 days	14–21 days
Hard callus	14–21 days	21–42 days	42–90 days
Remodeling	3 months	1 year	2 years to epiphyseal closure

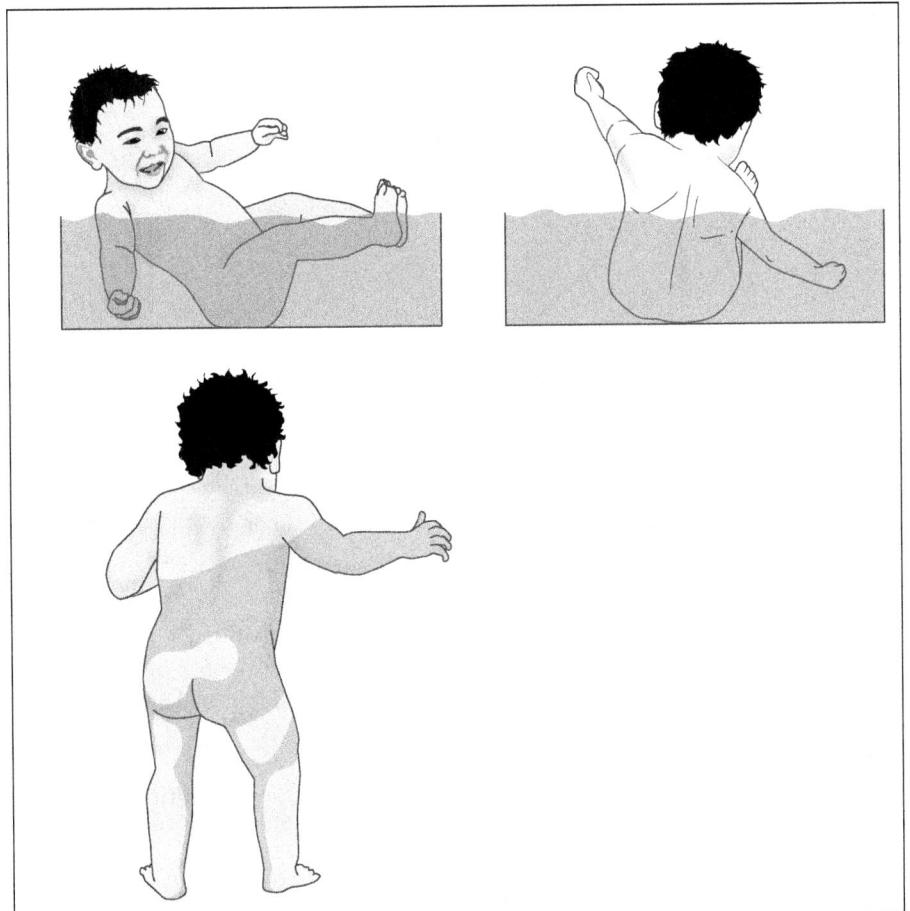

FIGURE 18.2: Immersion burn in doughnut pattern. Note the sparing of the buttocks that were forcibly held against the comparatively cooler surface of the tub

Source: Reprinted from Chiocca, E. M. (2021). *Advanced pediatric assessment* (3rd ed.). Springer Publishing Company.

- Some children present with lacerations that may look like rope burns on the wrists, ankles, torso, or neck.
- Physical trauma that occurs to the nervous system may be severe. Infants who present with nonaccidental head trauma may have subdural hematoma after violent shaking of the infant. Ophthalmology examination will reveal retinal hemorrhages that are a classic sign for abusive head trauma in infants.

- Blunt trauma that occurs to the head may cause skull fractures with hematomas. Blunt trauma to the abdomen may present with internal bleeding, abdominal pain.

Diagnostics

Skeletal survey will confirm if previous injuries have occurred and support the healthcare clinician's suspicion.

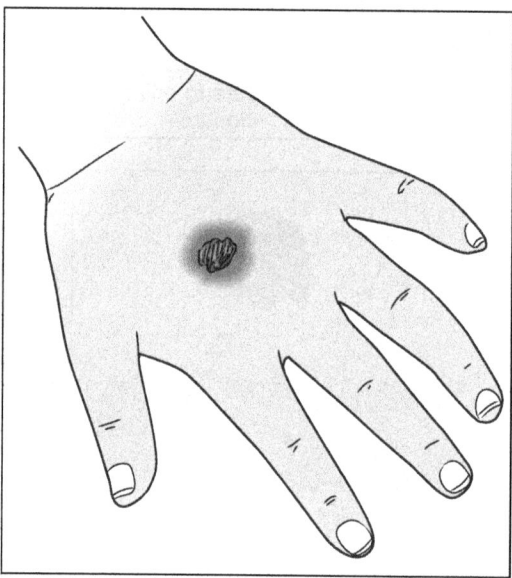

FIGURE 18.3: Cigarette burn

Source: Reprinted from Chiocca, E. M. (2021). *Advanced pediatric assessment* (3rd ed.). Springer Publishing Company.

Nursing Interventions

- Identifying and reporting injuries that do not fit the description of how it was caused is mandatory since healthcare clinicians are mandatory reporters.
- Providing a safe environment for the child depending on developmental age and response will assist with building trust.
- If a high suspicion for physical abuse, consult social work.
- Treat any life-threatening injuries immediately and stabilize the patient first before notifying authorities.

Special Considerations

- Be aware of bleeding disorders and cultural practices that may show marks and bruising (e.g., cupping, coining) that could resemble physical abuse.
- Authorities will come to the bedside of the patient and will take pictures of the injuries. Provide a safe environment for the child and explain the process in developmentally appropriate terms.
- **Identify patients at risk:**
  - Patients who have frequent visits to various emergency departments with varying physical injuries
  - Parents/caretakers who have delayed seeking treatment for a physical injury

- Parents/caretakers' description of the injury is vague and inconsistent with the injury pattern
- Families with a history of substance use disorders, alcohol abuse, mental illness, or adults with a history of physical abuse

Discharge Planning; Patient and Family Education

- Follow-up care is extremely important for families at risk.
- Discharge teaching will be specific to the physical injury; for example, burn injuries will require wound dressing care.
- Teaching may occur to foster parents/caretakers if child does not go back to the family home.

SEXUAL ABUSE

Description

- Child sexual abuse is defined as "any completed or attempted (noncompleted) sexual act, sexual contact with, or exploitation (noncontact sexual interaction) of a child by a caregiver" (Leeb, 2008).
- Child sexual abuse includes many types of sexual acts, including rape, sexual assault, incest, and exploitation of children.
- In general, child victims of sexual abuse do not disclose the abuse and rarely show symptoms.
- Victims of sexual abuse are often reluctant in disclosing the sexual act; they often feel guilty and ashamed of the behavior.

Assessment

- Early recognition is challenging.
- Many children victims of sexual abuse have normal findings on physical exams.
- In some cases, victims of sexual abuse may have some or all of the symptoms listed in the following.

Physical Signs may or may not be apparent; absence of physical abuse does not exclude child sexual abuse.
- Difficulty walking
- Difficulty sitting
- Bruising or tearing around the genital area
- Vaginal discharge, pruritus, and bleeding
- Sexually transmitted infections
- Genital pain
- Incontinence
- Abdominal pain
- Fecal incontinence
- Constipation

Behavioral Signs
- Regression (bedwetting, thumb sucking)
- Inappropriate sexual behavior
- Avoiding removal of clothing
- Excessive knowledge about sexual topics

- Depression
- Anxiety

Emotional Signs
- Aggressiveness
- Change in eating habits (e.g., eating disorders)
- Excessive fearfulness
- Self-harming behavior
- Withdrawal
- Sleep disturbances

Diagnostics

- Diagnostic evaluation should be done by a multidisciplinary team (experienced clinicians) who are knowledgeable and trained to detect signs and symptoms of sexual abuse.
- The diagnostic should be based on:
  - **Interview of the child** (based on the child's development level):
    - Determine if the child has behavioral or developmental problems.
    - Determine sexual development of the child and if it is appropriate to the child's age.
    - Use free recall open-ended questions using anatomical dolls.
    - Use "how" questions to elicit evaluative information.
    - Avoid urging the child to talk about the abuse.
  - **Parent/caregiver interview** (separately from the child to avoid the child being influenced by what the child hears from parent/caregivers):
    - Address relationship issues between the parent/caregivers and the child.
    - Determine parent/caregivers' own history of abuse.
    - Address parent/caregivers concerns.
  - **Medical and psychological history.**
- **Physical examination should include:**
  - Anogenital examination for children who have anogenital complaints (photo and video documentation preferred) as it allows forensic consultation without further examination.
  - Examine the child in both supine and the knee to the chest position.
  - If intravaginal trauma is suspected, vaginoscopy should be done under general anesthesia.
- Vaginal swab for girls and swab from the urethra for boys for chlamydia or gonorrhea.
- Urine analysis.
- Screening for sexually transmitted illness (STI) is not necessary as it depends on the nature of the abuse and the prevalence of STI in the population (note, STI may be asymptomatic).
- **Check for STI if**
  - child experienced penetration;
  - abuser is a stranger;
  - abuser has STI;
  - sibling or relative has STI;
  - child lives in a community with high STI; and/or
  - child has already diagnosed with STI.

Nursing Interventions

- Provide a private environment to the child.
- Receive accurate and complete history.
- When possible, assign Sexual Assault Nurse Examiner (SANE) nurses to the patient.

- Examine the child within 1 to 7 days if it is nonurgent evaluation (when the child discloses sexual contact occurred more than 2 weeks ago, and when the child has no medical or psychological needs).
- Examining the child immediately when the situation is urgent (child says assault occurred within the previous 72 hours and complains of pain, has bleeding, and has suicidal intentions).
- Treat physical injuries, if any.
- Ensure the child's safety (separate from the abuser, remove from home, place the child in an alternative setting).
- Collect the child's clothing (to retrieve DNA).
- Replace child's clothing with clean outfit.
- Emphasize to the child that they have not done anything wrong.
- Consult with child advocacy center and other centers to develop a multidisciplinary approach to evaluate and treat the unique needs of each child victim of sexual abuse.

Special Considerations

- Prevention of child maltreatment is part of every healthcare clinician's responsibility.
- Screen (asking standard questions) all presenting children.
- Recognize families at risk (substance [drug and alcohol] misuse, parent/caretakers who were victims of abuse themselves, poverty, single parents, adolescent parents, child with disability, preterm child, and child with chronic illness).
- Refer families at risk to counseling services.
- Educate new parents about the consequences of child maltreatment on their child.
- Report suspicions to child protective services.

Discharge Planning; Patient and Family Education

- When sexual abuse is confirmed, plan for putting the child in foster care placement as soon as legal disposition has been decided. (Foster home is a drastic solution, however, necessary when the child's life is in danger.)
- Encourage children to express their feelings.
- Explain to the child the reasons for sending them to foster care (not a punishment).
- Support the family and teach them the appropriate ways of parenting.

BIBLIOGRAPHY

Adams, J. A., Kellogg, N. D., Farst, K. J., Harper, N. S., Palusci, V. J., Frasier, L. D., Levitt, C. J., Shapiro, R. A., Moles, R. L., & Starling, S. P. (2016). Updated guidelines for the medical assessment and care of children who may have been sexually abused. *Journal of Pediatric and Adolescent Gynecology, 29*(2), 81-87. https://doi.org/10.1016/j.jpag.2015.01.007

Adshead, G., Brooke, D., & Mitchell, I. (Eds.). (2001). *Munchausen's syndrome by proxy: Current issues in assessment, treatment and research: current issues in assessment, treatment, and research* (1st ed.). Imperial College Press.

Cicchetti, D. (2016). Socioemotional, personality, and biological development: Illustrations from a multilevel developmental psychopathology perspective on child maltreatment. *Annual Review of Psychology, 67*, 187-211. https://doi.org/10.1146/annurev-psych-122414-033259

Gaudin, J. M. Jr., & U.S. Department of Health and Human Services. (1993). *Child neglect: A guide for intervention*. U.S. Department of Health and Human Services, Children's Bureau.

Glaser, D. (2020). Fabricated or induced illness: From "Munchausen by Proxy" to child and family-oriented action. *Child abuse and Neglect, 108*, 104649. https://doi.org/10.1016/j.chiabu.2020.104649

Hornor, G. (2014). Child neglect: Assessment and intervention. *Journal of Pediatric Health Care, 28*(2), 186-192. https://doi.org/10.1016/j.pedhc.2013.10.002

Jacobi, G., Dettmeyer, R., Banaschak, S., Brosig, B., & Herrmann, B. (2010). Child abuse and neglect: Diagnosis and management. *Deutsches Arzteblatt International, 107*(13), 231. https://doi.org/10.3238/arztebl.2010.0231

Leeb, R. T. (2008). *Child maltreatment surveillance: Uniform definitions for public health and recommended data elements*. Centers for Disease Control and Prevention, National Center for Injury Prevention and Control.

Mencio, G., & Swiontkowski, M. (2015). *Green's skeletal trauma in children* (5th ed.). Elsevier/Saunders.

Pekarsky, A. R. (2020). *Overview of child maltreatment (child abuse)*. Merck Manual: Professional Version. https://www.merckmanuals.com/professional/pediatrics/child-maltreatment/overview-of-child-maltreatment

Rape Abuse Incest National Network. (2021). *Warning signs for young children*. www.rainn.org

Rodgers, M. C. (2016). *Wong's essentials of pediatric nursing* (10th ed.). VitalSource Bookshelf version.

Rosado, N., Charleston, E., Gregg M., & Lorenzo, D. (2019). Characteristics of accidental versus abusive pediatric burn injuries in an urban burn center over a 14-year period. *Journal of Burn Care and Research, 40*(4), 437–443. https://doi.org/10.1093/jbcr/irz032

U.S. Department of Health and Human Services. (2020). *Child Maltreatment 2018: Summary of key findings*. www.acf.hhs.gov

U.S. Department of Health and Human Services Children's Bureau. (2019). *Child Maltreatreatment 2019*. www.acf.hhs.gov

Vrolijk-Bosschaart, T. F., Brilleslijper-Kater, S. N., Benninga, M. A., Lindauer, R. J., & Teeuw, A. H. (2018). Clinical practice: Recognizing child sexual abuse—what makes it so difficult? *European Journal of Pediatrics, 177*(9), 1343–1350. https://doi.org/10.1007/s00431-018-3193-z

KNOWLEDGE CHECK

1. A 10-month-old infant presents to the emergency department with a broken arm. The caregiver's story is inconsistent with the type of fracture sustained. As the nurse caring for this patient, what diagnostics should be performed?

    A. CT scan of the head
    B. Skeletal survey
    C. Urinalysis
    D. Complete blood count (CBC) with differential

2. A 4-year-old child admitted for asthma complains about soreness and pain in the abdomen and back. Upon further inspection, the nurse notices bruises with varying degrees of healing on the buttocks and lower abdomen. What is the nurse's first priority?

    A. Contact the authorities to report suspected child abuse.
    B. Notify social work to investigate suspected child abuse.
    C. With the child present, interrogate the caregiver regarding how the bruises were obtained.
    D. Notify the charge nurse that child abuse is expected to have occurred to the patient.

3. A 3-month-old infant arrives on the floor with altered mental status and fever. The caregiver present is demonstrating behavior that is consistent with altered mental status related to substance use. The child has a low-grade fever with no source noted and the caregiver is complaining about how irritable the infant has been over the past 2 days. The infant is at risk for which syndrome?

    A. Nonaccidental head trauma
    B. Seizures
    C. Mitochondrial syndrome
    D. Alcohol-related birth defect

4. A child is brought to the pediatrician's office for a recurring rash across the bridge of the nose. There are no other findings. This is the third time the mother has reported this rash. She is concerned and would like more invasive testing for allergies to occur. An older sibling has also presented with this rash in the past, characterized by raised papules, almost reminding the nurse of a burn. It has been determined after an extensive investigation that the mother has been putting hydrochloric acid across the noses of her children. This is an instance of which form of child maltreatment?

    A. Sexual abuse
    B. Psychological abuse
    C. Factitious disorder
    D. Child neglect

5. A 4-year-old child admitted to the hospital with failure to thrive and dehydration complains of hunger and thirst when the mother is not in the room. What is the most appropriate intervention?

    A. Allow the child to eat and drink as much as they want
    B. Offer food in small portions when the mother is not in the room
    C. Offer food in small portions when the mother is present in the room
    D. Offer the mother information on food that assists with weight gain.

KNOWLEDGE CHECK

1. **Correct Answer: B) Skeletal survey.** A child under the age of 1 who receives an injury that is inconsistent with how the injury occurred has a high suspicion for physical abuse. A skeletal survey will confirm if previous injuries have occurred and support the healthcare clinician's suspicion. A CT scan of the head, urinalysis, or a CBC with differential will not give definitive proof of suspected physical abuse.

2. **Correct Answer: B) Notify social work to investigate suspected child abuse.** Nurses are mandatory reporters and should involve social work early to investigate. Authorities should be contacted by the child protective team and social workers involved. Parents/caretakers and the child should be separated for the interrogation.

3. **Correct Answer: A) Nonaccidental head trauma.** An infant admitted with altered mental status and has a caregiver present who is also altered should create a high suspicion for nonaccidental trauma, specifically, abusive head trauma that is caused when a caregiver shakes the infant. Seizures, mitochondrial syndrome, and alcohol-related birth defect are all conditions that are not related to the presenting assessment.

4. **Correct Answer: D) Factitious disorder.** Pediatric falsification illness/factitious disorder by another—also known as Munchausen by proxy—can occur by the parent/caretaker causing physical harm that does not raise suspicions initially. Physical abuse may also be part of this disorder. This is not an example of sexual abuse, psychological abuse, or child neglect.

5. **Correct Answer: B) Offer food in small portions when the mother is not in the room.** There is a concern for refeeding syndrome in children with failure to thrive due to starvation. Allowing the child to eat small, not large, portions without the mother present, when there is a suspicion of abusive behavior in relation to pediatric falsification syndrome, will assist with the confirmation of this disorder when the child eats without difficulty and then begins to gain weight. When abuse is suspected, it is not advised to give the mother information on food that assists with weight gain, or to give the child food while the mother is in the room.

6. A 6-year-old child is admitted to the unit for abdominal pain, purulent vaginal discharge, and painful urination. The clinician is suspecting chlamydia trachomatis infection. To confirm the diagnosis of chlamydia, which diagnostic test should the nurse expect the clinician to order?

    A. Nucleic acid amplification test
    B. Vaginal swab
    C. CBC
    D. Polymerase chain reaction test

7. A 10-year-old child reveals that his grandmother tells him, "It is ok to let me touch your private area." The nurse suspects child sexual abuse; the patient has no signs and no complaints. What is a priority intervention for the nurse?

    A. Discuss the incident with the child's parent/caretaker
    B. Contact the police and report the case
    C. Report the case to child protective services
    D. Admit the child to the unit for further investigation

8. A 7-year-old child walks in to the asthma clinic for a routine checkup. The child says: "I am hungry. I had nothing to eat for 2 days." The nurse checks the asthma prescription refills and sees that the child's prescription has not been filled for the past year. Based on this information, which is the most appropriate diagnosis for this child?

    A. Factitious disorder
    B. Failure to thrive
    C. Child neglect
    D. Physical abuse

9. The emergency department nurse is caring for an 8-year-old child suspected of child maltreatment. The nurse reports the case to local authorities. Which nursing action is the most important?

    A. Document the findings accurately in the patient's chart
    B. Refer the parents/caretakers to a support group
    C. Assign a different nurse so that the child gets to know all the staff.
    D. Put a TV show on to distract the child.

10. An 11-year-old child reveals that her dad goes to her bed every night and starts touching her genital areas. The child is suspected of being a victim of sexual abuse. When assessing the child, which symptom should the nurse expect to see?

    A. Retinal hemorrhage
    B. Encopresis
    C. Nuchal rigidity
    D. Bulimia nervosa

KNOWLEDGE CHECK

6. **Correct Answer: B) Vaginal swab.** Screening and diagnosis of chlamydia are based on two tests, a urine test and a swab. The nucleic acid amplification test, the polymerase chain reaction test, and a CBC will not confirm the diagnosis of chlamydia.

7. **Correct Answer: C) Report the case to child protective services.** Reporting the case to child protective services is the priority as a mandatory reporter. When sexual abuse is confirmed, plan for putting the child in foster care placement as soon as legal disposition has been decided. A foster home is a drastic solution, however, necessary when the child's life is in danger. The child may not be admitted, but further investigation will be warranted.

8. **Correct Answer: C) Child neglect.** The child had nothing to eat for the past 2 days and the prescription has not been filled for the past year; therefore, this is a case of child neglect, and the nurse should investigate and determine the reasons for the neglect. Factitious disorder/Munchausen by proxy is a pattern of behavior that a caregiver does to create a physical or psychological illness that requires attention from medical professionals. There is no evidence in the question to indicate failure to thrive or physical abuse.

9. **Correct Answer: A) Document the findings accurately in the patient's chart.** The nurse should document findings accurately in the patient's chart for legal purposes. Documentation on the chain of custody form should include the names of persons collecting evidence, types of evidence, and date of collection. Referral to a support group and putting on television shows for the child is not the most important nursing action. It is important for the primary nurse to continue to provide care for the pediatric patient.

10. **Correct Answer: D) Bulimia nervosa.** Bulimia nervosa is an eating disorder that is one of the signs and symptoms of sexual abuse victims. Retinal hemorrhage, encopresis, or nuchal rigidity are not associated with sexual abuse.

CHAPTER 19

Emergencies, Trauma, and Poisonings

Genevieve Turner and David Jack

INTRODUCTION

Unfortunately, sometimes the family is faced with a pediatric emergency that requires emergent and skilled care delivery. This chapter will focus on those injuries, illnesses, and conditions that could be critical or life threatening and requires immediate action and/or intervention. Consider the following **ABCDE** acronym for stabilization.

Assessment and Stabilization

- Recognition of life-threatening illness or injury is one of the most important goals of emergency care. Rapid thorough assessment and recognition for threats to life and/or limbs.
- Airway:
  - Is airway intact?
  - Can the patient speak clearly?
  - Check for airway obstruction.
    - Sounds, stridor, gargling
  - Ensure c-spine precautions if necessary.
- Breathing:
  - Ventilation
    - Assess bilateral breath sounds.
    - Assess for tension pneumothorax.
      - Assess for need for chest tube.
    - Assess for need for intubation.
  - Oxygenation
    - Assess pulse ox, arterial blood gases (ABGs)/venous blood gases (VBGs).
    - Provide supplemental oxygen as needed.
- Circulation:
  - Look for bleeding/hemorrhaging; apply pressure. Insert large-bore intravenous (IV) catheter (at least 16 gauge).
  - Evaluate for sufficient pulses in all four extremities.
- Disability:
  - Assess level of consciousness using **AVPU** method.
    - Alert
    - Voice response

- Pain response
- Unresponsiveness
  - Limb movements should be inspected to evaluate potential signs of lateralization.
  - Pupillary light reflexes should be evaluated and blood glucose measured.
- Environmental/exposure:
  - With dignity in mind, expose body areas by removing clothing; note conditions such as trauma, bleeding, skin reactions (rashes), needle marks.
  - Feeling the skin or using a thermometer (when available), estimate body temperature.

CARDIAC ARRHYTHMIAS

Description/Nursing Interventions

- Bradycardia—heart rate (HR) ↓ 60 beats per minute, may have poor perfusion
  - **Causes of bradycardia:** Hypoxia, poisoning, electrolyte disorders, infection, sleep apnea, drug effects, increased intercranial pressure (ICP)
    - **Intervention:** Treat the cause.
      - Initiate chest compression.
- **Tachycardia:** ↑ HR
  - **Common causes:** Tissue hypoxia, hypovolemia, fever, metabolic stress, pain, poisons, toxins, drugs, anemia, injury, anxiety, tension pneumothorax, tamponade, thromboembolisms
    - **Intervention:** Treat underlying cause.
      - Vagal maneuvers, cardioversions, or pharmacologic treatment
  - **Cardiac arrest:** Tissue ischemia; CPR
  - **Post-resuscitation management:** Identifying and treating organ system dysfunction, correct tissue perfusion and cardiovascular function, correction of metabolic and acid-base function and hypothermia

EXTREMITY EMERGENCIES

Description

- A fracture is a disruption or break in the continuity of bone.
- Most fractures occur by trauma; other causes are due to a disease process, such as cancer or osteoporosis (pathologic fracture).
  - **Types:**
    - **Open:** The skin is broken and bone exposed.
    - **Closed:** The skin is intact over the site.
    - **Complete:** The break goes completely through the bone.
    - **Incomplete:** The break occurs partly across a bone shaft (often the result of bending or crushing forces applied to a bone).
- Fractures are identified according to the direction of the fracture line.
  - **Types:**
    - Linear
    - Oblique
    - Transverse
    - Longitudinal
    - Spiral fractures

- Fractures can be classified as displaced or nondisplaced.
  - **Displaced fracture:** The two ends of the broken bone are separated from each other and out of their normal positions.
    - **Types:**
      - Comminuted (more than two fragments)
      - Oblique
  - **Nondisplaced fracture:** The bone fragments stay in alignment.
    - **Types:**
      - Transverse
      - Spiral
      - Greenstick

Assessment

- Immediate localized pain.
- Decreased function.
- Inability to bear weight or use the affected part.
- Obvious bone deformity may be present.

Diagnostics

- X-ray
- CT scan, MRI

Management

- Fracture Reduction
  - Manual traction
  - **Closed reduction:** The nonsurgical, manual realignment of bone fragments to their anatomic position
    - Traction and countertraction are manually applied to the bone fragments to restore position, length, and alignment.
    - **Traction, casting, splints, or orthoses (braces):** Used after reduction to maintain alignment and immobilize the injured part until healing occurs.
  - Skeletal traction
  - **Open reduction:** Correction of bone alignment through a surgical incision
    - Includes internal fixation of the fracture with wires, screws, pins, plates, intramedullary rods, or nails.
    - Generally used when bone fragments are displaced and difficult to align as seen in comminuted fractures and transverse fractures, where the clinician will realign the bones through an open reduction internal fixation (ORIF). Once the bone fragments are aligned, a traditional cast or splint will be used to immobilize the bone.
  - **Fracture immobilization:** Uses casts, braces, splints, immobilizers, and external and internal fixation devices
- Open Fractures
  - Surgical debridement and irrigation
  - Tetanus and diphtheria immunization
  - Prophylactic antibiotic therapy

Emergency Management of Fractured Extremity

- Initial
  - Treat life-threatening injuries first.
  - Control external bleeding with direct pressure or sterile pressure dressing and elevation of the extremity.
  - Assess neurovascular condition distal to injury before and after splinting.
  - Elevate injured limb if possible.
  - Do not try to straighten fractured or dislocated joints.
  - Do not manipulate protruding bone ends.
  - Apply ice packs to affected area.
  - Obtain x-rays of affected limb.
  - Give tetanus prophylaxis if there is a break in skin integrity.
  - Mark location of pulses to aid repeat assessment.
  - Splint fracture site, including joints above and below fracture site.
- Continuous Monitoring
  - Assess vital signs, level of consciousness, O_2 saturation, neurovascular condition, pain.
  - Assess for compartment syndrome (excessive pain, pain with passive stretch of the affected extremity muscles, pallor, paresthesia, with late signs of paralysis and pulselessness).
  - Assess for fat embolism syndrome (FES).
    - Dyspnea, chest pain, temperature elevation

EYE INJURIES

Description

- Open globe rupture: Full thickness caused by blunt trauma.
  - Open globe laceration, possible intra-ocular foreign body; full thickness injury caused by sharp objects
- Closed globe: Does not have full thickness loss.
- Ocular chemical burns require emergency evaluation and treatment to prevent permanent vision loss.

Nursing Interventions

- Avoid eye manipulation (will increase intraocular pressure).
- If open globe is present, do not give eye drops.
- Place eye shield.
- Consult ophthalmologist.
- Initiate sedation, analgesics, antibiotics.
- Treatment of ocular chemical burns:
  - Remove debris.
  - Measure pH.
    - pH ↓ 6.5 or ↑ 7.5: Irrigate with water or saline until a neutral pH is attained.
    - **Normal ocular pH is 6.5 to 7.5**, thus if not in this range irrigation must continue. Sometimes **this process may take hours and require up to 10 liters of fluid.**
- Orbital Compartment Syndrome (OCS):
  - **Treatment:** Requires lateral canthotomy and lateral cantholysis

INHALATION INJURY

Assessment

- Gather history.
  - The time and nature of the toxin.
  - Was the toxin ingested or inhaled?
  - Assess for nausea, vomiting, abdominal pain, neurologic changes, disorientation.
  - ↓ or ↑ respiratory rate (RR).
  - ↓ or ↑ thermoregulation.
  - Pupillary contraction or dilation.

Nursing Interventions

- **Blood tests:** Chemistry, ECG, liver function tests, urine and blood toxicology.
- Specific antidotes depending on toxin.
- Activated charcoal (to bind with chemical substance in the bowel). Not used for iron overuse.
- Whole bowel irrigation with polyethylene glycol electrolyte solutions.
- Dialysis as needed.
- Notify poison control center.

PEDIATRIC LIFE-THREATENING RESPIRATORY ILLNESSES

Description

- Respiratory illnesses are common conditions that often require emergency treatment. Individual modalities are available in pediatric emergency department for the care of children with three common respiratory illnesses:
  - Bronchiolitis, croup, and asthma (covered in Chapter 6)

Anaphylaxis Emergency Treatment

Potentially fatal condition

Assessment

- Airway, Breathing, Circulation (ABC).
- Assess for angioedema on lips, tongue, oral pharynx.
- Assess for glottic swelling (ask patient name).
- Assess skin for urticaria or angioedema.

Initial Management

- Removal of the cause
- Administration of epinephrine
  - Intramuscular preferred method
    - May be repeated at 5 to 15 minutes intervals
- Administration of oxygen (8–10 L/minute); intubation if stridor or upper airway compromise
- Resuscitation with IV fluids (large bore gauge)
  - NSS bolus 20 mL/kg over 5 to 10 minutes
- **Albuterol (salbutamol):** For bronchospasm not improved by epinephrine

RESPIRATORY EMERGENCIES

Description

- Respiratory distress/failure; can be caused by hypoxemia

Assessment

- Assess for increase in RR and increased respiratory effort.
- Children with hypoxia initially compensate by increasing respiration rate and respiration effort.
- Initially, child will become tachycardia to increase cardiac output.
  - Assess for changes in skin color (cyanosis), agitation, anxiety, lethargy, and coma.
  - **Assessment:** Increase or decrease RR and effort, ≤ or ↓ HR, cyanosis, poor or absent aeration.
    - Assessment of tissue hypoxemia
      - **Early signs:** Tachypnea, tachycardia, nasal flaring, retractions, agitation, pallor, fatigue
      - **Late signs:** Cyanosis, slow RR, Brady, altered mental status

PEDIATRIC PEARLS

- If respiratory arrest progresses to cardiac arrest:

  Airway: Open, clear.
  Breathing: Provide oxygen, assist in ventilation, intubation if needed.
  Circulation: HR, rhythm, palpable pulses, IV access.
  Common Causes of Respiratory Failure: Pulmonary edema, resp infections, stridor, pulmonary effusion.
  Intervention: Support to restore adequate oxygenation and ventilation.

SHOCK

Description

- Inadequate delivery of oxygen and nutrients to the tissues
- Early recognition and early treatment to prevent respiratory failure

Assessment

- Compensatory mechanisms will be stimulated to maintain blood pressure.
  - Prioritized to maintain blood flow to the brain and heart. Increase HR leading to tachycardia, increase systemic vascular resistance to shunt blood flow to the vital organs leading to cool pale skin and weak pulses, abdominal vascular will constrict leading to decreased blood flow to kidneys and intestines.
  - Decreased urine output. Hypotension is a late sign of low cardiac output.
  - Can lead to pulmonary failure and cardiac arrest.

Nursing Interventions

- Restore oxygen delivery to the tissues.
  - High concentration oxygen
  - Advanced ventilation continuous positive airway pressure (CPAP) ventilation

- Volume status.
- Reduce oxygen demand.
- Consider sedation.
- Correct metabolic imbalances, correct hyper/hypokalemia, treat metabolic acidosis.

TRAUMA EMERGENCIES

Description

- Head injuries
  - Blunt head trauma is the most common reason for ED visit.
  - Traumatic brain injury (TBI) can lead to death and disability in children.

Assessment

- Depressed skull fractures
- Cerebrospinal fluid (CSF) leakage from ears and eyes
- Raccoon eyes, Babinski's sign, posturing, changes in Glasgow Coma Scale (GCS), vomiting

Nursing Interventions

- Avoid hypotension and hypoxia; can lead to increased mortality.
- Elevate head of bed (HOB) 30 degrees.
- Head position neutral.
- Seizure prophylaxis.

Diagnostics

Noncontrast enhanced cranial CT is the method of choice to detect a possible TBI (to decrease radiation exposure).

PEDIATRIC PEARLS

- Trauma does not cause hypotension, check for other sources.
- Pediatric patients compensate for larger volumes of blood loss. May not exhibit signs of hypovolemia until ≤25% loss.
- **Tachycardia may be the only sign of bleeding:** Don't wait until child exhibits hypotension.
- Recognition that all cardiac arrest events are not identical is critical for optimal patient outcome, and specialized management is necessary for many conditions (e.g., electrolyte abnormalities, pregnancy, after cardiac surgery).
- Post-cardiac arrest care is a critical component of the Chain of Survival and demands a comprehensive, structured, multidisciplinary system that requires consistent implementation for optimal patient outcomes.
- Syrup of ipecac is no longer used to induce vomiting after accidental ingestion.

BIBLIOGRAPHY

American Heart Association. (2020). *Guidelines for CPR and ECC.* https://ahaic.heart.org/guidelines-2020

Campbell, R. L., & Kelso, J. M. (2020). Anaphylaxis: Emergency treatment. *UpToDate.* Retrieved March 14, 2021, from https://www.uptodate.com/contents/anaphylaxis-emergency-treatment

Canares, T. L., Tucker, C., & Garro, A. (2014). Going with the flow: Respiratory care in the pediatric emergency department. *Rhode Island Medical Journal, 97*(1), 23–26.

Gardiner, M. F. (2021). Overview of eye injuries in the emergency department. *UpToDate.* Retrieved March 15, 2021, from https://www.uptodate.com/contents/overview-of-eye-injuries-in-the-emergency-department

Harding, M. M., Kwong, J., Roberts, D., Hagler, D., & Reinisch, C. (2019). *Lewis's medical-surgical nursing: Assessment and management of clinical problems* (11th ed.). Mosby.

Kindler, L. L., & Polomano, R. C. (2017). Pain. In S. L. Lewis, S. R. Dirksen, M. M. Heitkemper, & L. Bucher (Eds.), *Medical-surgical nursing* (10th ed., pp. 114–139). Elsevier.

Panchal, A. R., Bartos, J. A., Cabañas, J. G., Donnino, M. W., Drennan, I. R., Hirsch, K. G., Kudenchuk, P. J., Kurz, M. C., Lavonas, E. J., Morley, P. T., O'Neil, B. J., Peberdy, M. A., Rittenberger, J. C., Rodriguez, A. J., Sawyer, K. N., Berg, K. M., & Adult Basic and Advanced Life Support Writing Group. (2020). American Heart Association guidelines for cardiopulmonary resuscitation and emergency resuscitation and emergency cardiovascular care. Part 3: Adult basic and advanced life support: 2020 American Heart Association guidelines for cardiopulmonary resuscitation and emergency cardiovascular care. *Circulation, 142*(16_Suppl_2), S366–S468. https://doi.org/10.1161/CIR.0000000000000916

Shah, K. H., & Hajicharalambous, C. S. (2020). *Trauma guide: Beginner's approach to the trauma bay* (1st ed.). EMRA.

Velez, L. I., Greene Shepherd, J., & Goto, C. S. (2020). Approach to the child with occult exposure. *UpToDate.* Retrieved March 28, 2021, from https://www.uptodate.com/contents/approach-to-the-child-with-occult-toxic-exposure

KNOWLEDGE CHECK

1. A 4-year-old is brought to the emergency department for a possible drug overdose. The child is lethargic and confused. Their vital signs are as follows: an HR of 106 bpm, an RR of 14 per minute, and a blood pressure reading of 76/34. What is the nurse's highest priority?

   A. Draw serum blood gas
   B. Prepare for airway maintenance and gas exchange
   C. Draw blood serum for chemistries
   D. Insert a foley catheter to monitor renal function

2. An infant is brought into the emergency department to be evaluated for stridor. Which intervention is most likely to keep the 6-month-old calm during the assessment?

   A. Distract the infant with songs
   B. Give the infant a soft cuddly toy
   C. Encourage the parent to hold the infant
   D. Remove the pacifier to auscultate audible sounds

3. Which of the following fractures would most likely require an open reduction with internal fixation (ORIF) repair of the fracture?

   A. A linear fracture of the humerus that is stable and well aligned
   B. A greenstick fracture of the ulna
   C. A comminuted fracture of the tibia with displaced pieces
   D. A stress fracture of the calcaneus

4. A 7-year-old comes into the emergency department with a large amount of bleeding from his right lower leg. The nurse applies pressure to the wound. What is the next step?

   A. Start an IV
   B. Elevate the extremity
   C. Check blood pressure
   D. Determine the cause of injury

5. A 3-year-old presents in the emergency department with confusion, drooling, and difficulty swallowing. How would this condition be classified?

   A. His condition is non-urgent
   B. His condition is semi-urgent
   C. His condition is urgent and needs attention within 1 to 2 hours
   D. His condition is emergent and needs attention within 10 to 20 minutes

6. A 9-year-old is brought into the emergency department after getting hit in the head with a softball. The patient complains of a headache and vomiting. Which signs may indicate increased cranial pressure?

   A. Clear nasal and ear drainage
   B. Bradycardia and pupil changes
   C. Decreased blood pressure and pulses
   D. Tachycardia and irregular respirations

KNOWLEDGE CHECK

1. **Correct Answer: B) Prepare for airway maintenance and gas exchange.** Airway maintenance and gas exchange are the highest priorities as this child is demonstrating signs of hypoxia, which can include lethargy and confusion. The RR is well below the expected developmental parameters of a preschooler, which are 20 to 25 breaths per minute. Unsure of what the child overdosed on, potential further suppression of their respiratory center may occur thus supporting the current need for airway support and gas exchange maneuvers. Drawing serum blood gas, drawing blood serum for chemistries, and inserting a foley catheter to monitor renal function are all common interventions but are not considered a priority at this time.

2. **Correct Answer: C) Encourage the parent to hold the infant.** 6-month-olds begin to know familiar faces, may resist separation, and become stressed. Distracting the infant with songs, giving the infant a soft cuddly toy, and removing the pacifier to auscultate audible sounds, although appropriate measures are not as likely to gain the child's cooperation as having them be with their caregiver.

3. **Correct Answer: C) A comminuted fracture of the tibia with displaced pieces.** An ORIF repair is generally indicated when adequate alignment cannot be achieved, as in a comminuted fracture of the tibia with displaced pieces. If fracture displacement is great enough to not allow for adequate alignment, operative management should be chosen. A linear fracture, where there is a break in the bone, but it does not move the bone, usually is managed by closed reduction and casting. A greenstick fracture, which is common in children, results in a partial-thickness fracture where only cortex and periosteum are interrupted on one side of the bone but remain uninterrupted on the other. A stress fracture (also called hairline fracture) occurs mostly on the legs and feet. It is a result of repetitive movement and occurs when athletes suddenly increase the frequency or intensity of workouts such as running or jogging. Rest, elevation, and ice are common treatment modalities for stress fractures.

4. **Correct Answer: B) Elevate the extremity.** Elevating the extremity will mitigate blood loss. Determining the cause of injury is not an imperative at this time and can be addressed after. Checking the blood pressure and starting the IV are important, but will not stop the bleeding, which is the pressing issue.

5. **Correct Answer: D) His condition is emergent and needs attention within 10 to 20 minutes.** Drooling and difficulty swallowing are classical signs of acute epiglottis and considered an emergent situation. The child is demonstrating signs of respiratory distress and needs attention.

6. **Correct Answer: B) Bradycardia and pupil changes.** The nurse should recognize Cushing reflex (vasopressor response, Cushing reaction, Cushing effect, and Cushing phenomenon) which is a physiologic nervous system response to acute elevations of intracranial pressure. Cushing's triad consists of widened pulse pressure (increasing systolic, decreasing diastolic), bradycardia, and irregular respirations. Clear drainage from nose or ears may be CSF. Decreased blood pressure and pulses may indicate hemorrhage or dehydration.

7. An 18-month-old is brought to the emergency department after an accidental iron ingestion. What is the priority nursing action?

    A. Initiate dialysis
    B. Administer activated charcoal
    C. Give oral syrup of ipecac
    D. Initiate gastrointestinal decontamination

8. The nurse is conducting a safety presentation aimed at preventing concussions in children. Which of the following information should the nurse include in the presentation?

    A. Abstain from participating in sports until adolescence
    B. Refrain from crossing at intersections where traffic lights are present
    C. Use of helmet when skiing or snowboarding
    D. Children are less likely to get a concussion than adults

9. A parent of a 4-year-old calls the emergency room triage and states her child was stung by a honeybee and is unsure of what to do. The child is crying but has no respiratory distress or signs of anaphylactic shock. Tenderness, inflammation, and the stinger are noted. What is the most appropriate initial action that the triage nurse should direct the parent to do?

    A. Call the Emergency Response number 911
    B. Remove the stinger by gently scraping the skin
    C. Apply a cold compress with some baking soda
    D. Administer oral antihistamine

10. The pediatric nurse is planning a safety campaign to educate parents and child-care workers. Which of the following populations would benefit from a sleep safety program based on their developmental stage?

    A. Infants
    B. School-aged
    C. Tweens
    D. Adolescents

KNOWLEDGE CHECK

7. **Correct Answer: D) Initiate gastrointestinal decontamination.** Gastrointestinal (GI) decontamination is indicated for those who ingest a life-threatening poison. Dialysis is indicated for management of acute poisoning if poisoning is severe, such in rhabdomyolysis, and if there is no alternative therapy, and/or in patients with altered elimination pathways, such as those with renal or hepatic failure. Oral syrup of ipecac is no longer used, and activated charcoal is not used for iron overuse.

8. **Correct Answer: C) Use of helmet when skiing or snowboarding.** Studies have shown that wearing a helmet reduces one's risk of serious brain injury and death as a result of a fall or collision, as most of the impact energy is absorbed by the helmet rather than by the head and brain. Therefore, it is important to include the instruction to use a helmet when participating in appropriate activities like skiing or snowboarding, where falling is common. Although participating in sports puts children at higher risk for head trauma and concussion, it does not mean that a child should abstain from these activities until adolescents. Children are more likely than adults to get a concussion. It is not necessary for children to refrain from crossing intersections where traffic lights are present.

9. **Correct Answer: B) Remove the stinger by gently scraping the skin.** Removing the stinger is important, as the stinger will continue to release venom into the skin tissues. Following removal of the stinger, applying a cold compress with baking soda and administering oral antihistamines can reduce the inflammation. Mixing 1/4 of a cup of aluminum-free baking soda with one to two teaspoons of water together, and then apply the paste to the area that was stung is believed to help neutralize the acidity of the sting and mitigate inflammation. A discussion of an allergic and anaphylaxis presentation should be discussed with the parent. If allergic signs and anaphylaxis develop, then 911 should be called.

10. **Correct Answer: A) Infants.** There is an estimated 3,500 infants that die each year in the United States during sleep because of unsafe sleep environments. Sudden infant death syndrome (SIDS) and sudden unexplained infant death (SUID) occur in infants usually less than 1 year old in which the cause was not obvious. These deaths often happen during sleep in or in the baby's sleep area. The pediatric nurse should have an understanding and knowledge of sleep-safe environments and SIDS/SUID-risk-reduction strategies. According to the Children Safety Network, school-aged children (ages 5–9) should have topics such as fire safety, pedestrian safety, respect for self and others, booster seats, and so on. Tweens (ages 10–14) topics would likely be stranger danger, gang violence, bullying, seatbelt safety, and so on. For adolescence (ages 15–19), consider topics such as safe driving, date safety, babysitting classes, cyberbullying, and so on.

CHAPTER 20

Palliative and End-of-Life Care

Maryann Godshall

"Palliative care no longer means helping children die well, it means helping children and their families to live well and then, when the time is certain, to help them die gently."
—Mattie Stepanik, 2017

DESCRIPTION

Although death rates have dropped dramatically with the increase of life-saving technology and pharmacology, many children are living with chronic illness and disabilities. These children and families live under considerable stress, undergo numerous procedures, and may require high-tech care. When the treatments are no longer successful or "working," the decision must be made when to stop care. This must be approached in a holistic way. There are three similar yet different ways of caring for these children who have no medical options available to prolong their life. They are palliative care, hospice care, and end-of-life care.

Palliative Care

Palliative care provides support for children facing life-threatening illnesses or life-threatening conditions. The care is focused on enhancing and promoting the quality of life that remains and making them comfortable under these circumstances. This integrates physical, psychological, social, and spiritual care (Godshall, 2016). It is appropriate at any stage of illness and beneficial when provided at the same time of treatments of curative or life-prolonging measures. It is based on the needs of the patient; they are the focus and at the center of the decision. It gives them bereavement support, helps with decision-making to produce a plan for care that is right for the child and the family/caregiver(s), assesses their goals of care and preferences, and determines how to achieve them. It can be offered in a variety of care settings: the home, hospital, skilled nursing facility, or hospices (End-of-Life Nursing Education Consortium [ELNEC], 2018).

Life-limiting conditions are those for which there is no reasonable hope of cure and from which children will die. Some conditions cause progressive deterioration, meaning that the child becomes increasingly dependent on parents and caregivers. **Life-threatening** conditions are those for which curative treatment may be feasible but may fail (Together for Short Lives, 2018).

Hospice Care

Hospice care is a form of healthcare that provides palliative (comfort) care across a variety of settings based upon the philosophy that dying is the normal cycle of life. Hospice promotes the concept of "living until you die." Hospice is usually instituted if a child has six months or less to live. Once hospice is initiated, the care team assists the family in deciding the best place for the child to spend their final days. Most children prefer to die at home surrounded by family. The concept of home hospice is growing as an alternative to dying in the hospital (Godshall, 2016). Hospice can be instituted while undergoing palliative care.

End-of-Life Care

End-of-life care occurs when it is determined the end is near (usually in about less than 6 months). Care measures can be started to help the child die peacefully and without any pain. This care must recognize that each child and family have unique needs at this time. End-of-life care also must be easily accessible in the desired setting. It is a holistic approach looking at the physical, social, psychological, and spiritual needs of the family. Sometimes quality of life can be enhanced by providing respite for those who are caregivers. The home is usually the desired site but wherever the site is, encourage the family to include familiar items in the care of the child, like a favorite toy, blanket, picture, or other items of importance to the child. It is important that care measures be flexible to facilitate a good experience (Godshall, 2016).

Special Considerations

The concept of death and perceptions vary depending on the child's developmental age. These stages and interventions are listed in Table 20.1. One important fact to be emphasized is people should tell children the truth about death considering their developmental age and level of understanding.

CULTURAL DIVERSITY: CULTURAL PRACTICES

It is important for the nurse to be aware of any special religious, cultural practices, or rituals for the family. Also important is to know the right support person to help facilitate the cultural care of the dying child. By knowing this and including it, this can facilitate the dying process and make it meaningful. Implement special ceremonies or passage rites whenever possible. This can include prayer, having spiritual objects, burning a candle, applying ointments to the skin, music, silence, or chanting. Being present and not avoiding the situation is most important. Always ask; do not assume you know what is best for every family (Godshall, 2016).

TABLE 20.1: Developmental Stages, Understanding, and Interventions for Death

	Comprehension	Reactions	Interventions
Infant	No real comprehension of death.	React to separation from parent and change in routine.	Encourage parents or caregiver to remain close to infant.
Toddler	Death has very little meaning. Death is not permanent. Death is understood by changes in lifestyle.	May continue to act as everything is normal and the person is still alive. They react to parental anxiety and sadness.	Maintain normal environment and rituals. If parent has died, establish a constant caregiver for the child. Implement primary nursing.
Preschool	View death as temporary or reversible, as in cartoons. They do not see death as permanent.	They feel they may have caused the death through their actions, such as misbehavior, words, and feelings.	Use concrete language and images while avoiding cliches that can inhibit the grief process such as the deceased went on a long journey. Death should not be explained as "sleep," as the child will then fear going to sleep.

(continued)

TABLE 20.1: Developmental Stages, Understanding, and Interventions for Death *(continued)*

	Comprehension	Reactions	Interventions
School age	Understand that death is final and that it is universal. They understand that a loved one will not return. They may develop a deep sense of sadness and loss upon learning of someone's death. They may fear their own death related to the uncertainty of what will happen to them after they die. Fear of the unknown may be the child's main source of anxiety and fear related to death.	They may think people die because of some wrongdoing on the part of the deceased. Develop fears of their parents dying and continue to feel guilty if a loved one dies.	Encourage children to talk about their feelings. Encourage parents to honestly answer questions instead of avoiding them. Encourage parents to remain with their children as much as possible. Have parents share that they are sad and it is all right. Prepare them for post death services, what to expect.
Adolescent	Think abstractly about death, philosophize about it, and ponder their own lack of existence. Perceives death as distant, at the far end of a long life. But when someone they know dies, they will seek support from peers.	Some become fascinated with death and reflect on their own funeral by fantasizing on how others will feel and react.	Encourage support from their peers. Structure hospital admission to allow for maximal self-control and independence. Answer their questions honestly and treat them as mature adults. Respect their needs for privacy and solitude if they desire.

Source: Data from Children's Hospital of Philadelphia. (2021). *A child's concept of death.* https://www.chop.edu/conditions-diseases/childs-concept-death; Docherty, S., Brandon, D., Superdock, A., & Barfield, R. (2019). Impact of chronic illness, disability, or end-of-life care for the child and family. In M. J. Hockenberry, D. Wilson, & C. C. Rodgers (Eds.), *Wong's nursing care of infants and children* (11th ed.). Elsevier; Goldman, L. (2016). *Adults can help children cope with death by understanding how they process it.* https://theconversation.com/adults-can-help-children-cope-with-death-by-understanding-how-they-process-it-58057; Lally, M., & Valentine-French, S. (2021). *Developmental perceptions of death and death anxiety, lifespan development.* https://courses.lumenlearning.com/suny-lifespandevelopment/chapter/developmental-perceptions-of-death-and-death-anxiety/.

PROVIDING GUIDANCE FOR THE ANTICIPATED PROGRESSION OF DISEASE PROCESS

It is most important that the healthcare team be honest with the anticipated progression of the condition, treatment options, and outcomes of care. While you do not want to take away hope, one needs to be completely honest with options. The healthcare team should present to the child and family all treatment options while allowing time for them to process the information and ask questions. It is extremely important to never take away hope but giving false hope is not beneficial to moving forward with decisions that need to be made so that the child has a good death. Having a good, painless death is an extremely important nursing task. Providing honesty to both the child and family of realistic recovery and outcomes is the most important thing so that when the decision comes to change from curative care to palliative care, it can be made smoothly. Daily or weekly healthcare team meetings is of great benefit at making an informed and customed plan of care for each child.

Children must be provided with honest and accurate information as well. It is important to provide this information at an age-appropriate level so they can understand. Information should be clear and simple to understand. It is important to ask the parents how and when they would like their child to be told of their disease process and pending death. Guidance should be provided to not completely keep the child in the dark as to their prognosis.

THE GRIEVING PROCESS

As soon as a caregiver and family are made aware of a child's terminal condition, the family's life changes. Grief can be an emotional response as well as a physical one. During the grieving process, the nurse's care changes to include the entire family. This is particularly so if the child will be dying in the hospital. Paying attention to the parents or caregiver and family with particular attention to the siblings. Some experiences families or caregivers might go through are:

- Feelings of guilt
- Emotionally distancing oneself
- Crying
- Feeling responsible for the impending death
- Hostile reactions
- Inability to focus or complete daily tasks
- Searching for what they might have done differently
- Being hypervigilant over the child's care
- Not sleeping
- Not eating

One of the theorists on stages of grief and death and dying is Kubler-Ross (1983). She described the five stages most accurately. These stages can apply to the child, caregivers, and family.

Denial and Isolation

This stage is marked by feelings of numbness, disbelief, and shock. Denial is a way of protecting the child and family from emotional pain that is too much to bear all at once. They deny it or distance themselves from it. The nurse needs to recognize this and encourage the family to slow down, take it easy, and focus on self-care. Gradually help the family move to acceptance of the given prognosis.

Anger

This can be one of the most difficult phases to deal with. At this point, the child and family have developed an awareness that they are going to die. They search for a reason. Feel it is unfair. Why me? They may displace anger on each other or the healthcare team. They may blame God or their higher power and experience a spiritual crisis. The nurse can involve the hospital chaplain or pastoral care to assist with this. The nurse also can encourage the child to express their anger through therapeutic play or art therapy. They can assist the family to find a positive outlet for the anger. A support group might be of benefit. Also encouraging physical exercise as an outlet. Family members are encouraged to write down their feelings and journal. Siblings may start acting out at school. Suggestions to make the school aware of what is going on so adequate resources can be initiated for them at school.

Bargaining

It is common for family members to question what they did to make this happen. They often pray or make deals with the universe; if their child is saved, they will go to church more, help the homeless, or do something else. This is normal for families to make bargains with themselves or

God to spare the child's life. It is a sense of dying hope. It is important for the nurse to talk about this and reinforce that sometimes things just happen, and it is no particular person's fault or in their control. During the grief stages, the priority role of the pediatric nurse is to support the child and family. Collaborating with other healthcare professionals, such as child life specialists, is very beneficial throughout this process.

Depression

When the illness can no longer be denied or bargained away, the child and/or family may start feeling profound sadness. This feeling is to be expected. The nurse must be alert to when this feeling may become clinical. For example, one may experience insomnia, excessive sleeping, inability to get out of bed, overwhelming anger or overt hostility, significant weight gain or loss, or nightmares. In these cases, professional help is needed and should be introduced.

Acceptance

When the child and family have accepted the illness and/or impending death, an emotional adjustment is made. They may still feel they are on an emotional roller coaster, but they have moved on to acceptance and are now left with trying to make meaningful use of the time that is left. They also will start planning perhaps palliative or hospice care. The nurse must understand and support this process (Godshall, 2016).

ASSESSMENT OF PHYSICAL MANIFESTATIONS OF DEATH

When a child is dying, each of their experiences is unique and should be treated as such. Assessment of the dying child should continue as normal. Frequency of assessment may be altered as death approaches. Some symptoms that might be displayed are:

- Sleeping more
- Decreased appetite
- Becoming less social
- Changing of vital signs (e.g., decreased or increased in the body's compensatory mechanisms)
- Irregular breathing
- Changing toileting habits (e.g., decreased bowel movements and voiding)
- Muscle weakness
- Decreasing body temperature and complaints of being cold
- Confusion

It is important to prepare the caregivers and family for these declining symptoms and make sure the child is as comfortable as possible. The declining physical changes can be interspersed with brief energy and spurts of energy. Emotional changes are varied, and some children may report seeing visions of angels or family members who have died. They may recall fond family events that were important to them. The children often try to reassure their parents by telling them they are ready and not afraid to die (Docherty et al. 2019).

SUPPORTING END-OF-LIFE DECISION-MAKING

Once it is determined that all viable treatment options are no longer helpful, a multi-disciplinary team meeting should be held to determine the course of action towards the child having a good and painless death. Certain aspects of family-centered care should be discussed and implemented, such as who wants to be present at the time of death, how to convert the hospital room into a feeling of home, and how to make death as comfortable as possible. A do-not-resuscitate (DNR) or now called allow natural death (AND) order should be written. The attending physician should review each point in this document very clearly. The child should be included in this decision process if they are old enough to understand. Once this decision is made, it MUST be respected and followed by all healthcare team members. Sometimes parents change their mind during an actual code situation. This is usually because they are afraid to let go and are not ready for the death. As soon as possible after this situation, the family and healthcare team should meet again to review the status and wishes of the family. Feelings should be explored as to why they may have had a change of heart. This happens sometimes, and nurses must support the caregiver or guardian through this tough time. All questions should be answered and reasons for their fear or change of heart explained. The introduction of a palliative care or hospice team should be implemented. They will guide the journey through this very upsetting time to facilitate a good death.

UNEXPECTED DEATH

It is hard enough preparing for a deterioration in condition and the expected death of a child. When a child is injured and dies unexpectedly, it is traumatic. The family has no time to prepare themselves or others for the death. Many feel guilt, blame, and remorse for not having done something to protect their child or to prevent the circumstance. Without proper support, the chance of complicated grief responses is high. Death as a result of a car accident or trauma often includes the decision to withdraw life-support care like a ventilator or bypass machine. These cases frequently are high stress and have ethical, religious, or moral issues. These families are less prepared for death. Nurses can support these families by giving accurate information about what will occur when withdrawal of treatment occurs. These situations may also include a discussion about organ donation (Dougherty et al., 2019).

MANAGING CARE NEEDS THROUGH THE DEATH PROCESS

One of the biggest concerns that both the child and caregivers have during the death process is if the child will experience any pain. This fear must be addressed, explained how pain will be controlled, and assurances given that the child will have adequate pain control so that pain is not an issue.

Most parents have never cared for a dying child. It is therefore important that the nurse help caregivers notice and handle both the emotional and physical changes that are present. Emotional changes include children reassuring their parents sometimes, seeing and/or talking about angels or music. They may have visions or dreams and share them. Assure the family this is normal. Physical changes can vary among children. A continuous physical decline can be interrupted with brief spurts of energy or periods of alertness. Many caregivers ask, "How long?" This is not a question we can definitively answer. Periods of sleeping more and not eating are common. Drinking is less and may only be a few sips. Urine output is decreased. The child may lose consciousness. Breathing may become shallow and intermittent. Many parents become upset during this process as their children may become blue and cool to the touch. It is important to prepare caregivers for this and assure them that you will remain present with them to help them navigate through this period. Create as loving an environment as possible (Dougherty et al., 2019). It is of upmost importance to include the siblings in navigating this process and be sure that they are not ignored or forgotten.

Psychosocial needs of the dying child are most important. The pediatric nurse needs to consider:

Time to be a child: Have the child engage in age-appropriate activities and play for the child.

Communication/listening/expression of fear and anger: A very important care item for the child is to have someone who they can talk to about their feelings, fears, and emotional responses like joy or anger. Simply listening to them is of utmost importance. This person can be anyone the child can relate to. Being alone at the time of death and if it will hurt are the most common fears. Also, if the child does not want to talk about death must be accepted as well. The nurse should be present and help both the child and the family to find someone they can talk to about their feelings.

Depression and withdrawal: We can validate that it is all right to feel sad. Some children will be so sad they withdraw from speaking and interacting. We can offer to provide someone to talk with if they want to. Utilize child life therapy for these situations. In the adolescent population, independence and control needs to be given to them. Physical changes can make a child dependent on others for simple tasks. This loss of control may result in withdrawal or depression. It is important that the nurse validate and say it is all right to have these feelings without forcing the person to talk. A trusting environment with the nurse and a familiar relationship is essential. This is true for the family as well.

Spiritual needs: These as well as cultural needs should be respected, facilitated, and provided for. Rituals that allow one to give thanks, express gratitude, or say goodbye are all ways to honor the transition of getting well to one of letting go or dying. Sometimes what and how much to tell the child may be based on cultural background.

Wish fulfillment: Some organizations provide a service of wish-fulfillment for children who are terminally ill. If possible, help the child to decide what their last wish might be. A trip to Disney World, a new computer or toy, meeting a sports star are all examples of wishes. These wishes provide a good memory for the child and the family that will be treasured after the death. The nurse should encourage and try to facilitate this process simply by suggesting it to the family.

Permission from a loved one to die: Some children hang on and seem to need permission from a loved one to die. Many children feel that if they die, their parents will be hurt or not be all right. Therefore, sometimes the parents or caregivers need to tell the child it is all right to die and assure them that they will be ok. Sometimes the parent is not able to give this permission. They view it as giving up. So, someone close to the dying child and parent may need to be the one to give the child this permission. This is documented in the adult dying population as well.

Comfort in knowing they are not alone in the dying process: This is the most common reassurance that the child needs, to know that they will not be alone when they die. Parents, caregivers, and loved ones need to reassure the child that they will be there when death occurs. This is sometimes a difficult promise to keep, but every attempt should be made to allow the parents or caregivers to be present and hold the child if they choose at the time of death. The presence at death benefits both the child and the parents or caregivers.

Limit setting: Parents need to continue to set appropriate limits on the child's behavior and not allow them to get out of control. The guilt they may experience should not influence their ability to parent. This will prevent the child from getting out of control with their feelings and actions as they proceed toward death (Stanford Children's Health, 2021).

AFTER THE DEATH

Time should be given for the family to view and hold the child for as long as they need. This is their chance to say goodbye. This is saying goodbye to all the hopes and dreams they had for their child as well as the immediate goodbye. Allowing the family to take part in rituals like the last bath should be offered. A remembrance packet should be created for the family. A lock of hair and a handprint or footprint impression in plaster is a beautiful reminder of the child who was lost. Psychosocial support and sharing of literature of parental loss support groups should be provided to the parent or caregiver as well.

ORGAN DONATION AND AUTOPSY

Most states have a mandated request for organ or tissue donation when a child dies. In most instances the family may inquire about the organ donation process or the physician may gently ask. The organ procurement staff will approach the family and answer all questions. Whenever possible, this request is made prior to the child's death. Written consent must be obtained prior to the initiation of any organ donation. Important to note is that this discussion of organ procurement should take place before death occurs in a private and quiet place in the hospital other than the child's room. Then the nurse who is experienced in this area can answer any family questions and have the organ procurement organizer present as well to help the family answer and understand all aspects of this process.

An autopsy is done for any unexplained, unintentional, or violent death that occurs. Other than that, an autopsy can be done at the request of the family. This procedure needs to be explained to the family and all questions asked. This does not interfere with the ability of the family to donate the body for organ procurement for research purposes if that is desired.

Pediatric donation differs from adult donation in that if they are under 18 years of age, the parent or legal guardian must give permission. Children who are under 18 can sign up to be an organ donor when they get a driver's license, but the parents must make the donation decision and give consent (Health Resources and Services Administration [HRSA], 2021).

Body size and donation: The size of the body and the organs are considered when matching donors to recipients. That is why very small children most often receive donations from other young people, although older children and adults can often match. Sometimes, children can receive donations of partial organs such as a piece of a liver or lung (HRSA, 2021).

Caring for the Child Who Has Become an Organ Donor

Once the family has had an opportunity to say goodbye to their child, caring for the child until the time of donation can be an emotional time for the bedside nurse. The nurse needs to put those feelings aside and keep the child's organs well-perfused. The nurse works closely with the organ procurement organization (OPO). The direct care or orders typically transition from the intensivist to the OPO. Attention must be paid to maintaining the airway, adequate organ and tissue oxygenation and perfusion, normothermia, hydration, electrolyte balance, preventing infection, coagulopathic, and further complications. Diagnostic tests may be ordered as well as important blood gas analysis. When it is time to take the child to the operating room (OR) for the organ procurement, the critical care nurse prepares for transport to the OR by placing the child on a portable cardiac monitor and requesting respiratory therapist to provide ventilator support for transport to the OR (O'Leary, 2018).

This is a difficult time for all involved and support for nurses caring for the children going for organ donation is most important. This support needs to go past the day of donation. Nurses can support each other and are often most helpful to those caring for children under these stressful times.

CARING FOR THE CAREGIVER

It is most important to mention that caring for children who are dying is one of the most difficult things a nurse may ever encounter. It is important to have some education in caring for dying children. Also helpful is a team approach and having involved physicians agree about the direction of pediatric end-of-life care. Good communication and including parents in the decision-making process are paramount. Facilitating a good death experience is to allow family member's adequate time to be alone with a pediatric patient after they have died (Khraisat et al., 2017). Being present in the moment, involving the team in decision-making, and all (caregivers, family, and patient) being on the same page is most important when dealing with a child's death. These situations over and over can become stressful for the nurse. Don't forget to take time for yourself. Talk about difficult deaths with colleagues, support each other, and take time away to refresh and regain your own emotional strength. If possible, give the nurse caring for a dying child a lighter assignment so they can spend more time with the child and family, assuring the child a good death experience. This is key in the prevention of emotional and compassion fatigue. Take breaks, eat regularly, and get adequate sleep. Journaling your feelings, exercising, having a hobby, practicing meditation, and practicing yoga are good ways to provide self-care. Take good care of your patient but take equally good care of yourself.

BIBLIOGRAPHY

Children's Hospital of Philadelphia. (2021). *A child's concept of death*. https://www.chop.edu/conditions-diseases/childs-concept-death

Docherty, S., Brandon, D., Superdock, A., & Barfield, R. (2019). Impact of chronic illness, disability, or end-of-life care for the child and family. In M. J. Hockenberry, D. Wilson, & C. C. Rodgers (Eds.), *Wong's nursing care of infants and children* (11th ed.). Elsevier.

End-of-Life Nursing Education Consortium. (2018). *Preparing graduate nursing students to ensure quality palliative care for the seriously ill and their families*. https://www.aacnnursing.org/Portals/42/ELNEC/PDF/Graduate-CARES.pdf

Godshall, M. (2016). Caring for the child with chronic condition or the dying child. In S. L. Ward & S. M. Hisley's (Eds.), *Maternal child nursing care* (2nd ed., pp. 1386–1410). FA Davis.

Goldman, L. (2016). *Adults can help children cope with death by understanding how they process it*. https://theconversation.com/adults-can-help-children-cope-with-death-by-understanding-how-they-process-it-58057

Health Resources & Services Administration. (2021). *Organ donation and children*. https://www.organdonor.gov/about/donors/child-infant.html

Khraisat, O. M., Alakour, N. A., & O'Neill, T. M. (2017). Pediatric end-of-life care barriers and facilitators: Perception of nursing professionals in Jordan. *Indian Journal of Palliative Care*, 23(2), 199–206. https://doi.org/10.4103/0973-1075.204232

Kubler-Ross, E. (1983). *On children and death*. McMillan.

Lally, M., & Valentine-French, S. (2021). *Developmental perceptions of death and death anxiety, lifespan development*. https://courses.lumenlearning.com/suny-lifespandevelopment/chapter/developmental-perceptions-of-death-and-death-anxiety/

O'Leary, G. (2018). Deceased donor organ donation: The critical care nurse's role. *Nursing 2020 Critical Care*, 13(4), 27–32.

Stanford Children's Health. (2021). *Psychosocial needs of the dying child*. https://www.stanfordchildrens.org/en/topic/default?id=psychosocial-needs-of-the-dying-child-90-P03055

Together for Short Lives. (2018). A guide to children's palliative care. In *Supporting babies, children and young people with life-limiting and life-threatening conditions and their families* (4th ed.). https://www.togetherforshortlives.org.uk/wp-content/uploads/2018/03/TfSL-A-Guide-to-Children%E2%80%99s-Palliative-Care-Fourth-Edition-5.pdf

KNOWLEDGE CHECK

1. Which of the following is an accurate statement when considering providing pain relief for a dying child?

   A. Do not provide opioid analgesia so the child is more awake and can interact with their family.
   B. A child becoming addicted to opioid medications is a factor that should be considered when providing pain relief to a dying child.
   C. Adequate pain relief should be provided around the clock with pro re nata (PRN) medications available for breakthrough pain.
   D. To ensure good pain relief, all children, regardless of age, should be put on a continuous drip or patient-controlled analgesia pump of opioids as death approaches.

2. It is important for the pediatric nurse to consider factors related to a child's developmental understanding of death when a family member dies. What factor would be related to a preschooler's concept of death?

   A. Death is viewed as temporary, not permanent.
   B. Preschoolers have a concrete understanding of death.
   C. The preschooler may continue to act as if everything is still alright when a family member dies.
   D. Preschoolers are more sensitive to changes in lifestyle when a family member dies.

3. At which stage of development are children first able to understand that death is permanent?

   A. Toddler
   B. Preschool
   C. School-age
   D. Adolescent

4. Which of the following responses can be experienced by parents or caregivers of children who are dying?

   A. Binge eating
   B. Sleeping all the time
   C. Hypervigilance over the child's care
   D. Lack of empathy

5. When providing supportive care for a terminal pediatric patient, which of the following is an appropriate nursing intervention?

   A. Allow the parents to visit twice a day so the child can get adequate rest.
   B. Follow the hospital visitation policy of only visiting between 6 pm and 8 pm daily.
   C. Refer to the child as your son or your daughter instead of their name to show respect.
   D. Be aware of how children view or understand both their own death and the death of others.

6. A parent refuses to visit their adolescent child who is dying from cancer. The teen has accepted the diagnosis and is ready to die. Which Kubler-Ross stage of death and dying might the parent be experiencing?

   A. Anger
   B. Denial
   C. Bargaining
   D. Acceptance

1. **Correct Answer: C) Adequate pain relief should be provided around the clock with PRN medications available for breakthrough pain.** Children commonly fear that dying will hurt. It is most important that the child has adequate pain relief provided around the clock with as-needed medications for breakthrough pain. Answer A is not correct because pain medication is needed. The child will not become addicted to opioid medications. Not all children will be put on a drip or PCA pump during the dying process.

2. **Correct Answer: A) Death is viewed as temporary, not permanent.** The preschooler views death as temporary or reversible, as in cartoons. They do not see death as permanent. Answers C & D are related to the toddler's concept of death—act as if everything is still alright and is more sensitive to changes in lifestyle when a family member dies.

3. **Correct Answer: C) School-age.** The school-aged child is able to understand that death is final and that a loved one will not return. They may become fearful if they die at this stage because of the uncertainty of what will happen to them after they die. Nursing support and honesty should be provided. Toddlers and preschoolers will likely believe that death is temporary, or reversible.

4. **Correct Answer: C) Hypervigilance over the child's care.** Becoming hypervigilant over the child's care is a typical reaction of parents or caregivers of children who are dying. Anger, hostility, not eating, not sleeping, and empathy would also be considered common.

5. **Correct Answer: D) Be aware of how children view or understand both their own death and the death of others.** A nurse should understand the child's developmental age and concept of death. Unlimited parent and family visitation within reason should be allowed. The nurse should refer to the child by name to convey personalization and caring.

6. **Correct Answer: B) Denial.** The parent may be unable to accept the diagnosis and impending death. Avoidance and denial is their way of dealing with the situation. The nurse should give them time for themselves but encourage them to visit and spend time with their child as soon as possible.

7. A nurse is caring for a dying child. What physical symptoms might they expect to see as the child nears the end?

    A. Consistent periods of alertness
    B. Irregular respirations with some pausing
    C. Warm skin and cap refill of one to two seconds
    D. An increased need to urinate

8. Which statement is accurate when a nurse is discussing the process of pediatric organ donation?

    A. Assure the parent that all children can be an organ donor regardless of their disease process.
    B. The nurse should approach the family about organ donation when they see death is imminent.
    C. Consent for organ donation is not needed in the event of a sudden traumatic injury like a motor vehicle crash.
    D. The organ procurement agency should contact the family about organ donation.

9. A single parent is expressing feelings of guilt over not being able to take off work and spend more time with their dying child due to household obligations. What would be an appropriate comment to say to the parent?

    A. "I think you should take a leave without pay as you will never get this time back with your child."
    B. "Can't you talk to your boss about getting time off, your child is dying!"
    C. "I understand this can be very hard. We will try to spend as much time with your child as we can in your absence."
    D. "It is ok to work as I understand it keeps you busy and your mind off your dying child."

10. Which of the following is an important point to consider for the nurse taking care of a dying child?

    A. Stay late after the shift so the family knows you really care.
    B. Give the nurse caring for a dying patient a full patient assignment.
    C. Have a glass of wine or cocktail to relax after experiencing a child dying.
    D. Practice self-care and satisfy emotional needs in order to adequately take care of patients.

7. **Correct Answer: B) Irregular respirations with some pausing.** Most commonly, irregular respirations will be exhibited in dying pediatric patients. Cheyne-Stokes respirations of increased rate with prolonged pauses of apnea may occur. It is not common for these patients to exhibit an increased need to urinate, consistent periods of alertness, nor warm skin and cap refills of one to two seconds.

8. **Correct Answer: D) The organ procurement agency should contact the family about organ donation.** The OPO should be the entity to contact the family about organ donation. They have conducted studies showing that more people are willing to donate when contacted by the OPO. They present organ donation in a uniform and consistent manner. It is inappropriate for the nurse to confront the family about their child's organ donation arrangements

9. **Correct Answer: C) "I understand this can be very hard. We will try to spend as much time with your child as we can in your absence."** The nurse would want to empathize and convey understanding of the single parents' situation. Advising the parent to leave without pay or confront their boss or implying that the parent is avoiding the child on purpose are all examples of accusatory or judgmental tactics which are inappropriate for the nurse to employ.

10. **Correct Answer: D) Practice self-care and satisfy emotional needs in order to adequately take care of patients.** The nurse should use always use positive self-care practices, but especially when taking care of a dying child. Examples of such practices are: mediation, yoga, getting good sleep, taking breaks, eating regularly, talking with friends or colleagues about the patient's situation, being kind to each other, and so forth.

CHAPTER 21

Professional Responsibilities and Ethics

DiAnn Ecret

INTRODUCTION TO PROFESSIONAL RESPONSIBILITIES IN NURSING

Professional standards of nursing practice seek to provide clarity to the attributes of what defines the professional nurse. It is the responsibility of each nurse to practice within the standards or scope of their nursing role, population, and specialty (American Nurses Association [ANA], 2010). This is especially true in regard to understanding and adhering to national, state, and professional codes of nursing conduct in the care of children. Maintaining professional relationships, adhering to professional codes of conduct, and understanding nursing ethics competencies are essential standards of professional practice for the pediatric registered nurse. Application of maintaining professional responsibilities and professional codes of ethics is an important element of ethics; the application of practical considerations of moral considerations in the everyday care of patients is a type of ethical deliberation known as applied ethics (Perrin & McGhee, 2018).

Professional Standards in Pediatric Nursing embraces the ANA's national standards that seek to "protect, promote, and optimize the health and abilities of children from newborn age through young adulthood" (ANA, 2010). Utilizing a patient- and family-centered care approach, pediatric nurses strive for the prevention of illness and injury, restoration of health, and maximizing comfort in health conditions at the end of life. The nurse applies the nursing process through diagnosis, treatment, and management of the child's condition, while consistently advocating in the care of children and families. Pediatric nurses need to be aware of the State Nurse Practice Act in the state where they work.

HIPAA is another professional responsibility for all registered nurses, not only pediatric nurses. HIPAA stands for Health Insurance Portability and Accountability Act. This act was put in place to ensure patients have health insurance at a time of unemployment and to protect certain personal health information through confidentiality and privacy rules when it comes to healthcare and its services. Refer to the website for more information at www.hhs.gov/hipaa/index.html. It is essential to maintain confidentiality and privacy about patients when discussing care with the interprofessional team. Remember to not discuss personal health information with others not caring for the patient or in public areas. However, you need to be aware that in situations regarding patient safety where the patient is at risk of harming self or others, or if abuse is involved, then you can share the information with the proper authorities.

Another population to take into consideration for your professional responsibilities are **emancipated minors**. Emancipated minors take on adult responsibilities before reaching the age of maturity (usually 18 years old); they are responsible for their own care, not their parents such as in the case of marriage before the age of 18. Check on your state's definition of an emancipated minor.

It is important to keep in mind our roles and responsibilities within the healthcare setting and foster professional boundaries. Nurses provide the best care possible, advocate for the patient, and respect their patient's dignity. It is not appropriate for nurses to achieve a personal gain (power) from patients and families at their expense (vulnerability) such as accepting gifts or spending more time than necessary with a patient (visiting patients on off-hours or on other unassigned units; National Council of State Boards of Nursing [NCSBN], 2018).

As RNs, we may have ethical/moral dilemmas with families refusing care for their children based on cultural beliefs, myths, miscommunication, and at end of life for a child. It is an RN professional responsibility to use the nursing process at the time and assess the family's knowledge and listen to their explanations for refusing care. It may be that the RN only needs to educate the family further about the care plan or there may be a need for legal intervention to provide appropriate care to the child.

Bioethics is a relatively new field of ethics that sought to consider moral foundations, moral norms, and moral character in regard to the careful deliberation, considerations, and actions in medical professions, advances in technology, complex scientific considerations, such as issues at the beginning of life, at the end of life, and allocation of scarce resources.

INTRODUCTION TO NURSING ETHICS

Values, ethics, and advocacy are the key elements of nursing ethics. Nursing ethics specifically focuses on the application of moral action in relationship with patients and often embraces foundational principles of the ethics of caring while also functioning in the organizational and interdisciplinary functioning of bioethical standards. The nursing profession practices within the complexity of bioethical principlism, which include autonomy, beneficence, nonmaleficence, and justice (Beauchamp & Childress, 2019). Additionally, nursing significantly contributes to the ethical dialogue of what ethical practices mean in healthcare through the skillful navigation that raises standards: honesty, advocacy, veracity, relationship development, cultural competence, communication, and care (Butts & Rich, 2020).

Honesty in nursing requires truthfulness, following through with commitments, actions, and behaviors while caring for patients; honesty must also carefully, rationally, and diligently seek commitment and integrity of all actions (Butts & Rich, 2020). Advocacy supports patient autonomy, seeks to act for the benefit of the patient, and seeks the promotion of health and well-being for patients and communities (Butts & Rich, 2020). Veracity requires truthful communication, without withholding difficult conversations; it is always necessary to be transparent with uncertain facts and to never withhold the truth from patients, despite how difficult the news may be for the patient. Veracity for the nurse may require particular communication with the physicians to ensure that paternalism is avoided. Cultural competence, communication, relationship development and care further the knowledge of ethical responsibilities through implementation of the ANA's *Code of Ethics for Nurses*. This is a fluid document that continuously seeks to ensure the respect of one another and each patient that the nurse encounters.

PRINCIPLES OF BIOETHICS: RESPECT FOR AUTONOMY, BENEFICENCE, NONMALEFICENCE, AND JUSTICE

Fundamental principles of bioethics assert **respect for the autonomy** of individuals through individual rights associated with access of care, health education, and management of one's own trajectory of healthcare delivery (Beauchamp & Childress, 2019). Respect for autonomy aims to enhance individual decision-making in healthcare in order to promote patient's personal independence when making healthcare decisions. Respecting patient autonomy requires determination of an individual's ability for self-determination while having the capacity to make complex healthcare decisions. Self-determination requires that an individual has an adequate ability to understand information, is free from undo coercion of others, and ensures that there are no limitations that impair free choice in making healthcare decisions (Beauchamp & Childress, 2019). The presumption that an individual possesses competence occurs unless the person manifests incompetence. Therefore, determining capacity requires a careful analysis of potential incompetence. The standards of incompetence include the inability to verbalize or express preferred choices, the inability to comprehend a given situation or consequence, the inability to comprehend complex understanding of healthcare information, the inability to verbalize rational reasoning, the inability to reach a consistent decision, and/or the inability to verbalize comprehension of risks and/or benefits of intervention or treatment choices (Beauchamp & Childress, 2019).

Consequently, the nurse should understand that the elements of decisional capacity include the ability to understand relevant information, appreciate the medical situation, appreciate the possible consequences of treatment interventions, communicate free choice, and execute rational deliberation about one's own values as they relate to the clinician's recommendations about treatment options. Nursing is responsible for co-signing the consent, as a witness that ensures that the patient understands the treatment goals and that the patient autonomously consents to the treatment intervention. It is the role of the nurse to advocate for the promotion of informed and autonomous decision-making for individuals through the establishment of trusting relationships with the healthcare team. This process supports patient-and family-centered care goals that enhances the principle of self-determination, through relational support of family and the healthcare teams.

Elements of informed consent and surrogate decision-making become essential components of pediatric care. The elements of informed consent include voluntariness, competence to understand, reception of full disclosure of procedures, full disclosure of alternate procedures, and full disclosure of risks and benefits of all potential choices (Butts & Rich, 2020). Pediatric decision-making is generally left to the legal standards of surrogate decision-making by the child's guardian; implementing the "best interest standard," and the "standard of substitute judgment standard" requires similar but distinctly different considerations of care (Butts & Rich, 2020). Regarding informed consent, children 7 years of age or older with full cognitive capacity can agree/"consent" or offer **assent** (affirmation) for treatment or research participation.

The best interest standard requires that guardians seek to determine healthcare decision-making that considers the best probable benefit for the child, while fully evaluating the risks, burdens, and costs while also considering alternative treatment modalities (Butts & Rich, 2020). Ensuring autonomy and best interest standards intertwines the bioethical principle of respect for autonomy and the principles of nonmaleficence and beneficence. The standard of substitute judgment involves the guardian to consider treatment preferences that the child expresses or prefers, hence constantly seeking the respect of autonomy, despite legal determination of individual autonomy in the pediatric care setting. With the implementation of patient- and family-centered care, standards of substitute judgment for emotionally mature and rational pediatric patients has resulted in increased participation in their plan of care with guidance from the clinicians and guardians. Considering the respect and dignity of the child by clinicians carefully engages the relational autonomy of the patient through the active support in family-centered care paradigms for children who experience serious health illnesses and disabilities (Butts & Rich, 2020; Barnsteiner et al., 2014).

The principle of beneficence requires that the nurse is consistently seeking the welfare of individuals, communities, and populations; the nurse advocates for the benefits of the patients, those that they care for. Beauchamp and Childress define beneficence as action that ensures kindness, mercy, charity, and friendship of the "other" (2019). Nurses contribute to the welfare of others by protecting and defending the rights of others, preventing harm from occurring to others, seeking to remove conditions that may cause harm to others, helping persons with disabilities, and seeking to rescue persons in danger (Beauchamp & Childress, 2019).

In order for the nurse to consistently provide actions of beneficence for those who they care for requires an understanding of ethical competencies and moral integrity. Butts and Rich in *Nursing Ethics: Across the Curriculum and Into Practice* assert that ethical competencies in nursing practice have three major areas of distinction (2020). The three categories of nursing competencies include moral integrity, communication, and concern. Moral integrity includes elements of honesty, wisdom, truth-telling, truthfulness, benevolence, and moral courage. Communication includes effective listening and mindfulness, and concern includes cultural sensitivity, advocacy, and understanding of social influence for the benefit of the good (Butts & Rich, 2019).

The quality-of-life assessment made by healthcare providers is often made regarding professional determination of desired benefits regarding the wellbeing and outcomes of the medical care sought for a patient; hence the perceived determination of a quality of the life of the child. However, medical quality is an entirely different entity than an individual patient's quality of life assessment. Medical quality is an evaluation of the medical services rendered to another versus the individual patient's assessment of their own quality of life. This is an important distinction. Medical quality evaluates the degree that a healthcare system or service provides and supports the complexity of care for patients, ensuring the best outcomes (Frezza, 2019). However, the patient's own quality of life assessment requires that the healthcare provider and the nurse carefully utilize the best interest standard and the substitute judgment standard. Healthcare provider's determination of pediatric quality of life is often considerably lower than that of the patient. Health-related quality of life (HRQL) research consistently shows that children report a higher quality of life than their parents and healthcare providers (Butts & Rich, 2019). Therefore, adequately assessing the benefits of treatment and objectively determining the quality of life for children cannot adequately determine harms and benefits of over quality of life determinations. It remains important that nursing advocates for the preferences of patient and family decision-making.

The principle of nonmaleficence is the principle that exemplifies the professional obligation to "do no harm" to others (Beauchamp & Childress, 2019). Beauchamp and Childress (2019) stress the importance of making the distinction between the principle of beneficence and nonmaleficence so as to make the distinction between helping patients obtain the good while seeking the welfare of another, and to implement actions that "help" the other (beneficence) versus the principle of nonmaleficence which requires the obligation to "not" harm the other. Not harming the other highlights the essential imperative to avoid the infliction of harm to another, while also not imposing undue risks and harms (Beauchamp & Childress, 2019). The principle of nonmaleficence requires the clarity of distinguishing the concept of harms through an evaluation of moral rules that reflect the standards of due care. Moral rules that specify nonmaleficence include do not kill, do not cause pain or suffering, do not deprive others of common good, do not slander against another, and do not cause offense (Beauchamp & Childress, 2019). Therefore, nonmaleficence identifies healthcare issues that can involve neglect, paternalism, futility of care, withholding and withdrawing treatments.

Negligence is described as the absence of "due care" or the departure of appropriate nursing actions or behaviors that differ from the reasonable or prudent care of professional norms (Beauchamp & Childress, 2019; Butts & Rich, 2019). It is also the nurse's professional and moral responsibility to report abuse and neglect of children; maltreatment of children includes neglect and physical abuse. It is the responsibility of the nurse to assess and report any suspected abuse. Nurses are considered mandatory reporters and thankfully, most laws provide legal protection for nurses who report in good faith of suspected pediatric abuse or neglect (Butts & Rich, 2019).

Paternalism is likely to occur when the healthcare provider and the clinical team experiences value conflicts with the surrogate decision-making of the adults who are responsible for the choices of care made for their children; paternalism often occurs if the healthcare providers disregard parental decision-making in the management of care for the child. The deliberate withholding of information, the deliberate refusal to provide access to healthcare resources and education because the healthcare provider feels that the self-determination of the patient or the patients' families impairs quality of life or "feels" like there are better treatment options is considered paternalism. Elements of paternalism often include discrepancies between medical judgment, pediatric quality of life, or futility of care issues and considerations.

End-of-life decision-making in pediatrics requires compassionate considerations of the child and the child's family and a thorough analysis of each case's particular circumstances. Withholding treatment or not starting interventions for children who are medically fragile and imminently dying are oftentimes not considered obligatory treatments for certain circumstances; however, withdrawing treatment or stopping interventions that involve life-sustaining interventions when a child is imminently dying is much more likely to cause moral distress for providers and families alike. Beauchamp and Childress attest to the reality that "stopping" treatment interventions at the time of death are momentously laden with feelings of imminent causality of contributing to the death of the patient (2019). The conversations that determine the decision to sustain treatments and remove treatments must be carefully considered for each child's particular circumstances and should be expertly evaluated to ensure autonomy, self-determination, surrogate decision-making, beneficence, and nonmaleficence.

When continued medical and healthcare management is deemed an impossibility, futility of care conversations are often initiated by the healthcare team. Futility of care is recognized through a strong probability that continued treatment interventions are completely unlikely to produce positive health outcomes; oftentimes, healthcare workers and nurses experience moral distress in providing futile care to a pediatric patient, knowing that the care may cause undue suffering and ill effects for the child (Jonsen et al., 2015). Healthcare providers of care and nurses are not obligated to provide endless and continuing care that is deemed futile care; this determination must utilize sound clinical judgments (Butts & Rich, 2020). In complex pediatric decision-making scenarios for medically fragile children who experience acute, chronic, debilitating, and complex life-sustaining diagnoses, the determination of futility can become exceedingly complex. The best way to navigate through these complex decision-making scenarios is to initiate the hospital's ethics consultation process. The goals of ethics consultation are to improve patient care, improve treatment and services, and improve outcomes through the comprehensive analysis of the ethical questions, assess and determine patient's particular circumstances, assess and evaluate value tensions between all stakeholders, and promote communication and dialogue that respects the dignity of the child.

Consequently, the nurse is obligated to carefully reflect upon all elements of care practices that seek to advance the ethical delivery of care and outcomes for children and their families. Special considerations to maintain patient confidentiality are essential. Sustaining the trust of children, families, and populations is the nurse's professional responsibility. This includes careful adherence to state practice laws and privacy rules. Applied ethics in nursing requires wholeness of character, the pursuit of a higher purpose, and a special understanding that the moral integrity of the nurse requires obligations to act, to be, and to become the kind of person that seeks to do the right thing consistently in the care of children, families, and the community (Butts & Rich, 2020).

BIBLIOGRAPHY

American Nurses Association. (2010). *Nursing: Scope and standards of practice* (2nd ed.). American Nurses Association Nursing Knowledge Center.

Barnsteiner, J., Disch, J., & Walton, M. (2014). *Person and family centered care*. Sigma Theta Tau International Publications.

Beauchamp, T., & Childress, J. (2019). *Principles of biomedical ethics* (7th ed.). Oxford University Press.

Beauchamp, T., Walters, L., Kahn, J., & Mastroiannim, A. (2014). *Contemporary issues in bioethics* (8th ed.). Wadsworth Cengage Learning.

Butts, J. B., & Rich, K. (2020). *Nursing ethics: Across the curriculum and intro practice* (5th ed.). Jones and Bartlett Learning.

Frezza, E. (2019). *Medical ethics: A reference guide for guaranteeing principled care and quality*. Taylor & Francis Group.

Jonsen, A., Siegler, M., & Winslade, W. (2015). *Clinical ethics: A practical approach to ethical decisions in clinical medicine* (8th ed.). McGraw Hill Education.

Lo, B. (2020). *Resolving ethical dilemmas: A guide for clinicians* (6th ed.). Wolters Kluwer.

National Council of State Boards of Nursing. (2018). *A nurse's guide to professional boundaries*. https://www.ncsbn.org/ProfessionalBoundaries_Complete.pdf

Perrin, K., & McGhee, J. (2009). *Ethics and conflict* (2nd ed.). Jones and Bartlett Publishers.

U.S. Department of Health and Human Services. (2021). *Health information privacy*. https://www.hhs.gov/hipaa/index.html

KNOWLEDGE CHECK

1. What does the abbreviation HIPAA stand for?

   A. Health Insurance Portability and Accountability Act
   B. Health Insurance Privacy and Accountability Act
   C. Human Integrity Privacy and Accountability Act
   D. Health Insurance Portability and Autonomy Act

2. What statement **most** accurately describes the definition of veracity?

   A. The nurse applies equal division of time and resources amongst all patients that are cared for on a unit
   B. The nurse answers the patient's questions without withholding information
   C. The nurse actively seeks to "do no harm" to the patient
   D. The nurse is faithful to the ANAs' *Code of Ethics*

3. What is the role of the RN in the process of obtaining informed consent for a surgical procedure?

   A. Nurses must assist with explaining the procedure to the patient and obtain the original consent signature from the patient on the form
   B. Nurses do not need to participate in the informed consent process, this is solely the responsibility of the physician
   C. Nurses must ensure the patients understand the procedure and serve as a witness for the patient's signature
   D. Patients do not need to complete or sign a consent form for surgery

4. Which bioethical principle is adhered to, and is considered in the practical application of respect for a patient's self-determination during the informed consent process?

   A. Social justice
   B. Transparency
   C. Double effect
   D. Autonomy

5. When a nurse's actions aim to prevent the patient from harm, the nurse is applying which bioethical principle?

   A. Beneficence
   B. Autonomy
   C. Distributive justice
   D. Nonmaleficence

6. A fellow nurse coworker has been caring for a pediatric patient in the pediatric intensive care unit for several weeks. The child was transferred to the rehabilitation unit last month and will not be discharged for 2 months. The coworker visits the patient and family off hours and brings toys to the child. What is important for nurses to understand regarding their roles and responsibilities in this situation?

   A. It is important for families to share updates with former nurses to cope with the situation.
   B. A psychiatric evaluation is necessary for this nurse to rationalize their behavior.
   C. The nurse understands that patients and families can be vulnerable in the hospital and should set professional boundaries by not visiting them on off hours.
   D. The nurse understands that there are no professional boundaries in pediatric nursing care.

1. **Correct Answer: A) Health Insurance Portability and Accountability Act.** HIPAA is another professional responsibility for all registered nurses, not only pediatric nurses. HIPAA stands for Health Insurance Portability and Accountability Act. This act was put in place to ensure patients have health insurance at a time of unemployment and to protect certain personal health information through confidentiality and privacy rules when it comes to healthcare and its services.

2. **Correct Answer: B) The nurse answers the patient's questions without withholding information.** Veracity refers to habitual truth-telling. It is recommended that healthcare providers habitually keep patients informed, relaying the truth of a patient's particular circumstances and health diagnosis without withholding information. It is important for the nurse to care for all patients in the clinical environment; however, it is not feasible for nurses to provide equal time and resources due to the varying circumstances and acuity of each patient's diagnosis. It may be necessary for the nurse to focus attention on different patient priorities. Nonmaleficence is the ethical principle of "do no harm." Although the nurse should strive to uphold each of the ANA's code of nursing ethics standards, this does not accurately describe the definition of veracity.

3. **Correct Answer: C) Nurses must ensure that the patients understand the procedure and serve as a witness for the patient's signature.** The nurse is required to serve as a witness to the informed consent process provided by the treating clinician; in addition, the nurse should assess for patient competency and "be responsible" for knowing that if the patient does not meet the capacity assessment criteria, then a surrogate decision-maker may be needed. If the nurse is unsure that the patient "understands the consent information," then the nurse should notify the provider and wait to sign the consent. Nurses do not obtain the original consent signature. Nurses can help answer questions with the physician or provider of care but they are not the exclusive educator regarding the physician's procedure. Nurses participate in the informed consent process and sign consent forms for surgery as a witness. Being a witness requires that the nurse is present during the consent process with the physician.

4. **Correct Answer: D) Autonomy.** Self-determination includes the ability of a person having the ability to "manage self." Autonomy refers to the ability of a person having the ability to self-govern. Both self-governance and self-management require the person to meet the requirements of competency. Social justice theory in healthcare relates to utilitarian theory, where the greatest good for the greatest number of people is the priority consideration. Transparency is associated with openness, honesty, and an ability of others to be able to see actions performed. The principle of double effect is an ethical decision-making process that carefully considers whether an action is good or bad by examining the intention of the agent performing the action, analyzing consequences of the action, and reviewing whether the agent has a grave reason for the action, while exercising care to avoid the unintended or bad action.

5. **Correct Answer: D) Nonmaleficence.** Nonmaleficence seeks to avoid harm for patients in healthcare. Beneficence requires that the nurse is consistently seeking the welfare of individuals, communities, and populations. Autonomy is related to self-determination and capacity to make one's own decisions. Distributive justice seeks equality in care.

6. **Correct Answer: C) The nurse understands that patients and families can be vulnerable in the hospital and should set professional boundaries by not visiting them on off-hours.** It is important to keep in mind nurse's roles and responsibilities within the healthcare setting and foster professional boundaries. Nurses provide the best care possible, advocate for the patient, and respect their patient's dignity. It is not appropriate for nurses to achieve a personal gain from patients and families at their expense, such as accepting gifts or spending more time than necessary with a patient by visiting patients on off-hours or on other unassigned units.

7. An adolescent with no known identification is brought alone to the emergency department by ambulance after a motor vehicle accident. The adolescent is unconscious with a head injury and other serious injuries. Treatment requires surgery but the healthcare provider is unable to get informed consent from the family. What should the nurse do?

    A. Ask the ambulance driver to call the police to get the family to sign consent.
    B. Contact social services to ask for a court order for surgery.
    C. Sign the informed consent on behalf of the patient.
    D. Prepare and transport the adolescent to surgery.

8. What are the goals of bioethics and ethics consultation?

    A. To initiate legal proceedings against healthcare workers for neglect
    B. To initiate a root cause analysis about poor healthcare practices
    C. To improve patient care, treatment, services, and outcomes
    D. To determine if patients are capable of making their own decisions

9. Which of the following scenarios describe patient and family decision-making in pediatrics?

    A. The child should always be the primary decision-maker about their care.
    B. The family should be involved in promoting and protecting the needs of the child when patient care is planned.
    C. The seriously ill child should be encouraged to consider their needs, without interference from family and healthcare providers.
    D. Children should never influence the trajectory of their own care.

10. A medically fragile child is ordered a do-not-resuscitate (DNR) order. A DNR order is an example of:

    A. Withdrawal of care
    B. Futility of care
    C. Negligence
    D. Withholding of care

7. **Correct Answer: D) Prepare and transport the adolescent to surgery.** Informed consent is not necessary in an emergent situation as seen in the patient presentation. Delaying emergency treatment to obtain informed consent may lead to more serious injuries and/or death. Having the police find out the identity of the patient and family and/or contacting social services to ask for a court order for surgery will delay this emergency treatment. Signing the informed consent on behalf of the patient is inappropriate.

8. **Correct Answer: C) To improve patient care, treatment, services, and outcomes.** The goals of bioethics and ethics consultation serve to improve patient care, treatment, services, and outcomes. Bioethics and ethics consultations do not initiate legal proceedings against healthcare workers and do not initiate root cause analysis about poor healthcare practices as a punitive investigation. The principle of autonomy is only one area in bioethics.

9. **Correct Answer: B) The family should be involved in promoting and protecting the needs of the child when patient care is planned.** A child's legal guardian is considered the primary decision-maker in pediatric care. The child does not have legal competence to make autonomous decisions without the interference of family and healthcare providers. Children should be treated with respect and dignity during complex healthcare decisions and parents and guardians are encouraged to consider the child's input on decision-making.

10. **Correct Answer: D) Withholding of care.** A DNR order is withholding of care. Discontinuing cardiopulmonary resuscitation would be an example of the withdrawal of care. Futility of care is recognized as a strong probability that continued treatment interventions are highly unlikely to produce positive health outcomes. Negligence is characterized by the absence of due care.

PART IV
Practice Exam

CHAPTER 22

Practice Exam

1. A hospice nurse notices new onset of altered mental status, suggesting brain involvement while caring for a 5-year-old child with cancer. What is the priority nursing intervention at this time?

   A. Suggesting pain medication and sedation for the patient
   B. Arranging for the patient to go to an acute care facility
   C. Education for the family about communication and safety for the patient
   D. Instruct the family that death is imminent and to call for clergy

2. Which is the most appropriate nursing intervention in caring for a child with a head injury?

   A. Keep the child in a flat position
   B. Elevate the head of bed (HOB)
   C. Allow the child to ambulate without assistance
   D. Maintain a stimulating environment

3. Which test is the most accurate in screening for the HIV antigen in infants and young children?

   A. CD4 lymphocyte or T cells
   B. Western blot or protein immunoblot
   C. Polymerase chain reaction (PCR)
   D. Enzyme-linked immunosorbent assay (ELISA)

4. What is the most appropriate nursing intervention for a child diagnosed with an anterior pituitary gland tumor and hyperpituitarism?

   A. Promote positive body image and self-concept
   B. Provide pre- and postoperative care
   C. Encourage open communication within the family
   D. Provide developmentally appropriate activities

5. What is the most common type of anemia in infants and children?

   A. Thalassemia
   B. Sickle cell anemia
   C. Aplastic anemia
   D. Iron deficiency anemia

6. The nurse is alert for which sign of a complication for a 12-year-old child who is in the immediate postoperative cardiac catheterization period?

   A. Bradycardia and normal sinus rhythm
   B. Capillary refill of <2 seconds and minor discomfort at catheter insertion site
   C. Presence of S1 and S2 with warm extremities
   D. Tachycardia with cool, clammy skin

7. A 4-month-old infant presents to the ER with intermittent, noisy breathing that gets worse with crying. What condition does the nurse suspect when examining this child?

   A. Croup
   B. Influenza
   C. Laryngomalacia
   D. Respiratory syncytial virus

8. What activities are appropriate for growth and development for a 16-year-old in a long-term care facility?

   A. Encourage activities with friends, such as visiting, phone calls and videoconferencing
   B. Permit usage of video games during daytime hours only
   C. Provide procedure videos and pictures of equipment expected to be used
   D. Provide books for reading as well as informational handouts and pamphlets

9. The nurse is concerned about helping the caregivers of an infant with cerebral palsy to set long-term goals for the family. These goals should be set with the understanding that

   A. Cognitive impairments require special education
   B. Progressive deterioration requires future institutionalization
   C. Unknown extent of the disability requires continual adjustments
   D. Diminished immune responses require protection from infection

10. A nurse is providing care to a school-aged child hospitalized for illness related to factitious disorder imposed on another (FDIA)/Munchausen syndrome by proxy (MBP). What characteristics of FDIA/MBP should the nurse recognize?

    A. The parent was abused as a child
    B. The parent often neglects the affected child
    C. The child is often overly anxious
    D. The child exhibits attention-seeking behavior

11. A parent brings their school-aged child to the pediatrician's office for a follow-up visit after being prescribed methylphenidate for attention deficit hyperactivity disorder (ADHD) 4 weeks ago. The parent tells the nurse, "Things have been a little better at school since she started the medication but at home my child doesn't seem to have much appetite. I sometimes find her up late at night when she should be sleeping." How should the nurse respond?

    A. "What specific rules do you have for bedtime?"
    B. "What does her teacher say about her performance in class?"
    C. "When do you usually give her the medication?"
    D. "Can you tell me what she had to eat yesterday?"

12. A nurse is providing care to a 13-year-old hospitalized with an oblique fracture of the fibula after a motor vehicle accident. The extremity was casted 10 hours ago. The nurse received report that the patient has reported being in constant pain, rating it 10 out of 10 on the pain scale even after receiving the prescribed analgesic 90 minutes ago. The nurse performs an assessment with the following results: a temperature of 99°F, a heart rate of 92 beats per minute (bpm), respirations of 24 per minute, and a blood pressure of 130/80. The patient reports that the pain is "achy" and his toes feel "tingly." The nurse notes that the toes are slightly pale and cooler in temperature than those of the unaffected extremity. What action should the nurse take next?

    A. Document the assessment findings as expected for this type of injury
    B. Ask the healthcare clinician to prescribe a stronger analgesic
    C. Notify the healthcare clinician of the assessment findings
    D. Utilize nonpharmacologic measures to help alleviate the pain

13. A 24-month-old child is hospitalized for suspected sepsis. The child has a rectal temperature of 102.1°F and is lethargic. The parent reports that the child had a low-grade temperature "off and on" over the past 3 days but otherwise seemed well until today when the child wouldn't eat and was listless. Which nursing intervention should the nurse prioritize?

    A. Administering antipyretics
    B. Educating the parents
    C. Administering antibiotics
    D. Obtaining laboratory specimens

14. A 3-year-old child is being evaluated for a recurrent respiratory tract infection, the third one in three months. The child has been treated with two courses of antibiotics. Past medical history includes a hospitalization for bacterial pneumonia 1 year ago. The nurse should expect which next step in treating this child?

    A. A prescription for an additional course of oral antibiotics
    B. Hospitalization for intravenous antibiotic therapy
    C. A focused assessment on the immune system
    D. Begin intravenous immunoglobulin therapy (IVIG)

15. A nurse is assessing a 2-year-old child during a visit to the pediatrician's office. The child has had intermittent bouts of vomiting and diarrhea. The nurse suspects the child may have celiac disease. Which question should the nurse ask the caregiver to help confirm that suspicion?

    A. "Has anyone else in the family experienced these symptoms?"
    B. "What does your child's diet look like on a given day?"
    C. "Have you noted any blood in your child's stool?"
    D. "In relation to meals, when does your child experience vomiting?"

16. A nurse is receiving a report on a mother whose newborn has been diagnosed with a cleft palate. Which statement by the reporting nurse about the mother's past medical history indicates a risk factor for cleft palate?

    A. "The patient has had four prenatal visits."
    B. "The patient is being treated for a seizure disorder."
    C. "This is the patient's sixth pregnancy."
    D. "The patient developed gestational diabetes."

17. A nurse is providing care to a 3-year-old child hospitalized with pneumonia. The nurse notes the child has mild nasal flaring, retractions, a temperature of 100.1°F, and a respiratory rate (RR) of 30 beats per minute (bpm). The child coughs frequently and often whines or cries afterward. The child is receiving IV fluids and antibiotics as part of the treatment regimen. The child's parent is at the bedside. To further address the child's condition, what is the best action for the nurse to take next?

    A. Administer an analgesic as prescribed
    B. Administer an antipyretic as prescribed
    C. Encourage the parent to cuddle the child
    D. Utilize the Wong-Baker FACES Pain scale

18. A nurse is providing care to a 5-year-old child hospitalized with a lower respiratory infection. The child is tachypneic and wheezes are auscultated bilaterally. The nurse understands that the child's symptoms are attributed to which aspect of the child's respiratory system physiology?

    A. The diameter of the trachea
    B. An increased number of alveoli
    C. A cylindrical larynx
    D. A lower metabolic rate

19. In what stage of Kubler-Ross is an 8-year-old terminal patient when yelling and throwing things at the nurse?

   A. Anger
   B. Denial
   C. Bargaining
   D. Depression

20. What is the priority intervention for a child who was found with an empty bottle of acetaminophen tablets within 45 minutes?

   A. Initiate gastric lavage right away
   B. Implement warm intravenous fluid bolus
   C. Start chelation therapy as soon as possible
   D. Administer N-acetylcysteine rapidly

21. Which immunoglobulin crosses the placenta?

   A. IgD
   B. IgE
   C. IgM
   D. IgG

22. The nurse understands the body system most affected by metabolic disorders is

   A. Cardiovascular
   B. Respiratory
   C. Neurologic
   D. Gastrointestinal

23. When caring for a child experiencing hypercyanotic episodes, the nurse knows the priority intervention is:

   A. Provide supplemental oxygen and assist child to a squatting position
   B. Decrease intravenous fluids to maintain only a keep vein open (KVO) status
   C. Administer hydromorphone every 2 to 3 hours for pain
   D. Relieve symptoms with a cool compress applied to the forehead

24. The nurse is caring for an 8-year-old following a routine tonsillectomy. Which finding should be reported to the healthcare clinician immediately?

   A. Respiratory stridor
   B. Unwillingness to swallow
   C. Drooling of blood-tinged saliva
   D. An axillary temperature of 99°F

25. What nursing activities would improve the patient's body image and facilitate feelings of autonomy and dignity for a hospitalized adolescent?

   A. Insist that the patient uses the bedpan or urinal
   B. Perform personal hygiene activities for the patient
   C. Regardless of facility policy, allow the adolescent to wear their own clothing
   D. Offer to assist with grooming activities as the patient specifies

26. A nurse is educating the family about long-term care for a child diagnosed with a seizure disorder after a vagus nerve stimulator (VNS) has been placed. The nurse should inform them that the child should eat a diet featuring:

    A. Dairy and meat products
    B. Plant-based food items
    C. Foods low in carbohydrates
    D. Fruits, vegetables, and legumes

27. A school nurse is assessing a 7-year-old child who is seen with reports of a headache. This is the third time in recent weeks that the child has been to see the nurse for some type of somatic complaint. Each time the child shows up shortly before dismissal and requests to lie down for a while. At dismissal time, the child always seems reluctant to leave. What initial action should the nurse take?

    A. Refer the child for evaluation of the somatic complaints
    B. Express concern to the child's teacher about the behavior
    C. Ask the child if they are afraid of someone at home
    D. Contact child protective services to investigate the family

28. A nurse is assessing a 17-year-old female during a routine clinic visit. The patient is well dressed and pleasant in attitude. Vital signs are within normal parameters except for a slightly lower blood pressure. The patient is 5' 6" tall and weighs 110 pounds which is six pounds less than at her last visit four months ago. When asked about her menses, the patient states that her periods have been sporadic, and that the last one was 2 months ago. The nurse is concerned about the patient's weight loss and amenorrhea. What initial action should the nurse take to gain more insight into the patient's health status?

    A. Ask the patient if she is sexually active
    B. Consult a dietician about the patient's nutritional status
    C. Ask the patient what she thinks about her weight loss
    D. Have serum lab specimens drawn to check for anemia

29. A parent of a 5-year-old male expresses concern to a nurse about the child's gait. The parent states, "He seems really clumsy and always walks on his tiptoes." The nurse notes that the child stands with his shoulders back and abdomen pushed forward. The nurse suspects the child may have Duchenne muscular dystrophy (DMD). What action should the nurse take to further assess the child?

    A. Assess muscle strength by having the child toss a ball
    B. Ask the child what type of sports he enjoys playing
    C. Have the child stand up from a sitting position on the floor
    D. Ask the parent at what age the child began to walk

30. A nurse has provided teaching to a caregiver on at home fever management. Which statement by the caregiver provides the best indication that teaching was effective?

    A. "If a child has a fever and is very irritable, acetaminophen can be given."
    B. "A tepid sponge bath is the best option to reduce fever in children."
    C. "A temperature greater than 100.4°F requires an antipyretic be given."
    D. "Aspirin is a safe option to use to reduce fever in children."

31. A 6-year-old female is being treated for her third urinary tract infection (UTI) in 8 months. Both the child and caregiver report consistently using proper hygiene for toileting. Which procedure is the most likely next step in evaluating this child?

    A. Intravenous pyelogram (IVP)
    B. Renal biopsy
    C. Urodynamic study
    D. Voiding cystourethrogram (VCUG)

32. A 3-month-old infant presents to the clinic for a well-child visit. The caregiver reports that the infant often vomits small amounts of feedings one to two times per day. On assessment the infant's weight, length, and head circumference are all age appropriate, and the infant shows no signs of a respiratory infection. Based on the assessment findings, which is the infant's likely diagnosis?

    A. Celiac disease
    B. Gastroesophageal reflux
    C. Gastroesophageal reflux disease
    D. Hypertrophic pyloric stenosis

33. A 12-year-old patient presents to the emergency department with reports of pain in the lower right abdomen and vomiting that has worsened over the past 3 hours. The nurse assesses the patient and notes guarding of the abdomen and rebound tenderness on palpation. Initially the pain was assessed as a 10 on a scale of 1 to 10, but the patient now reports the pain as having resolved. What is the most appropriate next step?

    A. Continue to monitor the patient's status
    B. Document the change in the patient's pain level
    C. Request an order for an antiemetic
    D. Notify the healthcare clinician of the change in pain level

34. A nurse is providing care to a child hospitalized with an asthma exacerbation. The nurse is reviewing recent blood gases with the following results:

    pH: 7.32
    PaO_2: 70 mmHg
    $PaCO_2$: 49 mmHg
    HCO_3: 27 mEq/L

    What inference can the nurse make based on these results?

    A. These results are within normal parameters
    B. The child is experiencing respiratory acidosis
    C. The child is experiencing respiratory failure
    D. The child is experiencing respiratory alkalosis

35. A nurse is creating a plan of care for a hospitalized preschooler. What should the nurse consider when providing care to a preschool child?

    A. Expect the child to exhibit regression behaviors
    B. Maintain a strict schedule to assist the child in adapting to surroundings
    C. Recognize play as an opportunity for the preschooler to address fears
    D. Explain procedures only to parents to avoid adding stress to the preschooler

36. What home referrals should be made to assist a family and patient diagnosed with a terminal illness and has less than 6 months to live?

    A. Physical therapy
    B. Rehabilitation center care
    C. Hospice, palliative care
    D. Occupational therapy

37. What should the nurse do first with an emergent open fracture to the leg?

    A. Administer intravenous antibiotics as ordered
    B. Attempt to straighten the fractured joints
    C. Apply direct pressure to the area of bleeding
    D. Mark location of pulses to aid repeat assessment

38. What is the priority nursing action after receiving an order for subcutaneous immunoglobulin (IG)? The order reads: administer 400 milligrams per kilogram of intravenous immunoglobulin therapy (IVIG) subcutaneously.

    A. Check the weight-based math for accuracy
    B. Have emergency intubation equipment available
    C. Contact the clinician for clarification of the order
    D. Obtain vital signs before and after the IVIG administration

39. A child newly diagnosed with type 1 diabetes mellitus is confused, lethargic, and has fruity-smelling breath. Which order from the primary healthcare clinician should the nurse question?

    A. Assess blood sugar every 2 to 3 hours
    B. Obtain either urine or serum for ketone testing
    C. Administer insulin regular as ordered by sliding scale
    D. Intravenous fluid based on weight and electrolyte values

40. Which parental statement indicates that a nurse's teaching of the need for a splenectomy for a child diagnosed with sickle cell anemia has been successful?

    A. "This surgery will cure the sickle cell anemia."
    B. "The amount of anemia will be better after this surgery."
    C. "My child will not have any more sickle cell crisis now."
    D. "The surgery will decrease the risk of infection for our child."

41. What assessments would the nurse expect while examining a 4-year-old child diagnosed with congestive heart failure?

    A. Spoon-shaped fingernails
    B. Plotting 5% or less weight on a growth chart
    C. Spastic activity of the child's extremities
    D. Wave like, uncoordinated body movements

42. What is the priority intervention for a child experiencing epistaxis?

    A. Elevate the head of the bed 30° and apply pressure to the nasal ridge
    B. Keep the child flat, apply pressure to the bridge of the nose, and apply warm compress
    C. High Fowler's position, head forward, pinch bridge of nose, and ice pack above pinched area
    D. High Fowler's position, tilt the child's head back and press on the nasal ridge

43. What is the best way for the nurse to assess the adolescent's eating pattern?

    A. Request the teenager draw the size portions normally prepared by the caregiver
    B. Question the adolescent about how many calories and types of foods normally eaten
    C. Ask the teenager to write down what they remember eating for the past week
    D. Have the teen leave with an assignment of keeping track of and writing down food intake for a week

44. A nurse is teaching the family the purpose of an EEG. The parent verbalizes understanding of the EEG when which statement is said?

   A. "This test will tell us if there is a mass in the brain."
   B. "The EEG measures activity of the brain."
   C. "This diagnostic exam measures the percent of normal brain tissue."
   D. "This exam will show the level of intracranial pressure."

45. During an assessment of a 20-month-old child, a nurse notes a small, partially healed, triangular-shaped burn on the back of the child's upper arm and another healed burn on the scapula. When questioned, the parent states that the child is clumsy and bumped into the iron. What action should the nurse take?

   A. Tell the parent to be more careful with an iron
   B. Ask the child what happened to his arm
   C. Ask the parent when the accident took place
   D. Contact social services to evaluate the situation

46. A community health nurse is preparing a presentation on attention deficit hyperactivity disorder (ADHD). Which risk factor associated with ADHD should the nurse include in the presentation?

   A. Female gender
   B. Lead exposure
   C. Large for gestational age at birth
   D. Having a specific gene

47. A nurse is providing care to a family who has just learned that their child has been diagnosed with osteogenesis imperfecta. One of the parents says to the nurse, "No one else in the family has this disorder. How could this have happened?" What is the nurse's best response?

   A. "This is a genetically inherited disorder so someone in your family must have had it."
   B. "This is a genetic disorder that can occur spontaneously without anyone in your family ever having it before."
   C. "There is no need to worry since your child has the mildest form of the disease and won't be affected much."
   D. "I understand your need to know why this happened but let's focus on your child's plan of care."

48. A 3-year-old child presents to the clinic with blister-like lesions around the mouth, nose, and chin that appeared 2 to 3 days prior. The nurse notes that some of the lesions are fluid filled with others having a honey-colored crust and reddened base. Which is the appropriate treatment option for this child?

   A. Mupirocin calcium cream
   B. Corticosteroid cream
   C. Permethrin cream
   D. Calamine lotion

49. A nurse is providing care for a 2-year-old hospitalized with hemolytic uremic syndrome (HUS). The nurse is reviewing the child's recent laboratory results. Which laboratory result should the nurse expect to see?

   A. Increased sodium level
   B. Decreased phosphate level
   C. Decreased creatinine level
   D. Decreased platelet level

50. A nurse is reviewing the radiologic report of a child diagnosed with Crohn's disease. Which finding should the nurse expect to read in the report?

    A. Pseudopolyps on the lining of the large bowel
    B. A cobblestone appearance to the bowel wall
    C. A dilated proximal colon with an empty rectum
    D. Superficial ulcers in the intestinal lumen

51. A 10-year-old child is hospitalized with moderate to severe dehydration secondary to an intestinal obstruction. As part of the treatment regimen, the child is receiving daily maintenance intravenous (IV) fluids. The nurse is calculating the hourly infusion rate using the formula for daily maintenance fluid requirement. What rate should the nurse set the infusion pump for this child who weighs 71 pounds? Round to the nearest whole number.

    A. 1746 mL/hour
    B. 73 mL/hour
    C. 86 mL/hour
    D. 134 mL/hour

52. A nurse has completed a focused respiratory assessment on a school-aged child with the following findings: breathing is labored with respirations 32 beats per minute (bpm); lung sounds are coarse crackles auscultated on inspiration along with expiratory wheezing; skin color is pale with bluish tinge around the mouth and under the eyes; productive cough with yellow mucus. Which assessment finding is most concerning?

    A. Respiratory rate
    B. Lung sounds
    C. Productive cough
    D. Skin color

53. A nurse is assessing a newborn during a home visit 1 week after birth. The newborn weighed 3.4 kg at birth. At 1 week of life the nurse should anticipate the newborn's weight to:

    A. Increase by 0.5 kg
    B. Increase by 1 kg
    C. Decrease by 0.34 kg
    D. Decrease by 0.85 kg

54. What is the priority nursing intervention for a nurse assisting parents whose child is being resuscitated?

    A. Encourage the parents to cry and start the grieving process
    B. Allow the parents to be present during the resuscitation
    C. Arrange for facility clergy to pray with the family
    D. Insist the parents avoid looking at the child

55. Which treatment is no longer recommended for accidental ingestion in children?

    A. Syrup of ipecac
    B. Gastric lavage
    C. Activated charcoal
    D. Dialysis

56. Which statement by an adolescent tells the nurse that education about impetigo needs further clarification?

    A. "I can give this to others and should be careful."
    B. "I can still go to school after starting the antibiotic medication."
    C. "The sores should be totally covered until they are completely gone."
    D. "I should soak and remove the crusts prior to using the prescribed ointment."

57. What is the most appropriate nursing intervention for a 7-year-old child with a hemoglobin A1C level of 7.4%?

    A. Assess a spot capillary glucose measurement
    B. Administer insulin using a sliding scale
    C. Immediately notify the primary healthcare clinician of the result
    D. Document the results recognizing this as developmentally appropriate

58. The nurse is aware of the need to maintain strict intake and output for a child post cardiac catheterization because

    A. Urine retention can occur as a result of the procedure
    B. Contrast materials used during the catheterization may cause diuresis
    C. This is a procedure which involves potential large amounts of blood loss
    D. Dehydration and low blood sugar is possible because of preoperative nil per os (NPO) status

59. What is a symptom of allergic rhinitis?

    A. Pus like drainage
    B. Bruises (shiners) under the eyes
    C. Shortness of breath
    D. Pharyngitis

60. During a well-child visit, a 13-year-old states, "I think I might have something wrong with me. I am more uncoordinated that I have ever been." Which response by the nurse is most appropriate?

    A. "We can do some neuroimaging and have some studies done to rule out your concerns."
    B. "Have you been prescribed glasses or hearing aids? Do you wear them?"
    C. "Physical development during this time is often fast and uneven. This is normal and can affect your coordination and physical abilities."
    D. "I understand this is very concerning. Tell me how many of your family have had brain tumors."

61. While conducting a routine examination of a 1-year-old child, the nurse notices the child does not react to a loud noise. What is the priority intervention at this time?

    A. Comprehensive assessment of cranial nerves
    B. Speak softly behind the child to see if the child turns toward the noise
    C. Family education of signs and symptoms of retinal detachment
    D. Referral to audiologist and parent/caregiver, family education of safety measures

62. The family of a seriously ill child asks the nurse to assist them in initiating palliative care for the child. Which is the best action for the nurse take?

    A. Provide information on new drugs/treatments in clinical trials
    B. Provide a referral for family counseling
    C. Organize a patient care conference
    D. Explain that palliative is initiated in the final months of life

63. A 22-month-old toddler presents to the clinic for a scheduled visit. The nurse completes an assessment and notes that the child does not make eye contact but constantly looks up at the ceiling. The parent tells the nurse that the child does that a lot especially with strangers. What is the most appropriate action for the nurse take?

    A. Ask the parent if the child makes eye contact with them
    B. Observe an interaction between the parent and child
    C. Agree that the child is probably shy around strangers
    D. Explain to the parent that the child's behavior is abnormal

64. A nurse is teaching a family how to care for their infant who has a Pavlik harness to correct hip dysplasia. Which statement made by the family requires additional teaching?

    A. "It is good to know that our baby will only need the harness for 3 weeks."
    B. "Any adjustment of the harness straps will be done by our healthcare clinician."
    C. "I have adjusted how I hold my baby in order to breastfeed comfortably."
    D. "We find that knee socks keep the harness from rubbing the baby's legs."

65. A 2-month-old premature infant is being discharged home. The infant is HIV+ but has gained adequate weight, is feeding well, and is otherwise stable. The mother tells the nurse, "I wonder about my ability to take care of my baby." Which is the nurse's best response?

    A. "You can always call us if you have questions, so don't worry."
    B. "There is no need to be concerned since your baby is not symptomatic."
    C. "Tell me what concerns you most about taking care of your baby."
    D. "Here is a list of community resources you can access for assistance."

66. The parent of an 8-week-old infant brings the child to the clinic for a well-child visit. The infant was diagnosed with a hypospadias at birth. The parent asks the nurse about having the infant circumcised. Which is the nurse's best response?

    A. "Normally, infants are circumcised 2 to 3 days after birth."
    B. "We can make arrangements for your child to be circumcised at his next visit."
    C. "Circumcision does not cause injury to the meatus in infants with hypospadias."
    D. "Circumcision is delayed until the hypospadias has been surgically corrected."

67. A nurse has identified a problem of imbalanced nutrition, less than body requirements for a child diagnosed with short bowel syndrome. Which intervention will best address this problem?

    A. Encourage the parents to serve high calorie snacks
    B. Promote a diet that includes complex carbohydrates
    C. Teach the parents how to administer enteral feedings
    D. Include loperamide as part of the medication regimen

68. A nurse is calculating the daily maintenance fluid requirement for a child who weighs 52 lbs. How many milliliters of fluid should the child receive per day?

    A. 1572 mL
    B. 1500 mL
    C. 1632 mL
    D. 2364 mL

69. A parent calls the nurse and says, "My child has been diagnosed with spasmodic laryngitis. What can I do to make him more comfortable?" What is the nurse's best response?

    A. "You can give your child acetaminophen for a high fever."
    B. "You should take your child to the hospital for evaluation."
    C. "We'll start your child on a course of antibiotics."
    D. "Use a humidifier or sit with your child in a steamy bathroom."

70. A nurse is assessing a 2-year-old toddler for adequate growth and development. The child has gained about four pounds over the past year. The nurse observes the parent trying to help the toddler copy circles in a book. In response, the toddler babbles at the parent while vigorously pushing the parent's hand away. Which is the nurse's most appropriate action?

    A. Document the assessment findings as expected for age
    B. Notify the healthcare clinician about the child's speech patterns
    C. Tell the parent that the child's behavior toward them is inappropriate
    D. Refer the child to an occupational therapist for help with gross motor skills

71. Which type of fracture occurs partly across a bone shaft (often the result of bending or crushing forces applied to a bone)?

    A. Open
    B. Complete
    C. Incomplete
    D. Closed

72. Which sign should the nurse recognize as a cardiac arrhythmia in a young child?

    A. Heart rate of 120 beats per minute (bpm)
    B. Capillary refill < 2 sececonds
    C. Heart rate < 60 bpm with poor perfusion
    D. Respiratory rate (RR) of 25 per minute

73. Which factor would alert the nurse to question an order of silver sulfadiazine 1% ointment for a child with a burn?

    A. The age of the child over 12 months
    B. The timing of the burn over 1 week prior
    C. The child has an allergy to pain medications
    D. The area of the burn being the facial region

74. A child is undergoing testing of thyroid function evaluating T4 and T3 function and serum levels of protein-bound iodine (PBI). What question specific to this situation should the nurse ask the family prior to this testing?

    A. "Does anyone in your family have thyroid problems?"
    B. "Have you had the child's eyes examined recently?"
    C. "Does the child use table salt on the food at meals?"
    D. "Has your child had a cold and ingested cough medicine recently?"

75. A nurse is administering a blood transfusion to a child diagnosed with aplastic anemia. What signs are most important for the nurse to recognize as a transfusion reaction?

    A. Transfusion reactions do not occur in children
    B. Rhinorrhea and sinus pressure
    C. Fever and tachycardia
    D. Hypotension and ankle edema

76. Which assessment finding would the nurse most likely expect to be documented for a child diagnosed with congestive heart failure?

    A. Bradycardia
    B. Clear breath sounds
    C. Falls asleep while eating
    D. Weight gain over expected amount

77. A child who is post-tonsillectomy vomits bright red blood. What should the nurse do first?

    A. Nothing, this is an expected outcome after tonsillectomy
    B. Position the child on their side
    C. Call the healthcare clinician
    D. Obtain an order for an antiemetic

78. The early signs of ventricular shunt malfunction for an infant are

    A. A tense fontanelle and vomiting
    B. Severe headache and a loss of memory
    C. Projectile vomiting, and changes in vision
    D. Low-pitched cry, dilated pupils, and constipation

79. A 5-year-old child presents with confusion, lethargy, and loss of previously achieved milestones. Laboratory results show anemia. The nurse suspects which diagnosis?

   A. Hydrocephalus
   B. Epilepsy
   C. Brain tumor
   D. Plumbism

80. A 10-year-old child has been diagnosed with a terminal illness. A nurse is at the bedside providing support and explaining end-of-life care to the child and family. What intervention should the nurse implement to support the child?

   A. Encourage the parent to include the child in any care decisions
   B. Send the parent from the room to give the child privacy to process the information
   C. Provide activities designed to distract the child from the situation
   D. Administer a sedative to relieve any anxiety the child may experience

81. An 8-year-old is sent to the school nurse for complaints of a stomachache. The child tells the nurse, "I don't like being here! It makes my stomach hurt. This schoolwork is too hard for me." Which is the nurse's most appropriate next step?

   A. Arrange a meeting with the child's parents and teacher to discuss the situation
   B. Ask the child what they had to eat to determine the cause of the stomachache
   C. Notify the child's teacher that the stomachache is due to anxiety about schoolwork
   D. Encourage the child to talk more about why they think schoolwork is too hard

82. A child is seen in the clinic for evaluation of a facial rash. The child is diagnosed with impetigo and is to be treated with oral cephalexin. The healthcare clinician has prescribed 160 mg every 8 hours for 7 days for the child who weighs 16 kilograms. The recommended dosage is 25 to 50 mg/kg/day in 3 to 4 divided doses. The nurse is to provide teaching to the family about the medication. What is the appropriate action the nurse should take?

   A. Contact the healthcare clinician to adjust the dosage
   B. Inform the healthcare clinician that the child is allergic to macrolides
   C. Educate the parent on the importance of finishing all of the medication
   D. Instruct the parent that cephalexin should be taken with food

83. Which statement best describes the recommendations for immunizations for children diagnosed and symptomatic with HIV/AIDS?

   A. Live attenuated vaccines are contraindicated for children infected with HIV
   B. The vaccine schedule is adjusted depending on the severity of the child's illness
   C. Administration of any routine vaccine will depend on the child's CD4 count
   D. The vaccine schedule is maintained but is adjusted for live attenuated vaccines

84. A 6-year-old presents to the emergency department with reports of fever, abdominal pain, and headache for 2 days. The parents also reported that the child had "blood in the urine." In completing an assessment, which question will most likely help determine the child's diagnosis?

   A. "What was your child's last meal?"
   B. "Has anyone else in the family been sick?"
   C. "Has your child had a sore throat recently?"
   D. "Is your child up to date on immunizations?"

85. A nurse is preparing to administer a nasogastric (NG) tube feeding to an infant. Before starting the feeding which intervention should the nurse prioritize?

    A. Assess bowel sounds
    B. Check for tube placement
    C. Measure gastric residual
    D. Measure abdominal circumference

86. A nurse is providing care for an infant diagnosed with chronic lung disease (CLD). The nurse has created a plan of care whose primary focus is lung function. What should the nurse identify as the secondary focus of the plan of care?

    A. Nutrition
    B. Fluid balance
    C. Growth and development
    D. Parental support

87. A nurse is providing care to an 8-year-old child hospitalized for a severe asthma exacerbation. As the nurse prepares the child for discharge, what should be the primary focus of the patient teaching plan?

    A. Avoidance of triggers
    B. Use of a peak flow meter
    C. How to take medications
    D. Improving the Asthma Action Plan

88. The parent of an 18-month-old calls the nurse expressing concern that the child is developmentally delayed. What is the nurse's best response?

    A. "What aspect of your child's development concerns you?"
    B. "Tell me about how your child interacts with others."
    C. "You will need to have your child evaluated by a specialist."
    D. "Can you bring your child to the office for evaluation?"

89. A nurse is caring for a child who fell at the school playground. Which sign is not an indication of a head injury?

    A. "Raccoon eyes"
    B. Macroglossia
    C. Depressed skull fractures
    D. Clear drainage from ears

90. What is the priority nursing assessment for a child in shock?

    A. Metabolic alkalosis
    B. Metabolic acidosis
    C. Tachypnea
    D. Respiratory alkalosis

91. Which prescription will the nurse question for a child exhibiting signs of tinea pedis?

    A. Soak the foot in warm water daily
    B. Administer antifungal cream daily for 14 days
    C. Cleanse the skin daily with antibacterial soap
    D. The child cannot return to school for 1 week

92. What is the best intervention for an adolescent with end-stage cancer?

    A. Have the child attend a meeting where the plan of care is discussed
    B. Discuss the progression of the disease with the proper clinical terminology
    C. Encourage the child to consider the family in the planning for the future
    D. Explain to the child and family what treatment continuation will include

93. A 6-year-old child diagnosed with cancer is scheduled for radiation therapy. What teaching about radiation therapy is important for the nurse to include in the care plan?

    A. Radiation markings can be washed off
    B. Apply lotion and creams to radiated area
    C. The child should not experience any pain during treatment
    D. Desquamation of the skin in the radiated area can occur

94. Which serum electrolyte level is the priority to be evaluated for a child who has been prescribed furosemide?

    A. Calcium
    B. Chloride
    C. Potassium
    D. Magnesium

95. The nurse is caring for a child who has had persistent otitis media effusions and is scheduled to have pressure equalizing tubes placed in 3 days. What should parents be taught to observe for after their child has a myringotomy?

    A. Purulent drainage from the ears
    B. An improvement in speech and communication
    C. A lack of response to noises of all volumes
    D. A reduction in response to verbal cues

96. The nurse is performing well-baby checks in a pediatric clinic. During physical examination of a 1-month-old infant, the nurse notices a dimple with a tuft of hair in the lumbar sacral area indicative of spina bifida. Which developmental delays does the nurse expect for this infant?

    A. Some degree of paralysis of the lower limbs is expected
    B. The infant is not expected to experience physical delays
    C. Muscles of the legs will be flaccid with some sensory loss
    D. There may be issues related to bowel and bladder control

97. A nurse knows that the difference between the pediatric and adult Glasgow Coma Scale (GCS) score is:

    A. The inclusion of cranial nerve assessment
    B. The number scale is slightly altered for each value
    C. The GCS is less likely to be used in pediatrics because it is not necessary
    D. The pediatric GCS allows for developmentally appropriate cues for altered level of consciousness

98. A 4-year-old child has been diagnosed with terminal cancer. The child's healthcare team met with the parents to discuss the child's prognosis and options for palliative and hospice care. After the clinician finished speaking, one of the parents asks, "So, we're going to try a different type of medication now, right?" How should the nurse interpret the parent's question?

    A. The parent misunderstood what the healthcare clinician said
    B. The parent has lost confidence in the healthcare team
    C. The parent is likely in denial about the child's prognosis
    D. The parent needs additional information about the child's prognosis

99. A 14-year-old female is seen for a routine visit. The nurse assesses the patient and notes that one shoulder seems slightly higher than the other. Further assessment using the Adam's forward bending test shows a slight curvature to the spine. When questioned, the patient denies having back pain. What implication do these assessment findings have for this patient?

   A. The patient will require further evaluation and testing
   B. The patient will be instructed to avoid carrying heavy backpacks
   C. The patient has severe scoliosis that requires surgery
   D. The patient has idiopathic scoliosis which will resolve as the patient grows

100. A child is scheduled to receive the inactive polio vaccine (IPV) during a well-child visit. The parent tells the nurse, "I don't know anyone who has had this disease. What would someone look like who had it?" Which is the nurse's best response?

   A. "A person who contracts polio may have symptoms that include fever, and swollen glands behind the ears and under the chin."
   B. "Polio is characterized by breathing or swallowing difficulty, severe muscle weakness, or floppy limbs."
   C. "Flu-like symptoms and an itchy sandpaper-like body rash are common occurrences in someone affected by polio."
   D. "People diagnosed with polio will have impaired mobility due to muscle wasting and muscle spasticity."

101. A school nurse is teaching a group of adolescent students about infectious mononucleosis. The nurse should include which information on how to avoid a potential complication?

   A. Saltwater gargles are recommended for a sore throat
   B. Contact sports should be avoided for several weeks
   C. It is important to avoid sharing eating utensils with others
   D. Frequent rest periods may be needed for up to 6 weeks

102. A nurse is providing teaching to a group of caregivers of children diagnosed with chronic kidney disease. Which statement by a parent indicates a good understanding of the dietary requirements associated with this disease?

   A. "Cabbage and cauliflower are two of our favorite veggies."
   B. "Hot dogs and hamburgers are our favorites during the summer."
   C. "My child will be happy to continue enjoying ice cream."
   D. "Peanut butter is a great source of protein for our family."

103. A nurse is discussing short bowel syndrome with the parents of a child newly diagnosed with the disorder. Which statement best describes the condition?

   A. Short bowel syndrome can result in bouts of diarrhea and constipation
   B. Children diagnosed with short bowel syndrome will develop a variety of complications
   C. Total parenteral nutrition (TPN) is a lifetime requirement for short bowel syndrome
   D. Short bowel syndrome causes nutrient malabsorption and electrolyte imbalance

104. A nurse is providing care to a child who was brought into the emergency department with a foreign object aspiration. The object has successfully been removed. Which action is most appropriate for the nurse to take next?

   A. Administer supplemental oxygen
   B. Monitor the child for signs of complications
   C. Teach the parents how to avoid foreign object aspiration
   D. Prepare the child's discharge instructions

105. A nurse suspects a child has developed a respiratory syncytial viral (RSV) infection. Which risk factor, if found in the past medical history, supports the nurse's suspicion?

    A. Birth occurred in the spring
    B. School-aged
    C. Female gender
    D. Breastfed for 6 months

106. A nurse is providing care to children during well-child visits at a pediatrician's office. Which child requires intervention by the nurse?

    A. A 4-year-old who wants his imaginary friend to get immunized too
    B. A toddler who has mastered bowel control but still has episodes of bedwetting
    C. A 13-month-old who is able to pull themselves up and cruise around furniture
    D. A 9-month-old who requires support to maintain a sitting position

107. A nurse is caring for a toddler who came to the emergency department with a possible drug overdose. Which is the priority intervention?

    A. Maintain a patent airway
    B. Monitor for infection
    C. Provide psychological support to the caregiver
    D. Obtain labs to assess renal function

108. Which medication will the nurse expect to be administered for maintaining cardiovascular perfusion to a child requiring resuscitation?

    A. Lidocaine
    B. Epinephrine
    C. Atropine
    D. Glucose

109. Which is an expected finding for an infant diagnosed with congenital hypothyroidism?

    A. Normal height on growth chart
    B. Hypertonia
    C. Hypoglycemia
    D. Macroglossia

110. Which assessment is the nurse least likely to observe in a patient with osteosarcoma?

    A. Severe bone pain
    B. Swelling of the area
    C. Redness of the extremity
    D. Ataxia or gait changes

111. What assessment should the nurse consider a priority when examining the circulation status of a toddler in the emergency department?

    A. Mobility
    B. Tympanic temperature
    C. Level of consciousness
    D. Heart rate on cardiorespiratory monitor

112. A nurse in the emergency department is caring for a 4-month-old infant diagnosed with congenital heart defects. The infant has had prolonged nausea and vomiting for 3 days and is dehydrated. The nurse understands dehydration puts a child with cardiac history at higher risk for which condition?

    A. Cerebrovascular accident
    B. Supraventricular tachycardia
    C. Physiologic jaundice and kernicterus
    D. Neurologic conditions such as seizures

113. The nurse is providing education for the family with several children under the age of 9 about risk factors for otitis media. What is the greatest risk factor for developing otitis media?

    A. Activities involving water such as swimming and showering
    B. Bacteria entering the Eustachian tube
    C. Long, narrow, flat Eustachian tubes in children
    D. Ear drum damage due to attempts to clean the ear

114. A child falls to the floor having a seizure. Which intervention does the nurse initiate when providing care to the patient during the seizure?

    A. Go to the nurses' door of the room to call for help
    B. If incontinent, cover the patient with a blanket or sheet
    C. Protect the patient from injury related to seizure movement
    D. Remove or loosen any tight clothing around the neck or waist

115. A nurse assesses a child with a neurologic condition by passively flexing the neck. The child flexed their hips and knees in response to this movement. The nurse recognizes this assessment as

    A. Developmentally appropriate
    B. A significant Kernig's sign
    C. Abnormal posturing
    D. Brudzinski's sign

116. A 20-month-old child is suspected of having developmental delays and has been referred to an early intervention program. The child's caregiver asks the nurse how the program will help their child. Which statement best describes early intervention programs?

    A. Early intervention programs are special education classes for children with disabilities
    B. These programs are designed to provide respite care for caregivers with children with special needs
    C. The programs are intended to enhance the development of infants and toddlers who are at risk for or who have developmental delays or disabilities
    D. They are individualized educational programs (IEP) designed to meet the educational needs of infants and toddlers

117. A nurse is providing care for an adolescent following a femur fracture. The patient has been placed in skeletal traction. The nurse should consider which principle about positioning when taking care of this patient?

    A. The patient's buttocks should be slightly elevated off the bed
    B. The affected limb should be extended and maintained in a straight line
    C. The hip on the affected side should be flexed slightly with the knee suspended in a sling
    D. The hip and leg should be flexed at 90° while the lower leg is placed in a boot

118. A school-aged child presents to the emergency department with reports of a sore throat, hoarseness, loss of appetite, and difficulty swallowing that has developed over the past 3 days. On assessment the nurse notes a temperature of 100.4°F, heart rate 104 beats per minute (bpm), and respirations of 28 per minute. The child also has a thick greyish coating on the tongue, tonsils, and pharynx, and swelling about the neck. Based on these findings the child has been admitted to the hospital for treatment. The nurse anticipates the child's treatment regimen will include:

    A. Strict droplet precautions, antitoxins, and antibiotics
    B. Respiratory isolation, antipyretics, and oral fluids
    C. Droplet precautions, cool mist humidifier, and intravenous fluids
    D. Standard precautions, seizure precautions, and muscle relaxants

119. An 8-year-old presents to the clinic for a sick visit with reports of a sore throat, fever, and nausea and vomiting for the past 36 hours. The nurse performs an assessment with the following results: temperature of 102.6°F; a bright red appearance to the tongue; an inflamed pharynx and tonsils with white specks; a fine, reddened, rough-textured rash on the trunk and extremities. What is the most likely diagnosis for this child?

    A. Fifth disease
    B. Rubeola
    C. Roseola infantum
    D. Scarlet fever

120. A nurse is providing care for a child hospitalized with acute renal failure. The child has been prescribed several medications as part of the treatment plan. Which medication should the nurse question?

    A. Furosemide
    B. Nifedipine
    C. Polystyrene sulfonate
    D. Gentamycin

121. A nurse is administering a gavage feeding to a premature infant. Which action should the nurse take to promote growth and development during feedings?

    A. Give the infant a pacifier
    B. Position the infant on the right side
    C. Burp the infant during the feeding
    D. Elevate the head and shoulders 30°

122. A nurse is providing care to a child suspected of having epiglottitis. The child has inspiratory stridor on auscultation, has tachypnea, dystonia with a sore throat, and is febrile. Which nursing action is the priority?

    A. Administer an antipyretic
    B. Offer a popsicle to soothe the throat
    C. Place the child in a supine position
    D. Keep the child as calm as possible

123. A nurse is performing an assessment on a 20-month-old male child during a sick visit to the pediatrician. The caregiver reports that the child has had some nasal congestion for the past 2 to 3 days and developed a harsh, hoarse cough in the last 36 hours. The child has a temperature of 99.8°F, is alert, and is restless. Based on this information which is the most likely cause of the symptoms?

    A. Pneumonia
    B. Asthma
    C. Bronchiolitis
    D. Laryngotracheobronchitis (LTB)

124. A nurse is providing anticipatory guidance on infant growth and development to a parenting class. Which toys should the nurse suggest to promote the development of an 8-month-old infant?

   A. Soft toys with bright contrasting colors
   B. Stuffed animals with button eyes
   C. Toys with large buttons or knobs to manipulate
   D. Dolls that can be dressed and undressed

125. What is the priority action when assessing a stable child with no respiratory distress after an insect sting in the ER?

   A. Apply a cardiac monitor ready for defibrillation
   B. Immediately administer emergency medications
   C. Assess the child's skin for dermatologic reaction
   D. Find out if any medications were administered prior to coming to the ER

126. Which assessment finding is not considered a sign of shock in a child?

   A. Weak thready pulses
   B. Temperature of 36.9°C/98.4°F
   C. Cool clammy skin
   D. Altered level of consciousness

127. What is the immediate, priority treatment for an adolescent diagnosed with acromegaly (hyperpituitarism)?

   A. Assess the self-concept of the patient
   B. Administer octreotide acetate as ordered
   C. Ascertain the patient's developmental age
   D. Family education of expected treatment options

128. Which laboratory test result does the nurse initially expect to be low for a child diagnosed with iron deficiency anemia?

   A. Serum ferritin
   B. Serum iron level
   C. Transferrin saturation
   D. Total iron-binding capacity

129. Which medication is expected to be given primarily in large amounts to achieve a therapeutic level to children diagnosed with congestive heart failure?

   A. Furosemide
   B. Dobutamine
   C. Theophylline
   D. Digitalis

130. Laboratory tests are ordered for a child suspected of having Kawasaki disease. Which laboratory results confirm this suspicion?

   A. Elevated hemoglobin levels
   B. Decreased white blood cell count
   C. Negative C-reactive protein (CRP) levels
   D. Elevated erythrocyte sedimentation

131. The nurse in the clinic is teaching parents of a toddler diagnosed with conjunctivitis. Which responses by the parents require further instruction?

    A. "Applying warm compresses can help with symptoms along with medication."
    B. "I am thinking my child could possibly have caught this at school."
    C. "Allergies and conjunctivitis are similar in how they present symptoms."
    D. "It is great that only one child has this. The other family members won't get this."

132. A 13-month-old child is being treated in the emergency department (ED) for febrile seizures. Clinical data most relevant to evaluate the effects of the prescribed medication, acetaminophen (Tylenol) is

    A. Pain scale of 2
    B. Absence of seizures
    C. Temperature of 98.6°F
    D. Therapeutic drug level

133. A community health nurse is giving a presentation on child abuse to a neighborhood group. What information should the nurse include?

    A. Children will often tell the truth when asked if they have been abused
    B. Sexual abuse can only be perpetrated on a child by an adult
    C. Management of the effects of child abuse often includes palliative care
    D. Persons unknown to the victim are frequently the perpetrators of abuse

134. A 9-month-old infant, born at 26 weeks gestation, is seen in the clinic. What should the nurse consider when assessing the infant for attainment of developmental milestones?

    A. Developmental milestones will be consistent with those expected of a 9-month-old
    B. Developmental milestones will be consistent with those of a 6-month-old
    C. The infant will always be behind in attaining growth and development milestones
    D. By the age of 12 months, the infant will be on target for developmental milestones

135. A 7-year-old presents to the clinic for a follow-up visit on a fractured left ulna. The child has a short cast that has been in place for 2 weeks. On assessment, the nurse notes several colorful drawings on the cast, along with some softened indentations that are soiled. The child is able to freely move his fingers. The fingers are pink with normal capillary refill. The child reports having minimal discomfort in the arm. The nurse can fit two fingers between the cast and the child's arm. Based on the assessment findings, what is the best action for the nurse take?

    A. Reinforce the importance of keeping the cast clean
    B. Compliment the child on the cast's colorful decorations
    C. Determine what is done to protect the cast while bathing
    D. Ask about the type of activities the child engages in

136. A nurse is providing teaching to the family of a child diagnosed with a community-associated methicillin-resistant *Staphylococcus aureus* (CA-MRSA) infection. What is most important for the nurse to convey during the teaching session?

    A. The importance of compliance with the medication regimen
    B. Avoid sharing personal items with other family members
    C. Recognition of the signs of worsening disease
    D. An understanding of the risk factors for transmission

137. A family consisting of three siblings is seen in the pediatrician's office to receive scheduled immunizations. The siblings are aged 4, 7, and 11. The 7-year-old was recently diagnosed with systemic lupus erythematosus (SLE). The oldest child will receive the Tdap and meningococcal vaccine. The other two children are due for the MMR and DTaP vaccines. How should the nurse proceed in administering the vaccines?

   A. Administer each child's vaccines as scheduled
   B. Omit the MMR vaccine for the 7-year-old
   C. Omit the meningococcal vaccine for the 11-year-old
   D. Omit the MMR vaccine for the 4- and 7-year-olds

138. A 6-year-old child presents to the clinic for a sick visit with reports of fatigue, intermittent nausea and vomiting, and poor appetite for the past 4 days. On assessment, the nurse notes that the child has lost five pounds since the previous visit 4 weeks ago. The child also has right upper quadrant tenderness on palpation. The nurse notifies the healthcare clinician of the assessment findings. Which finding is most concerning?

   A. Weight loss
   B. Upper quadrant tenderness
   C. Intermittent nausea and vomiting
   D. Lack of appetite

139. A 3-year-old child presents to the emergency department with reports of intermittent abdominal pain, vomiting, and lethargy. The caregiver reports that the pain occurred suddenly and has worsened over the past few hours. During an assessment, the nurse notes that the abdomen is distended, and the child vomits approximately 150 mL of bilious fluid. Based on this information the child is likely to be diagnosed with which condition?

   A. Gastritis
   B. Gastroenteritis
   C. Bowel obstruction
   D. Impacted bowel

140. A 3-year-old child is seen in the pediatrician's office for a sick visit. The nurse completes an assessment with the following findings: temperature 103°F, respiratory rate (RR) 32 beats per minute (bpm), and inspiratory stridor is heard on auscultation. The child is sitting in a tripod position, is refusing to lie down, and reports having a sore throat. The nurse suspects the child has developed epiglottitis. Which assessment finding best supports the nurse's suspicion?

   A. Respiratory rate
   B. Temperature
   C. Sore throat
   D. Inspiratory stridor

141. A nurse is providing care to a 10-month-old infant newly diagnosed with cystic fibrosis (CF). The infant was born at 34 weeks gestation and was considered small for gestational age (SGA). The infant has required continuous respiratory support in the form of supplemental oxygen and bronchodilators. The infant is currently being gavage fed fortified breast milk, but the mother is hoping to start breastfeeding as soon as possible. In preparing the family for discharge, what is the best action for the nurse to take?

   A. Have the social worker provide options for community support
   B. Ask the nutritionist to review the infant's nutritional requirements with the parents
   C. Teach the parents to maintain the infant's pulmonary hygiene
   D. Work with the case manager to organize a patient care conference

142. Which nursing action is a priority after the administration of epinephrine to a patient experiencing anaphylaxis?

    A. Notify the primary healthcare clinician
    B. Administration of a bronchodilator
    C. EKG and cardiac monitoring
    D. Frequent assessment of vital signs

143. What is the nurse's best response to a question about how to test for a child's food allergy?

    A. Perform an allergen skin test
    B. Test an elimination diet and assess for decreased symptoms
    C. Obtain serum antibodies evaluation after allergen exposure
    D. Administer intradermal injection of extract of various foods, one at a time

144. Which recommendation is most appropriate for children diagnosed with enzyme deficiencies?

    A. Low sodium, high fiber, high protein foods
    B. Restricted diet depending on the amino acid
    C. A diet rich in herbs and natural foods
    D. Dietary foods high in carbohydrates and dairy

145. What diagnostic test will the nurse expect to be ordered to confirm a suspected neuroblastoma for a 1-year-old child?

    A. Urine catecholamine metabolites
    B. Absolute neutrophil count (ANC)
    C. Serum electrolyte levels
    D. Complete blood count

146. What is the priority information for the nurse to include when educating parents about a cardiac catheterization?

    A. Children are usually not scared because it doesn't hurt
    B. The diet will be advanced as tolerated until bowel sounds return
    C. The child will sleep for several hours till the anesthesia wears off
    D. The child will have a pressure dressing where the incision was made

147. Which statement by a parent indicates further instruction is needed after teaching about post-cardiac surgery care for a newborn?

    A. "My baby will need to be constantly fed and for a long time after the surgery."
    B. "My baby seems to be satisfied after feeding and will wait a few hours before feeding again."
    C. "Pumped breast milk can be given to the baby after the surgery even though the baby will need intensive care."
    D. "A doctor said the baby may need assistance in the form of a feeding tube after the procedure. But maybe the baby won't need it?"

148. The nurse is educating the family of an 11-year-old child about alcohol, tobacco, and issues of peer pressure. Which education is the priority for this family?

    A. Forbid the child to have peers who use tobacco or consume alcohol
    B. Encourage open communication and discuss the effects of alcohol and tobacco use
    C. Do not allow smoking or consumption of alcohol in the house
    D. Secure all tobacco and alcohol products so that only adults have access

149. An infant diagnosed with hydrocephalus is scheduled for surgery. What is the priority nursing intervention in the preoperative period?

   A. Test the urine for protein
   B. Reposition the infant frequently
   C. Provide a stimulating environment
   D. Assess rectal temperature every 15 minutes

150. A 3-month-old infant is seen in the clinic for a well-child visit. The infant is very fussy, and the mother seems frustrated trying to quiet the infant. The mother tells the nurse, "I don't know how much more I can stand. This baby just won't stop fussing!" Which is the best intervention for the nurse to implement?

   A. Enroll the mother in parenting classes
   B. Refer the infant for developmental problems
   C. Assess for the presence of a support system
   D. Have the mother wait in the waiting room

151. A 4-year-old child has exhibited changes in sleep and appetite and has shown disinterest in activities formerly found enjoyable. Today, the parents have brought the child to the mental health clinic to be evaluated for depression. The parents ask the nurse what is likely to occur during this visit. What should the nurse tell the parents?

   A. "The child will be placed in a group setting with other same-age children."
   B. "The therapist will want to work with all of you as a family during this visit."
   C. "The therapist will use therapy to change your child's behavior and thinking."
   D. "The therapist will use play to encourage your child to express her feelings."

152. A 15-year-old is being discharged after surgery to correct a slipped capital femoral epiphysis (SCFE). The nurse is providing discharge instructions for home care. Which piece of information is important for the patient and family to consider?

   A. Weight bearing is not allowed for at least 6 weeks
   B. There is a potential for developing avascular necrosis (AVN)
   C. A wheelchair will need to be used for the first 2 weeks
   D. Toe touch weight bearing with crutches is allowed

153. A 6-year-old child presents to the emergency department with reports of increasing pain in the right lower extremity. The child walks with a pronounced limp and rates the pain an eight on the FACES pain scale. The nurse notes tenderness and warmth on palpation of the tibia. The parents and the child deny falls or any other trauma to the leg. When asked about recent illnesses, the parents state that the child had a cold a week ago and had chickenpox 2 weeks ago. A complete blood count shows an elevated white cell count, and an x-ray of the extremity shows soft tissue swelling around the bone. Based on this information what is the most appropriate next step in the child's care?

   A. The child will receive an orthopedic consult
   B. The child will be admitted for intravenous antibiotics
   C. The child will be discharged home after receiving an analgesic
   D. The child will be instructed in the safe use of crutches

154. A child is receiving intravenous immunoglobulin therapy (IVIG) as treatment for X-linked agammaglobulinemia. Which action is important for the nurse to consider when administering IVIG?

   A. Ensure the infusion rate is based on mg/kg/minute
   B. Monitor for adverse reactions every 30 to 60 minutes
   C. Discontinue the infusion for discomfort at the IV site
   D. IVIG may be piggybacked with other intravenous fluids

155. A 2-year-old child is being evaluated for suspected Hirschsprung disease. The parent reports that the child has infrequent bowel movements, usually occurring once or twice per week, and has a poor appetite. The nurse assesses the child and notes a distended abdomen. On exam, the rectum is found to be empty but afterward the child has an explosive bowel movement. Which assessment finding is most indicative of this disease?

   A. Distended abdomen
   B. Poor appetite
   C. Infrequent bowel movements
   D. Rectal exam

156. A child diagnosed with severe dehydration is to receive 20 mL/kg boluses of Lactated Ringers solution as part of a rehydration regimen. The child weighs 36 pounds. How many milliliters should the nurse administer in each bolus? Round to the nearest whole number.

   A. 16 mL
   B. 327 mL
   C. 1 L
   D. 164 mL

157. A child diagnosed with cystic fibrosis (CF) has also been diagnosed with failure to thrive. The nurse providing care for the child recognizes that this new diagnosis is most likely related to which aspect of the pathophysiology of CF?

   A. Tenacious sputum production
   B. Altered electrolyte balance
   C. Pancreatic enzyme insufficiency
   D. Hypersecretion of gastric acid

158. A child is hospitalized for treatment of an exacerbation of cystic fibrosis (CF). The nurse has identified several patient goals in the plan of care. Which goal should the nurse prioritize?

   A. Maintains adequate nutrition
   B. Demonstrates adequate coping skills
   C. Demonstrates ease of breathing
   D. Exhibits no signs of infection

159. Which assessment finding is considered a late finding in respiratory distress?

   A. Tachycardia
   B. Tachypnea
   C. Nasal flaring
   D. Cyanosis

160. Which parental statement about a child with a shellfish allergy would require the nurse to implement further teaching?

   A. "I'm so happy this condition will get better with age."
   B. "Shrimp is one of the foods my child has to avoid."
   C. "We usually eat at home and do not go to restaurants much."
   D. "This allergy means we will have to learn more about food ingredients."

161. Which finding most likely indicates Cushing disease in an adolescent with long-term corticosteroid therapy?

   A. Hair loss
   B. An increase in height above expected amount
   C. An increase in calcium in the bones
   D. Rapid weight gain in a short amount of time

162. Which condition is the nurse most likely to suspect while examining a 28-month-old child exhibiting spontaneous nasal and oral bruising and bleeding without reported injury?

   A. Hemophilia
   B. von Willebrand disease
   C. Chronic iron deficiency anemia
   D. Disseminated intravascular coagulation

163. What statement by a caregiver warrants further assessment by a nurse when assessing a child with a cardiovascular concern?

   A. "We nap once a day. Sometimes the child doesn't want a nap, but I do."
   B. "I see my child squat when we take our morning walks."
   C. "My child is rarely out of breath and walks everywhere in a hurry."
   D. "My child is constantly moving and running."

164. The nurse is assessing the pain level for a child diagnosed with rheumatic fever. What is the priority intervention when the child indicates moderate to severe pain?

   A. Have the child verbalize how to use the patient-controlled anesthesia system
   B. Provide nonpharmacologic interventions before pain medications
   C. Administer pain medications such as salicylates
   D. Carefully log roll the child to a more comfortable position

165. A nurse is caring for a child with large adenoids and tonsils. Which laboratory test is a priority for the nurse to check before a tonsillectomy?

   A. Platelet count
   B. Erythrocyte sedimentation rate (ESR)
   C. C-reactive protein (CRP)
   D. Creatinine level

166. A child experiencing increased intracranial pressure (IICP) is exhibiting signs of decerebrate posturing. The nurse would expect the child to present with:

   A. Flexion and pronation of fingers
   B. Flaccid paresthesia of lower extremities
   C. Rigid extension and pronation of the arms and legs
   D. Abnormal flexion of the upper extremities and extension of the lower extremities

167. A school nurse has interacted with a 11-year-old student several times during the school year. The nurse suspects the student is being abused. Which statement by the child supports the nurse's suspicion?

   A. "I get headaches almost every day."
   B. "My sister is the favorite and has all the fun."
   C. "My dad says I'm not worth spending money on."
   D. "I'm not allowed to try out for any activities."

168. A medically fragile child is hospitalized for treatment of an infection. The parents are very involved in their child's care and plan for one of them to room in with the child every day. To ensure optimum care for the child, which intervention should the nurse prioritize?

   A. Develop a therapeutic relationship with the parents
   B. Maintain a routine close to the child's home routine
   C. Encourage parental participation in the child's care
   D. Update the parents on the child's condition and plan of care

169. A school-aged child has been diagnosed with Legg–Calvé–Perthes disease (LCP). Which statement best describes the projected treatment for this child?

   A. Treatment will depend on the disease severity and the child's age
   B. Pain relief and rest are the hallmark treatments for this disease
   C. Physical therapy is paramount to an optimal outcome for this child
   D. The child will require surgery and will use a walking aid until healing is complete

170. A 2-week-old neonate presents to the emergency department with reports of lethargy and poor feeding. The caregiver states, "My baby was fine yesterday but now sleeps all the time and won't nurse." The nurse assesses the neonate and notes a rectal temperature of 96.8°F, a heart rate of 172 beats per minute (bpm), and respirations of 70 per minute. The neonate has some nasal flaring, acrocyanosis, and responds minimally to flicking of the soles of the feet. The nurse believes the neonate has developed sepsis. What other information will provide the most insight into the neonate's condition?

   A. The neonate's immunization record
   B. The history of family exposure to illness
   C. The mother's perinatal records
   D. The neonate's genetic and metabolic screening

171. A 15-month-old toddler is scheduled to receive four vaccines during a well-child visit. Which is the best action for the nurse to take to administer the vaccines efficiently and safely?

   A. Mix two to three vaccines per syringe
   B. Utilize approved combination vaccines
   C. Administer one vaccine per extremity
   D. Administer two vaccines per day over 2 days

172. A nurse is providing care for a premature newborn in the intensive care nursery. The infant has been diagnosed with necrotizing enterocolitis (NEC). In order to monitor for signs of worsening disease, which assessment concept is most important for the nurse to perform?

   A. Nutrition
   B. Pain
   C. Renal status
   D. Skin integrity

173. A nurse is providing care to a child hospitalized for treatment of Meckel's diverticulum. The nurse understands that nursing care should include monitoring for which potential complication?

   A. Anemia
   B. Encopresis
   C. Vitamin D deficiency
   D. Inguinal hernia

174. A nurse is providing anticipatory guidance to a family whose child is prescribed pancrelipase as a treatment for cystic fibrosis (CF). What should the nurse tell the family?

   A. Administer the medication between meals
   B. Avoid administering with milk, antacids, or iron
   C. Tablets may be chewed if they cannot be swallowed
   D. Take a missed dose with the next scheduled dose

175. A nurse is teaching chest physiotherapy to the parents of a child diagnosed with cystic fibrosis (CF). Which is the best way for the nurse to evaluate the parents' understanding of the teaching?

　　A. Observe each parent as they perform the skill on the child
　　B. Guide each parent step-by-step as they perform the skill
　　C. Provide the parents with written step-by-step instructions
　　D. Ask each parent to verbalize their understanding of the teaching

CHAPTER 23

Practice Exam Answers and Rationales

1. **C. Education for the family about communication and safety for the patient.**

   Nursing interventions should be aimed at accommodating the change in the patient's status and maintaining safety. The scenario does not indicate the need either to sedate the patient, nor to move the child to an acute-care facility, nor does it indicate that death is imminent.

2. **B. Elevate the head of bed (HOB).**

   A proper nursing intervention for head injuries is elevating the HOB at least 30°, not in a flat position, to help decrease intracranial pressure if present. Other interventions include maintaining head in a neutral position especially if spinal injury, initiating seizure precautions, and maintaining a quiet, nonstimulating environment. Children should not ambulate without assistance.

3. **C. Polymerase chain reaction (PCR).**

   PCR tests directly for the HIV antigen and is the most predictive screening for HIV. Enzyme-linked immunoassay (ELISA) and the Western blot test detect the presence of HIV antibodies. The CD4 count is used as a measure of disease status and progression.

4. **B. Provide pre- and postoperative care.**

   This condition is treated using surgical intervention. The priority intervention will be providing pre- and postoperative care. Body image and family communication are secondary to the surgical intervention.

5. **D. Iron deficiency anemia.**

   A newborn usually has enough iron in reserve to last for the first 6 months of life. After that, children need iron incorporated into the diet. Thalassemia and sickle cell anemia are genetic disorders affecting red blood cells but not the most common type of anemia. Aplastic anemia is not the most common type.

6. **D. Tachycardia with cool, clammy skin.**

   Cold, clammy skin, increased heart rate, and dizziness are signs of hypotension that may be a complication after a cardiac catheterization. Decreased heart rate, syncope, and tachypnea would also be very concerning, but not necessarily a sign of an expected complication immediately. Expected findings would be a sinus rhythm (as arrhythmia would be a complication of a cardiac catheter), warm extremity with a brisk capillary refill would be expected. Minor pain at the insertion site is also expected and treated with acetaminophen

7. **C. Laryngomalacia.**

   Signs and symptoms of laryngomalacia include inspiratory stridor exacerbated by crying, feeding, or agitation. Croup is a bark-like cough. Influenza is systemic. Respiratory syncytial virus is unrelated to stridor (noisy breathing).

8. **A. Encourage activities with friends, such as visiting, phone calls, and videoconferencing.**

   This developmental stage of adolescence is most concerned with peers and social groups. Books, handouts, and pamphlets are not as interesting as videos for this group, and video games should not be restricted to daytime hours. Equipment to be used may be scary for the patient.

9. **C. Unknown extent of the disability requires continual adjustments.**

   Cognitive impairments require some adjustments but not necessarily special education as it is not specific. Cerebral palsy (CP) is not usually progressive in nature and doesn't require institutionalization. The immune system is separate from the neurologic system.

10. **A. The parent was abused as a child.**

    Characteristics of FDIA/MBP include the parent (often the mother) was a victim of child abuse and the parent has a history of mental health illness such as personality disorder or pathologic lying. In FDIA/MBP the parent does not neglect the child but is overly protective of the child. It is the parent, not the child who is often overly anxious or exhibits attention-seeking behavior.

11. **C. "When do you usually give her the medication?"**

    The nurse should ask when the child takes her medication since methylphenidate can cause insomnia and anorexia. Children on methylphenidate should also be monitored for hypertension, tachycardia, and weight loss. The parent should be instructed to give the medication in the morning with food to decrease the likelihood of insomnia and anorexia. Asking the parent about rules for bedtime, what the child had to eat, or what the child's teacher is saying about her performance are appropriate questions to ask during the visit. However, based on the parent's concerns, the nurse should determine when the child usually receives the medication.

12. **C. Notify the healthcare clinician of the assessment findings.**

    The nurse's assessment findings suggest early signs of compartment syndrome and should be relayed to the healthcare clinician immediately so that the patient can be evaluated. These are not expected assessment findings for this type of injury. While the vital signs might be elevated in response to the injury and the resulting pain, the color and temperature of the toes, and the tingly sensation are not normal findings and require intervention. Utilizing nonpharmacologic pain management and/or asking the healthcare clinician for a stronger analgesic are all inappropriate interventions that will hinder the patient from receiving the correct and proper care.

13. **D. Obtaining laboratory specimens.**

    The priority intervention should be to obtain laboratory specimens, including blood cultures. Antibiotics wouldn't be administered until blood cultures and other labs were obtained. Administering antipyretics and educating the parents regarding the child's condition are both important but the priority would be to obtain lab specimens in order to administer antibiotics.

14. **C. A focused assessment on the immune system.**

    The most appropriate next step is completing a thorough physical assessment paying special attention to signs of impaired immunity such as the presence/absence of lymph nodes and skin manifestations such as eczema. The child has already had two courses of antibiotics that weren't effective, so a more in-depth assessment is required before prescribing additional antibiotics or admitting the child to the hospital. IVIG therapy may be an appropriate intervention once the child has been thoroughly evaluated for an immunity deficiency.

15. **B. "What does your child's diet look like on a given day?"**

    Celiac disease is an immunologic disorder in which gluten products cause damage to the small intestine resulting in vomiting and diarrhea. Knowledge of the child's diet will help support the nurse's suspicions. Asking if anyone else has the symptoms may be an appropriate question but the answer won't support the nurse's suspicion of celiac disease. Bloody stools are associated with inflammatory bowel syndrome, not celiac disease. The timing of the child's vomiting in relation to meals will not help support the nurse's suspicions

16. **B. "The patient is being treated for a seizure disorder."**

    The use of anticonvulsants is associated with the development of cleft lip and cleft palate. The fact that the patient had just four prenatal visits does not preclude the development of a cleft palate. Multigravidity is not associated with cleft palate. Gestational diabetes occurs during the second half of pregnancy; a cleft palate will occur during the first 8 weeks of gestation.

17. **D. Utilize the Wong-Baker FACES Pain scale.**

    The crying and whining after coughing indicate the child is in pain. The nurse should assess the child's pain using the Wong-Baker FACES Pain scale. Before the nurse can administer an analgesic, the child's pain level should be assessed to determine the right type and the right amount of analgesic to administer based on the severity of the pain. An antipyretic would be administered for a fever of 100.4°F or greater. Having the parent cuddle with the child is appropriate but the nurse needs to directly address the pain by assessing the severity and then administering an appropriate analgesic.

18. **A. The diameter of the trachea.**

    A child's tracheal lumen is narrower than that of adults. Inflammation, edema, and/or mucus narrows the lumen even more causing symptoms related to a lower respiratory infection (wheezing, rales, and tachypnea). An increased number of alveoli is expected from 3 months of age up to age 8 when the child can have as many as 300 million alveoli, but this does not create wheezing or tachypnea in the child. The larynx of young children is funnel shaped, not cylindrical like older children and adults. The funnel shape results in a narrowing of the larynx. Children have a higher, not lower, metabolic rate than adults. This higher rate can result in children developing hypoxemia much faster than adults in the presence of any respiratory distress.

19. **A. Anger.**

    Anger includes feelings of rage or resentment, which can be manifested by a patient yelling or throwing things. Denial includes feelings of isolation. Bargaining occurs when a client and/or family pleads for more time to reach an important goal. Depression includes sadness, grief, and mourning for an impending loss.

20. **A. Initiate gastric lavage right away.**

    If the toddler ingested the pills within the last 60 minutes, a gastric lavage would be the preferred treatment. If the acetaminophen is in the bloodstream, N-acetylcysteine may be administered. Chelation therapy is meant for metal poisoning. IV fluid replacement is used to treat hypovolemic shock.

21. **D. IgG.**

    IgG comes from the mother through the placenta. Because of this, the newborn has passive immunity to antigens in which the mother has developed antibodies. The fetus lives in an antigen-free environment, so it produces only trace amounts of immunoglobulins, specifically IgM. IgA, IgD, IgE, and IgM do not cross the placenta. This means they require an antigenic challenge after birth for them to start producing. IgM reaches the adult level when the infant is 1 year of age.

22. **C. Neurologic system.**

    The nervous system is most consistently affected by metabolic disorders. The physical examination should focus on evaluating neurodevelopmental functions. Abnormalities commonly revealed include impaired states of alertness and arousal, tremors, posturing, clonic jerking, tonic spasms, or seizures.

23. **A. Provide supplemental oxygen and assist child to a squatting position.**

    Supplemental oxygen and squatting position decreases workload on the heart and helps with perfusion. A cool cloth does not reduce workload or help with perfusion. Morphine is preferred over hydromorphone and IV fluids are implemented, not changed to KVO status.

24. **A. Respiratory stridor.**

    Respiratory stridor signifies a problem with the airway and possible impending obstruction. Unwillingness to swallow may be from pain. Drooling of blood-tinged saliva is expected after tonsillectomy. An elevated temperature is expected after surgery; less than 100.5°F is not considered febrile.

25. **D. Offer to assist with grooming activities as the patient specifies.**

    Grooming activities and having control with determining self-care and offering choices facilitates body image, dignity, and autonomy for the patient. Eliminating choice for how to void or defecate, and performing personal hygiene activities does not foster dignity or autonomy for the patient. Nurses must follow the facility policy and procedure, wearing their own clothing may be a safety risk.

26. **C. Foods low in carbohydrates.**

    A ketogenic diet, or one extremely low in carbohydrates, has been found to be the most beneficial for these patients.

27. **C. Ask the child if they are afraid of someone at home.**

    The nurse should determine if there is a reason the child is reluctant to go home. The nurse should also recognize that the child's somatic complaints probably play a part in the child's reluctance to go home. The nurse could express concern about the child to the teacher, the nurse could refer the child to a healthcare clinician for evaluation of the somatic complaints, but neither measure should be the nurse's initial action. The nurse should contact child protective services if they have suspicions of abuse but the initial action should be to question the child about feeling safe at home.

28. **C. Ask the patient what she thinks about her weight loss.**

    The best initial action is for the nurse to question the patient about her thoughts on the weight loss. The patient's lower blood pressure, weight loss, and amenorrhea are potential signs and symptoms of anorexia. If the patient doesn't think anything is wrong with her weight loss or thinks she should lose more weight, in conjunction with the other assessment findings is strongly suggestive of anorexia. Asking the patient if she is sexually active is appropriate considering her amenorrhea, drawing lab specimens to check for anemia, and consulting a dietician are all appropriate actions, but initially the nurse should ask about the patient's thoughts on the weight loss.

29. **C. Have the child stand up from a sitting position on the floor.**

    Children with DMD have muscle weakness that won't allow them to rise from a sitting position on the floor in the usual fashion. Observing the child stand from a sitting position on the floor would elicit the Gowers sign which is a hallmark of DMD. To note the child's muscle strength, the nurse would use resistance testing. Asking what type of sports the child enjoys would give the nurse some idea of the child's activity level and asking the parent when the child began to walk would give the nurse a sense of how well the child meets developmental milestones but neither action addresses the suspicion of DMD.

30. **A. "If a child has a fever and is very irritable, acetaminophen can be given."**

    At home fever management includes administering acetaminophen to provide comfort if the child has a fever and is irritable. A tepid sponge bath is not the best option to reduce fever in children. This practice is considered controversial and, if used, care should be taken to ensure the bath does not induce shivering. Antipyretics should be used if the child demonstrates discomfort and irritability. Aspirin should never be given to children as it presents a risk for the development of Reye's syndrome.

31. **D. Voiding cystourethrogram (VCUG).**

    A VCUG is the most likely next step in diagnosing this child. The VCUG will show any structural defects and will be diagnostic for vesicourethral reflux (VUR). Eighty percent of those diagnosed with VUR are female and have a history of frequent UTIs. An IVP evaluates hematuria and screens for an obstruction or tumor of the kidney. A renal biopsy is diagnostic for renal disease or transplant rejection. Urodynamic studies evaluate dysfunctional voiding.

32. **B. Gastroesophageal reflux.**

    Gastroesophageal reflux is common in infants, is considered benign, is not associated with respiratory illness, and does not interfere with growth/development. Gastroesophageal reflux disease, a more serious disorder, is associated with respiratory illness, poor weight gain, and excessive crying. Hypertrophic pyloric stenosis results in projectile vomiting and affects infants beginning at 3 to 6 weeks of age. Celiac disease is an immunologic disorder in which gluten products cause damage to the small intestine and usually manifests when solid foods are introduced to the diet (around 4 months of age).

33. **D. Notify the healthcare clinician of the change in pain level.**

    Based on the assessment findings the patient likely has developed appendicitis. Sudden relief of the patient's pain is a sign of a ruptured appendix, a medical emergency that should be conveyed to the healthcare clinician immediately. Continuing to monitor the patient's status and documenting the change in the patient's pain level are appropriate interventions but are not what the nurse should do next. Requesting an order for an antiemetic is appropriate for someone who is vomiting but given the emergent nature of the patient's pain level, it is not the action the nurse should take next.

34. **B. The child is experiencing respiratory acidosis.**

    This child is experiencing respiratory acidosis. Respiratory acidosis manifests as a pH <7.35, PaO_2 <75, and $PaCO_2$ >45. Normal blood gas results would be pH 7.35 to 7.45, PaO_2 75 to 100 mmHg, $PaCO_2$ 35 to 45 mmHg, and HCO_3 24 to 28 mEq/L. Respiratory failure would manifest as pH <7.35, PaO_2 <50 mmHg, and $PaCO_2$ >50 mmHg. Respiratory alkalosis would manifest as pH >7.45, $PaCO_2$ <35 mmHg, and HCO_3 <24 mEq/L.

35. **C. Recognize that play is an opportunity for the preschooler to address fears.**

    The use of play can be a great opportunity for the preschooler to work through their fears of hospitalization. Regression behaviors would be expected more in a toddler as opposed to a preschooler. It is important to explain the plan of care and procedures not just to the parents but to the preschooler as well. The child would experience more stress by not knowing what is happening to them. The procedure explanation should be done in simple, concrete terms, being mindful of the words used due to the preschooler's magical thinking. The child's schedule should not be so strict as to deny any flexibility. The nurse should try to plan care around the child's usual home schedule for things such as mealtimes, bedtime, homework, and so on.

36. **C. Hospice, palliative care.**

    Hospice is palliative care provided to terminally ill persons and their families in the last 6 months of the client's life. It is not appropriate for the patient to go be referred to physical therapy, occupational therapy, or to a rehabilitation care center.

37. **C. Apply direct pressure to the area of bleeding.**

    It is important to treat life-threatening injuries first. Therefore, the nurse must control external bleeding with direct pressure or sterile pressure dressing and elevation of the extremity. After, the nurse should assess neurovascular condition distal to injury before and after splinting. The nurse must not try to straighten fractured or dislocated joints, nor manipulate protruding bone ends. Marking the location of pulses to aid repeat assessment occurs after the bleeding has been controlled.

38. **C. Contact the ordering clinician for clarification of the order.**

    After reviewing the prescription, the nurse would contact the healthcare clinician. IVIG can only be administered IV and should not be given subcutaneously or intramuscularly. Clarification is needed before the nurse proceeds. The nurse would need to weigh the client as this medication dosage is weight-based, but the nurse's priority is to contact the clinician for clarification. The client's vital signs only need to be assessed to determine a baseline prior to starting the medication.

39. **A. Assess blood sugar every 2 to 3 hours.**

    The client is experiencing diabetic ketoacidosis (DKA). It is characterized by drowsiness, dry skin, flushed cheeks and cherry-red lips, acetone breath with a fruity smell. The nurse would question only checking the glucose level every 3 hours as it should be assessed at least hourly to ensure the client's level does not fall more than 100 mg/dL (5.55 mmol/L) per hour. Fluid therapy is given to treat dehydration, correct electrolyte imbalances (sodium and potassium due to osmotic diuresis), and improve peripheral perfusion. Short-acting insulin such as regular is used for blood sugar correction. Urine or blood is evaluated to assess level of ketones.

40. **B. "The amount of anemia will be better after this surgery."**

    A splenectomy will not cure sickle cell anemia, but it will help limit the degree of anemia. It will have no effect on any crisis episodes. The spleen also plays a role in straining the plasma for invading microorganisms so that phagocytes and lymphocytes can destroy them. Without the spleen, the child is at greater risk for infection.

41. **B. Plotting 5% or less weight on a growth chart.**

    Signs of CHF in children include failure to gain weight; weakness; fatigue; restlessness; irritability; and a pale, mottled, or cyanotic color. Spastic movements indicate seizure activity or cerebral palsy. Wave-like, uncoordinated activity is also seen in cerebral palsy, and spooning of the fingernails are seen in iron deficiency anemia.

42. **C. High Fowler's position, head forward, pinch bridge of nose, and ice pack above pinched area.**

    Sitting up with head forward facilitates airway clearance, pressure to the anterior part of the nose helps occlude the bleeding vessels, and ice constricts vessels.

43. **D. Have the teen leave with an assignment of keeping track of and writing down food intake for a week.**

    Keeping a food diary can help to assess eating patterns and will help the adolescent become aware at the same time. Drawing portion sizes and recalling information about past meals or calories consumed may not be accurate.

44. **B. "The EEG measures activity of the brain."**

    An EEG is a test that measures the electrical activity of the brain and detects any abnormalities in the brain waves. It is not related to imaging and will not show a mass. The EEG does not show increased intracranial pressure (ICP) or measure brain tissue normal or otherwise.

45. **D. Contact social services to evaluate the situation.**

    The nurse should contact social services to investigate the situation further. The triangular shape of the burn indicates that just the tip of the hot iron came in contact with the child's arm. If the child bumped into the iron, there would likely be a more linear burn than just the triangular tip of the iron. Given the shape of the burn, it would be inappropriate for the nurse to just tell the parent to be more careful with the iron or to ask when the accident took place. The nurse could question the child about the injury but not in front of the parent as the parent's presence could inhibit the child's response.

46. **B. Lead exposure.**

    Exposure to lead along with prenatal alcohol use and cigarette smoking are risk factors for ADHD. ADHD is more prevalent in males than females. Prematurity and low-birth weight are risk factors for ADHD. There is no specific gene associated with ADHD, although it can run in families.

47. **B. "This is a genetic disorder that can occur spontaneously without anyone in your family ever having it before."**

    Osteogenesis imperfecta is a genetic disorder that can have an autosomal dominant or a recessive gene inheritance. It has also been known to be the result of a spontaneous gene mutation. Telling the family that it is a genetically inherited disorder so someone in the family must have it is not therapeutic, is accusatory, and is incorrect since the disorder can occur as the result of a spontaneous gene mutation. Telling the family that they should not worry, that their child has the mildest form of the disorder and won't be affected much is not true. Even though the child may have the mildest form of the disorder, the nurse has no way of knowing to what degree the child will be affected. That response also does not answer the parents' question. Although it is therapeutic to acknowledge the parents' need to understand how the child developed the disorder, the nurse should answer their question rather than direct them away from it.

48. **A. Mupirocin calcium cream.**

    The child's symptoms indicate impetigo, a bacterial skin infection caused by *Staphylococcus aureus*. Mupirocin calcium cream is used to treat impetigo. It is applied three to four times/day for 5 to 14 days. Calamine lotion can be used to provide comfort from the pruritus of a varicella infection (chickenpox). Corticosteroid cream is used to treat contact dermatitis and urticaria. Permethrin cream is used to treat scabies.

49. **D. Decreased platelet level.**

    Serum laboratory results associated with HUS include decreased platelets and anemia, which is reflective of the hemolytic aspect of the disease. An increased, not decreased, creatinine level is associated with the renal effects of HUS. A decreased sodium level and an increased phosphate level are reflective of the renal effects of HUS.

50. **B. A cobblestone appearance to the bowel wall.**

    Radiographic findings of Crohn's disease include a cobblestone appearance of the bowel wall secondary to the presence of longitudinal ulcers and transverse fissures. Other findings include deep ulcers in the intestinal wall and full thickness inflammation of the wall of the colon. Pseudopolyps and superficial ulcers are radiologic findings of ulcerative colitis. A dilated proximal colon is characteristic of Hirschsprung disease.

51. **A. 73 mL/hour.**

    Formula: 0 to 10 kg: 100 mL/kg/d (100 × kg)
    11 to 20 kg: 1,000 mL (for the first 10 kg) + 50 mL/kg/d for each additional kilogram from 11 to 20 kg
    >20 kg: 1,500 mL (for the first 20 kg) + 20 mL/kg/d for each additional kilogram over 20 kg
    Divide the total by 24 to get the hourly intravenous fluid rate.
    Convert the weight in pounds to kilograms: 71 lbs/2.2 kg = 32.3 kg;
    1500 mL + 20 mL/kg for each additional kg over 20 (20 × 12.3 kg = 246 mL)
    1500 mL + 246 mL = 1746 mL per day
    1746 mL/24 hours = 72.75 mL/hour round to 73 mL/hour

52. **D. Skin color.**

   The skin color is pale and the bluish tinge around the mouth and eyes indicates cyanosis which is a late sign of respiratory distress requiring immediate intervention. The labored breathing and respiratory rate (RR) indicate tachypnea, and along with the lung sounds and productive cough contribute to the child's skin color. But the cyanosis in and of itself is the most concerning finding.

53. **C. Decrease by 0.34 kg.**

   It is normal for newborns to lose 10% of their birth weight in the first week of life. Newborns will then regain their birth weight by 10 to 14 days of life. During the first week of life, newborns do not increase their weight by 0.5 to 1 kg but will lose up 10% of their birth weight. This newborn weighed 3.4 kg; 10% of 3.4 kg is 0.34 kg. A decrease of 0.85 kg is 25% of the newborn's birth weight and is not an expected finding.

54. **B. Allow the parents to be present during the resuscitation.**

   Allow the family to be present at both medical rounds and resuscitation is the priority; provide explanations of all procedures. The family should look at the child and be involved in the care. In times of impending death and loss, initiate spiritual comfort by calling the hospital clergy only if appropriate; offer to pray with the family only if appropriate. Have the parents participate in early and repeated care conferencing to reduce family stress. Encourage the grieving process for the parents as appropriate; the question is asking about the priority during resuscitation.

55. **A. Syrup of ipecac.**

   Syrup of ipecac is no longer used to induce vomiting after accidental ingestion. GI decontamination via gastric lavage is indicated for those who ingest a life-threatening poison. Dialysis is only advised if indicated, such as in rhabdomyolysis. Activated charcoal is not used for iron overuse or acetaminophen exposure (only if receiving treatment within 4 hours) but is still used in accidental ingestion.

56. **C. "The sores should be totally covered until they are completely gone."**

   Impetigo is an infectious bacterial infection. The crusts should be removed after soaking prior to applying topical medications. Leaving the lesions open to air will aid in healing. Children diagnosed with impetigo may attend school during treatment.

57. **D. Document the results recognizing this as developmentally appropriate.**

   The nurse would continue to monitor the client as this level is within range for this client's age. Hemoglobin A1C provides information regarding the long-term control of glucose levels. This age client should have an A1C less than 8% (0.08). There is no indication the nurse needs to assess the client's current glucose level. The nurse does not administer insulin based on A1C levels. The healthcare clinician does not need to be notified for a normal level.

58. **B. Contrast materials used during the catheterization may cause diuresis.**

   The contrast material has a diuretic effect, so the nurse assesses the child closely for signs and symptoms of dehydration and hypovolemia. Although blood loss can occur, this is not the reason for monitoring the child's fluid balance. Typically, food and fluid are withheld for 4 to 6 hours before the procedure.

59. **B. Bruises (shiners) under the eyes.**

   Signs and symptoms of allergic rhinitis includes presence of nasal congestion, clear rhinorrhea, itching, and allergic shiners (dark circles/bruises under the eyes). Pharyngitis would occur if there was a throat infection, not a sinus infection. The drainage from the infected sinuses will generally be thick but it is not purulent. Respiratory difficulty is not seen because only the sinuses are involved.

60. **C. "Physical development during this time is often fast and uneven. This is normal and can affect your coordination and physical abilities."**

For this age group (adolescent), it is developmentally appropriate due to physical growth changes to be uncoordinated. This information is not suggestive of brain tumors and the statement is not appropriate. The patient does not mention anything about visual or hearing difficulties. Neuroimaging is not the appropriate response to the patient statements. Further information should be gathered and the clinician will suggest further testing if warranted.

61. **D. Referral to audiologist and parent/caregiver, family education of safety measures.**

A 1-year-old child should react to noises, especially loud noises. Speaking softly is not appropriate because the child has already not reacted to a loud noise. Retinal detachment is visual, not related to hearing, and a comprehensive assessment of the cranial nerves is not necessary due to the assessment of a hearing issue.

62. **C. Organize a patient care conference.**

The nurse should organize a patient care conference for the family. This will allow the family to explain their reasons for wanting to initiate palliative care and help the team determine the family's needs. It would also introduce the family to healthcare team members who would be part of the palliative care team. Providing information on new drugs/treatments in clinical trials as well as referrals for family counseling could be part of an overall palliative care treatment plan but is not the action the nurse should take to initiate palliative care. Hospice care, not palliative care, is initiated in the final months of life. Palliative care can be initiated at any point during treatment.

63. **B. Observe an interaction between the parent and child.**

Observing the child and parent interaction will allow the nurse to see if the child makes eye contact with the parent. The lack of eye contact in a toddler could be an early sign of autism. The nurse could ask the parent if the child makes eye contact with them, but it would be better if the nurse sees it in real time. It would also allow the nurse to screen for other behavioral warning signs of autism such as resisting cuddling or hand flapping. While it might be true that the child's lack of eye contact is due to shyness around strangers, the nurse should assess the child further and not just agree with the parent. It is not appropriate for the nurse to tell the parent that the child's behavior is abnormal. The child should be evaluated more before making that determination.

64. **A. "It is good to know that our baby will only need the harness for 3 weeks."**

On average infants will wear a Pavlik harness for 3 months not 3 weeks, so the nurse should reinforce the correct time duration with the family. Saying that straps should only be adjusted by the healthcare clinician, that breastfeeding positions will require modification, and that knee socks will help avoid skin irritation from the harness are all accurate statements which do not require any intervention by the nurse.

65. **C. "Tell me what concerns you most about taking care of your baby."**

This therapeutic option allows the mother to elaborate on her concerns, giving the nurse an opportunity to answer questions and provide anticipatory guidance for the mother. Letting the mother know that the infant's healthcare team is available to her is appropriate. However, telling the mother that there is no need to worry or be concerned is nontherapeutic and does not allow her an opportunity to share her concerns. Although the infant is doing well, being HIV+ and premature puts the infant at risk for future illnesses and/or developmental problems. Providing a list of community resources is an appropriate intervention, but first the nurse needs to understand more about the mother's specific concerns.

66. **D. "Circumcision is delayed until the hypospadias has been surgically corrected."**

The penile foreskin may be used as part of the hypospadias repair, so circumcision is delayed until after surgery. It is true that under normal circumstances infants are usually circumcised within 3 days of birth but this infant's condition precludes the procedure at that time. Circumcision is contraindicated in the presence of a hypospadias in order to avoid injury to the meatus. In addition, depending on the severity of the defect, the foreskin could be used as part of the repair.

67. **C. Teach the parents how to administer enteral feedings.**

Enteral feedings and/or total parenteral nutrition (TPN) are needed to ensure adequate nutrition in a child diagnosed with short bowel syndrome. Encouraging high calorie snacks or a diet of complex carbohydrates will not supply adequate nutrition for this child due to the malabsorption characteristics of short bowel syndrome. Administering loperamide will help address the diarrhea associated with short bowel syndrome but won't ensure adequate nutrition.

68. **A. 1572 mL.**

Formula:
0 to 10 kg: 100 mL/kg/d (100 × kg)
11 to 20 kg: 1,000 mL (for the first 10 kg) + 50 mL/kg/d for each additional kilogram from 11 to 20 kg
>20 kg: 1,500 mL (for the first 20 kg) + 20 mL/kg/d for each additional kilogram over 20 kg
Convert the weight in pounds to kilograms: 52 lbs/2.2 kg = 23.6 kg:
1500 mL for the first 20 kg + 20 mL for each additional kg over 20 kg (20 × 3.6 = 72)
1500 mL + 72 mL = 1572 mL per 24 hours

69. **D. "Use a humidifier or sit with your child in a steamy bathroom."**

Spasmodic laryngitis is a form of croup that affects younger children, 3 months to 3 years of age, and is usually viral. It is characterized by a sudden onset of a barking cough that occurs at night. To provide comfort from the coughing, parents can use a humidifier or sit with the child in a misty bathroom. Febrility is not part of the manifestations of spasmodic laryngitis, so acetaminophen administration is not indicated. Spasmodic laryngitis is self-limiting and usually resolves within 3 to 5 days with at-home management. Unless the child's respiratory status worsens there is no need for the parent to take the child to the hospital. Since the cause is likely viral, antibiotics are not indicated.

70. **B. Notify the healthcare clinician about the child's speech patterns.**

A 2-year-old toddler should have a vocabulary of 40 to 50 words and the ability to form two- to-three-word sentences. Babbling at 2 years of age requires the nurse to notify the healthcare clinician for follow-up. A weight gain of four pounds within a year is within the average expected weight gain of three to five pounds/year for a toddler. Negativism is a normal part of a toddler's development which occurs as the toddler tries to exert their independence. At 2 years of age, toddlers can scribble, but do not have the fine motor skills to copy or draw a circle until 3 years of age. Except for speech, the other patient assessment findings are appropriate for a 2-year-old and do not require a referral to an occupational therapist or telling the parent that the child's behavior is inappropriate.

71. **C. Incomplete.**

Types of fractures: open, the skin is broken, and bone exposed; closed, the skin is intact over the site; complete, the break goes completely through the bone; incomplete, the break occurs partly across a bone shaft (often the result of bending or crushing forces applied to a bone).

72. **C. Heart rate < 60 bpm with poor perfusion.**

According to the Pediatric Advanced Life Support (PAL) guidelines, a heart rate below 60 with poor perfusion is considered a cardiac arrhythmia and chest compression is to be initiated.

73. **D. The area of the burn such as the facial region.**

   Silver sulfadiazine 1% is used for burns. This medication should not be used with sulfa allergy, nor applied to the face, nor used on an infant under 2 months of age. A child's allergy to pain medication, and the timing of the burn do not factor into the decision-making process when ordering the ointment.

74. **D. "Has your child had a cold and ingested cough medicine recently?"**

   Radioimmunoassay of T4 and T3 is a specific blood study to determine how much PBI is present in serum. Ask if a child has recently taken large amounts of cough medicine containing iodide before the study or the PBI level may be abnormally elevated. The small amount of iodine ingested from iodized salt does not affect PBI levels. Asking about family history is not a priority. Phenytoin, a common anticonvulsant medication prescribed for children with recurrent seizures, may displace thyroxine from binding globulin and further contribute to low PBI levels. Exophthalmos may occur but is not the priority.

75. **C. Fever and tachycardia.**

   Signs of transfusion reaction include fever, chills, urticaria, tachycardia or bradycardia, hypotension, headache, restlessness, dyspnea, abdominal pain, and oliguria.

76. **C. Falls asleep while eating.**

   Manifestations of heart failure include difficulty feeding or eating, becoming tired easily when feeding or eating, shortness of breath with exercise intolerance, crackles and wheezes on lung auscultation, tachycardia, and hypotension.

77. **B. Position the child on their side.**

   The nurse should first position the child on their side to prevent aspiration and then call the clinician. Vomiting bright red blood is a complication of tonsillectomy. An antiemetic may be ordered but is not the first priority.

78. **A. A tense fontanelle and vomiting.**

   Tense fontanelle and vomiting are early signs of ventricular shunt malfunction. Severe headache, loss of memory, projectile vomiting, changes in vision, low-pitched crying, dilated pupils, and constipation are all late signs of shunt malfunction and ICP. Loss of memory and changes in vision are difficult to assess in infants.

79. **D. Plumbism.**

   Anemia by itself does not relate to confusion and lethargy. The inclusion of neurologic impairment with anemia points to lead poisoning or plumbism. This is not seizure activity (not epilepsy), and this is not associated with the flow of cerebrospinal fluid (CSF) in the ventricles or a brain tumor which is rare in children.

80. **A. Encourage the parent to include the child in any care decisions.**

   The nurse should ensure the child is included in any care decisions. While privacy is important for any patient, children at this age need their parents to be close by to provide support. Distracting the child from the situation could deny the child opportunities to ask questions and/or express their feelings and concerns. Support from the child's parent and/or the nurse and providing opportunities to express feelings should be utilized to calm an anxious child before administering a sedative.

81. **D. Encourage the child to talk more about why they think schoolwork is too hard.**

   Providing the child with an opportunity to express concerns about schoolwork validates their feelings and gives the nurse insight into issues that can be shared with the child's teacher and parents. The nurse could ask the child what they had to eat but the child already told the nurse that coming to school makes their stomach hurt. Notifying the teacher that the child's stomachache is due to anxiety may be appropriate and arranging a meeting with the child's parents and teacher could be useful at some point, but the next step would be to address the child's concerns.

82. **C. Educate the parent on the importance of finishing the medication.**

    It is vital that the child finishes the full course of medication to ensure elimination of the bacteria. Failure to do so often results in a rebound infection and contributes to the creation of antibiotic-resistant organisms. There is no need to contact the healthcare clinician to adjust the dosage as it is correct. The clinician has prescribed 160 mg every 8 hours which is 480 mg/day (30 mg × 16 kg) which is within the recommended dosage. Cephalexin is not a macrolide but a cephalosporin. Cephalexin may be taken with or without food.

83. **D. The vaccine schedule is maintained but is adjusted for live attenuated vaccines.**

    Children who are HIV+ should stay on schedule for routine vaccines. However, administration of live attenuated vaccines will depend on the child's CD4 count. Severely immunocompromised children should avoid live attenuated vaccines but those with adequate CD4 counts may receive those as well as other scheduled vaccines.

84. **C. "Has your child had a sore throat recently?"**

    The child's symptoms, especially the hematuria, are consistent with post streptococcal glomerulonephritis. A question that would help determine the diagnosis would be to ask if the child has had a sore throat recently. Asking if anyone else in the family had been ill, if the child is up to date on immunizations, or about the child's last meal are all appropriate questions to ask during the assessment. However, asking if the child has had a sore throat will help to determine the child's diagnosis.

85. **B. Check for tube placement.**

    The priority nursing intervention prior to starting the feeding is to check the tube placement to ensure it is in the stomach and has not migrated up into the trachea. Assessing bowel sounds, measuring the abdominal circumference, and measuring gastric residual are all appropriate interventions the nurse does prior to a feeding but priority is checking the tube placement.

86. **B. Fluid balance.**

    Besides the infant's lung function, the nurse should prioritize the infant's fluid balance. The infant with CLD, also known as bronchopulmonary dysplasia (BPD), is at risk for fluid overload which can adversely affect lung function. This often requires administration of diuretics and daily weight monitoring. Nutrition, the infant's growth/development, and parental support are all important to the infant's plan of care, but other than oxygenation and lung function, fluid balance should be prioritized.

87. **A. Avoidance of triggers.**

    The primary goal of asthma treatment is to avoid exacerbations and allow the child to engage in normal everyday activities; therefore, the primary focus of the nurse's teaching plan should be the avoidance of any triggers that could bring on an asthma attack. This means the child and family should be taught to identify environmental/nonenvironmental triggers for that child. Learning how to take prescribed medications, how to use a peak flow meter, and improving an Asthma Action Plan are all important to the child's overall health. However, avoiding triggers to an asthma exacerbation should be the primary focus of the teaching plan.

88. **A. "What aspect of your child's development concerns you?"**

    Asking the parent what aspect of the child's development concerns them allows the nurse to further assess the situation, which will then determine whether the parent should bring the child to the pediatrician's office. Until the child has been evaluated by the nurse and/or the healthcare clinician and found to be developmentally delayed, there is no need for evaluation by a specialist. Asking the parent how the child interacts with others will not provide enough information to determine if the child is developmentally delayed.

89. **B. Macroglossia.**

    Macroglossia is not a sign of a head injury. Raccoon eyes, depressed skull fractures, and clear drainage from the ears are signs and symptoms of a head injury.

90. **B. Metabolic acidosis.**

    Shock can lead to prolonged bleeding, metabolic acidosis, decreased respiratory rates/failure, bradycardia, and cardiopulmonary arrest. Metabolic alkalosis, tachypnea, and respiratory alkalosis will not be found in children in shock.

91. **D. The child cannot return to school for 1 week.**

    The nurse would question the child being out of school for a week. While these infections are highly contagious, children can return to school once treatment is started. Tinea pedis can be treated with topical or oral antifungals or a combination of both. Topical agents, such as luliconazole, are used for 1 to 6 weeks, depending on the brand. Antibacterial soaps help reduce the risk of infection to the affected area.

92. **D. Explain to the child and family what treatment continuation will include.**

    The American Academy of Pediatrics (AAP) recommends informing the child and family of what to expect of further treatments and procedures, explaining the prognosis in a developmentally appropriate way to ensure the child's understanding, and endeavoring to gain the child's candid opinion of the proposed care plan as the best intervention. The AAP also recommends that decision-making for older children and adolescents should include the assent of the child or adolescent.

93. **D. Desquamation of the skin in the radiated area can occur.**

    Radiation therapy side effects and teaching include dry or moist desquamation followed by hyperpigmentation. Avoid use of lotions and creams. Educate to not remove skin markings for radiation fields. Child may have a sore throat, provide pain medication as needed.

94. **C. Potassium.**

    Furosemide is not a potassium-sparing diuretic. It is used to manage edema due to heart failure and for treatment of hypertension. Serum potassium levels should be evaluated in someone taking this medication.

95. **B. An improvement in speech and communication.**

    Ear tubes facilitate drainage and an improvement in hearing will often lead to an improvement in speech and communication. There should be an increase in response to verbal cues and noises of all volumes. Purulent drainage is not an expected finding and would indicate an infection.

96. **B. The infant is not expected to experience physical delay.**

    A dimple or tuft of hair signifies spina bifida occulta and is not associated with neurologic deficit. Some degree of paralysis of the lower limbs, flaccid leg muscles with sensory loss, and bowel and bladder control issues are related to myelomeningocele.

97. **D. The pediatric GCS allows for developmentally appropriate cues for altered level of consciousness.**

    The GCS is a standardized tool to assess degree of consciousness using three parts: eye opening, verbal response, and motor response. Additionally, the pediatric GCS takes into account developmental cues. Developmental considerations are not taken into account for the adult GCS. The pediatric GCS allows for this type of assessment for scoring. Cranial nerve assessment is not included in the GCS. The numeric scale is not altered between the two tools.

PART IV PRACTICE EXAM

98. **C. The parent is likely in denial about the child's prognosis.**

    Although the healthcare team has explained the child's prognosis, the parent seems to ignore what was said and asks the nurse about starting a different medication. The parent's statement does not reflect loss of confidence in the healthcare team but is in fact asking about different medications that can be used. The parent's statement reflects avoidance of the issue more so than a misunderstanding of what was said or a need for additional information.

99. **A. The patient will require further evaluation and testing.**

    The assessment findings point to a strong possibility that the patient has scoliosis, but a definitive diagnosis requires further evaluation and testing. Carrying heavy backpacks is not associated with a curvature of the spine. The nurse does not have enough information to determine whether the child has scoliosis, its severity, and/or if it would require surgery. The nurse does not have enough information to determine whether the patient has idiopathic scoliosis, and it is not true that idiopathic scoliosis will resolve as the patient grows. While it is true that curves less than 25% require no treatment, other treatment options depend on the severity of the curve, and the age at diagnosis.

100. **B. "Polio is characterized by breathing or swallowing difficulty, severe muscle weakness, or floppy limbs."**

    Paralytic polio is characterized by breathing and swallowing difficulty, severe muscle weakness, and muscle flaccidity which can affect the respiratory system resulting in respiratory arrest and death. Some early symptoms include fever, sore throat, headache, muscle stiffness, and tenderness. Some patients may not even have symptoms or know they are infected. Although fever may be an early sign of polio, swollen parotid lymph nodes are not an associated symptom. A sandpaper-like body rash is not a symptom associated with polio. People diagnosed with polio may have impaired mobility and muscle wasting but will have muscle flaccidity not spasticity.

101. **B. Contact sports should be avoided for several weeks.**

    Splenomegaly is common with mononucleosis so contact sports and strenuous activities are discouraged to avoid a ruptured spleen. Saltwater gargles are recommended as a comfort measure for a sore throat, frequent rest periods may be necessary due to fatigue that can last up to 6 weeks or more, and patients with mononucleosis should avoid sharing eating utensils to avoid passing the infection to others but these measures do not avoid complications of the disease.

102. **A. "Cabbage and cauliflower are two of our favorite veggies."**

    Leafy green vegetables such as kale, lettuces, and spinach are high in potassium and should be avoided in patients with chronic kidney disease. However, cabbage and cauliflower are both renal friendly vegetables low in potassium. Hot dogs are high in sodium, ice cream is high in potassium, and peanut butter is high in phosphorus. High sodium, potassium, and phosphorus should be avoided in patients with chronic kidney disease.

103. **D. Short bowel syndrome causes nutrient malabsorption and electrolyte imbalance.**

    Short bowel syndrome occurs when there is a significant length of the small intestine that is nonfunctioning or has been removed, resulting in nutrient malabsorption, intestinal flora overgrowth, and electrolyte imbalance secondary to diarrhea. Short bowel syndrome results in diarrhea but not constipation. It is true that short bowel syndrome places children at risk for a variety of complications but a higher predisposition to complications does not necessarily mean they will precipitate. It is not true that TPN is a lifetime requirement for short bowel syndrome. It is possible for children to stabilize enough to subsist on enteral feedings alone.

CHAPTERS 23 PRACTICE EXAM ANSWERS AND RATIONALES

104. **B. Monitor the child for signs of respiratory complications.**

    The most appropriate action for the nurse to take is to monitor the child for signs of respiratory complications such as increased work of breathing or stridor resulting from inflammation. Supplemental oxygen would not be needed unless the child developed signs of respiratory distress. Teaching the parents how to avoid foreign object aspiration and preparing the child's discharge instructions are both appropriate interventions for this child but neither are the actions the nurse should take next.

105. **A. Birth occurred in the spring.**

    Risk factors for RSV infection include birth occurring April through September due to the peaked incidence of the virus causing infection in winter and spring (September/October to April/May) months affecting infants. Risk factors for RSV include young children under age 2, not school-aged children, male gender, and lack of breastfeeding. Additional risk factors include prematurity, complicated congenital heart defects, immunocompromised, and exposure to tobacco smoke.

106. **D. A 9-month-old who requires support to maintain a sitting position.**

    By 7- to 9-months of age an infant should be able to sit unsupported, so this infant requires intervention by the nurse. It is common for a 4-year-old preschooler to have an imaginary friend and to want that imaginary friend to participate in his life. A toddler who is mastering toileting may still have episodes of bedwetting. By 12 months of age, an infant should be able to stand and support themselves while cruising around furniture.

107. **A. Maintain a patent airway.**

    Airway and breathing are the priority. Monitoring for infection, providing support, obtaining labs to monitor renal function are all common interventions but are not considered priority.

108. **B. Epinephrine.**

    The three most common inotropic agents used after an arrest are epinephrine, dopamine, and dobutamine. Epinephrine is the drug of choice for children during and immediately after resuscitation. Atropine is used to address symptomatic bradycardia that is unresponsive to ventilation and oxygenation. Glucose is used to treat hypoglycemia. Lidocaine is not used for blood pressure.

109. **D. Macroglossia.**

    Infants diagnosed with congenital hypothyroidism will present with impaired growth, hoarse or lack of cry, feeding problems, protruding abdomen, and macroglossia. Normal height on growth chart, hypertonia, and hypoglycemia are not expected in an infant diagnosed with congenital hypothyroidism.

110. **A. Severe bone pain.**

    Osteosarcoma typically is characterized by dull bone pain that may be present for several months, eventually progressing to limp or gait changes. The affected limb may exhibit erythema and swelling, warmth, and tenderness.

111. **C. Level of consciousness.**

    Assessing the level of consciousness should be priority when monitoring circulation status. Hypoxia causes changes in neurologic status such as dizziness and restlessness, and the nurse should identify these changes early. A change in the level of consciousness is a late sign. Mobility is not a priority in measuring circulatory status. Nurses must verify perfusion using nursing assessment and palpation, not solely by machines. Temperature does not evaluate circulatory status primarily.

112. A. Cerebrovascular accident.

If an infant with heart disease becomes dehydrated, the infant can develop thrombi from the increased amounts of red blood cells (RBCs) and the viscosity of the blood leading to a risk for a cerebrovascular accident (stroke). Jaundice would only occur if the liver was involved. Tachycardia and seizures can occur with dehydration but an infant with a congenital heart defect would be at a higher risk for a cerebrovascular accident.

113. B. Bacteria entering the Eustachian tube.

The Eustachian tube is the primary point of entry for bacteria to get into the middle ear. Water-related activities are associated with otitis externa, not media. Children have short Eustachian tubes and ear drum damage is not related to otitis media.

114. C. Protect the patient from injury related to seizure movement.

Safety is the main priority during a seizure, not incontinence. The patient should never be left alone. Clothing can be loosened after the seizure activity.

115. D. Brudzinski's sign.

Brudzinski's sign is tested by the child lying supine with the neck flexed. A positive sign occurs if resistance or pain is met. The child may also passively flex hips and knees in reaction, indicating meningeal irritation. Kernig's sign is tested by flexing legs at the hip and knee, then extending the knee. A positive report of pain along the vertebral column and/or inability to extend knee is a positive sign and indicates irritation of meninges. This assessment does not signify impending seizure activity with abnormal posturing, and it is not a normal developmental finding.

116. C. The programs are intended to enhance the development of infants and toddlers who are at risk for or who have developmental delays or disabilities.

These programs, some of which are state mandated, are designed to enhance the development of infant/toddlers who have been identified at risk for or who have developmental delays. They help to ensure these children are able to reach their maximum potential in later childhood. These programs are not designed to provide respite care for caregivers with special needs children but to enhance the caregivers' ability to support their child. These programs are not special education classes for children with disabilities. Their focus is on enhancing the development of infants and toddlers. IEPs are plans to enhance the education of preschool, elementary, middle, and high school students (some of whom who have special needs), not infants and toddlers.

117. D. The hip and leg should be flexed at 90° while the lower leg is placed in a boot.

This type of skeletal traction is called 90-90 and is used for femur and tibia fractures where a pin has been placed in the affected bone and traction applied. The buttocks are slightly elevated off the bed in Bryant's traction which is used for developmental dysplasia of the hip (DDH). Buck traction is a form of skin traction used for knee immobilization and hip fractures and the traction force is positioned with the affected limb extended and maintained in a straight line. Russel traction is a type of skin traction used for femur fractures where the hip is flexed slightly, and the knee is suspended in a sling.

118. A. Strict droplet precautions, antitoxins, and antibiotics.

This child likely has contracted diphtheria based on the hallmark manifestation of the thick grey coating on the tongue, tonsils, and pharynx as well as the edematous neck. Strict droplet precautions and administration of antitoxins and antibiotics would be the first-line treatment. Respiratory isolation, antipyretics, and oral fluids would be used in treating mumps. Droplet precautions, IV fluids, and a cool-mist humidifier would be part of the treatment regimen for a child hospitalized with scarlet fever. Standard precautions, seizure precautions, and muscle relaxants would be part of the treatment regimen for a child hospitalized with tetanus.

119. **D. Scarlet fever.**

The sore throat, inflamed pharynx, and the tongue's appearance are all consistent with scarlet fever. While rubeola, roseola, and fifth disease all have fever and rashes, the erythematous sandpaper-like rash is specific to scarlet fever. The fifth disease rash has a maculopapular lace-like appearance. The rubeola rash has an erythematous maculopapular appearance and the roseola rash is pinkish red, flat, and blanches when touched.

120. **D. Gentamycin.**

Gentamycin is an aminoglycoside, a nephrotoxic antimicrobial that should be used with caution. The nurse should question the order and request an alternative or an adjusted dose. Nifedipine is an appropriate drug to treat hypertension associated with acute renal failure. Polystyrene sulfonate is used to treat hyperkalemia associated with renal failure and furosemide is a diuretic used to inhibit sodium reabsorption and promote diuresis.

121. **A. Give the infant a pacifier.**

Giving the infant a pacifier during each feeding will promote normal growth and development by allowing exercise of the jaw through the sucking motion. Sucking the nipple will also help the infant to identify the action with feeding and the sensation of fullness. Other methods of promoting normal growth and development include cuddling, rocking, and talking to the infant during feeding. Positioning the infant on the right side should be done at the end of the feeding to promote gastric emptying. Burping the infant during and after the feeding prevents the build-up of air in the stomach and can help prevent regurgitation of the feeding. Elevating the head and shoulders during each feeding helps the formula stay in the stomach.

122. **D. Keep the child as calm as possible.**

The priority action the nurse should take is to keep the child as calm and quiet as possible. Epiglottitis is inflammation and swelling of the epiglottis which can cause airway obstruction and is considered a medical emergency. Keeping the child calm and mitigating crying can prevent further swelling which can lead to the need for intubation. To ensure safety, the child with epiglottitis should have nothing by mouth, as the child may have difficulty swallowing, therefore offering a popsicle is inappropriate. Placing the child in a supine position is inappropriate as airway occlusion can occur. The child should be allowed to assume a position of comfort (e.g., the tripod position or sitting upright on a parent's lap). Administering an antipyretic is appropriate for the child's plan of care but is not the priority action.

123. **D. Laryngotracheobronchitis (LTB).**

LTB, a form of croup, is an acute upper respiratory viral infection that affects children 6 months to 8 years of age (males more so than females). It is characterized by a hoarse brassy cough, stuffy nose, low-grade fever, dyspnea, and irritability. Pneumonia and bronchiolitis are both lower respiratory infections that present with tachypnea, retractions, nasal flaring, adventitious lung sounds, and varied febrility. Asthma is a chronic inflammatory disorder of the airway that usually occurs in children aged 5 years and up. It is characterized by hypersecretion of mucus and bronchoconstriction that can be brought on by various environmental and nonenvironmental triggers.

124. **C. Toys with large buttons or knobs to manipulate.**

Toys that have large buttons or knobs to manipulate would enhance development of infants 8 to 12 months of age. As infants grow, toys are geared to developing the motor skills and language skills that the infant or child is developing at the time. Soft toys with bright colors would promote the development of newborns. Stuffed animals with button eyes are a choking hazard for infants. Infants do not yet have the fine and gross motor skills to dress or undress a doll. Those types of dolls are more appropriate for older toddlers or preschoolers.

125. **D. Find out if any medications were administered prior to coming to the ER.**

The nurse would first determine if any medications have already been administered to this client. The client does not appear to be in distress based on the assessment and vital signs are considered normal in a stable client. The nurse would expect stridor, wheezing, hypotension, tachycardia, and shortness of breath—among other symptoms—in the client having an anaphylactic reaction. Since the client is stable, epinephrine is not indicated at this time.

126. **B. Temperature of 36.9°C/98.4°F.**

Signs of shock include a decreased level of consciousness, tachycardia, weak, thready pulses, and cool, clammy skin, not a temperature of 36.9°C/98.4°F.

127. **B. Administering octreotide acetate as ordered.**

Administering octreotide acetate as ordered is the priority intervention and treatment for acromegaly. Assessing the child's self-image, chronological or developmental level, and educating the family about expected treatment options are all appropriate but would not be considered the priority.

128. **A. Serum ferritin.**

Serum ferritin is decreased during the first stage of iron deficiencies. During the second stage, the lack of transport iron is identified primarily by a decrease in transferrin saturation. A decrease in serum iron and an increase in total iron-binding capacity are likely as well. The question asks for initial findings.

129. **D. Digitalis.**

The use of large doses of digoxin at the beginning of therapy to build up the blood levels of the drug to a therapeutic level is known as digitalization. During the 24 hours digitalization is occurring, the child should be on a cardiac monitor and the nurse should monitor the PR interval and a decreased ventricular rate. Dobutamine is not given in this manner. Theophylline is for asthma treatment and used primarily for exacerbations. Furosemide is a diuretic.

130. **D. Elevated erythrocyte sedimentation.**

With Kawasaki disease, the erythrocyte sedimentation rate (ESR) and the CRP level are elevated. The complete blood count (CBC) may reveal mild to moderate anemia and an elevated white blood cell count during the acute phase.

131. **D. "It is great that only one child has this. The other family members won't get this."**

Conjunctivitis is highly contagious. There are several reasons for irritation of the conjunctiva and allergies are one of them; symptoms of conjunctivitis and allergies can appear similar. Warm compresses will help with symptoms.

132. **C. Temperature of 98.6°F.**

The temperature of 98.6°F is directly related to the effects of the acetaminophen. The medicine was not given for pain, the seizures are related to the temperature, the acetaminophen did not reduce the seizure activity, but acted on the body temperature. Acetaminophen is not elevated with a serum blood level.

133. **C. Management of the effects of child abuse often includes palliative care.**

Palliative care is often part of the plan of care for victims of child abuse. Palliative care includes treatment of the child's symptoms as the result of the abuse (posttraumatic stress disorder [PTSD], anxiety, depression, pain) and care related to resulting injuries. Children often will not tell the truth when asked if someone has hurt them. Often, they will lie about being hurt to protect the perpetrator who is frequently a parent, relative, or someone else they know (teacher, coach), not a stranger. Sexual abuse is often perpetrated by an adult but can also be perpetrated by an older child or teenager on a younger child.

134. **B. Developmental milestones will be consistent with those of a 6-month-old.**

    The growth and development of infants born prematurely should take into account their adjusted age in order to perform a more accurate assessment. For this 9-month-old infant born at 26 weeks gestation (14 weeks or 3.5 months early), the adjusted age is 6.5 months old. So, in assessing the infant, the nurse would expect the growth/development milestones of a 6-month-old, not a 9-month-old. It is not true that the infant will always be behind in growth/development. An adjusted age would need to be considered until the child reached 2 to 3 years of age; therefore, it is not true that the child would be on target by age 12 months.

135. **C. Determine what is done to protect the cast while bathing.**

    Because of the soft indentations on the cast, the best action for the nurse to take is to ask what the child does to protect the cast while bathing. Getting the cast wet can cause softening of the cast and indentations. Those indentations can cause skin irritation and breakdown. The cast should be kept clean, and the nurse can reinforce that, but the best action is to address the softened areas on the cast. The nurse can ask about the child's activities and compliment him on the cast's decoration, but the best action is to address the softened areas on the cast as this will likely lead to complications.

136. **A. The importance of compliance with the medication regimen.**

    The most important instruction to convey is the importance of taking the full course of prescribed antibiotics. Finishing all the antibiotics will eliminate the infection from the child and will help slow the growth of antibiotic-resistant pathogens. Teaching the child to avoid sharing personal items will help stop the spread of infection but does not eliminate the infection. Recognizing signs of worsening disease and the risk factors for transmission are also appropriate health promotion teaching points and will help the family avoid reinfection but at this time it is most important for the child to be compliant with completing the course of antibiotics.

137. **D. Omit the MMR vaccine for the 4- and 7-year-olds.**

    The MMR vaccine contains a weakened but live virus and should not be administered to an immunocompromised child or anyone in that household. The nurse should not administer each child's vaccines as scheduled or omit the MMR just for the 7-year-old that is immunocompromised. The meningococcal vaccine is not a live vaccine, so it is safe for the 11-year-old to receive it and to be in contact with the immunocompromised sibling.

138. **B. Upper quadrant tenderness.**

    The most concerning finding is the upper quadrant tenderness which could indicate a liver disease, such as cirrhosis. Weight loss, intermittent nausea and vomiting, and a lack of appetite are also symptoms associated with early cirrhosis but could also be attributed to other disorders. All the symptoms require follow-up and should be brought to the healthcare clinician's attention, but the upper quadrant tenderness is most concerning.

139. **C. Bowel obstruction.**

    Bilious vomitus occurs in the presence of a bowel obstruction. Gastritis is associated with epigastric pain as opposed to abdominal pain. Gastroenteritis will present with abdominal pain, diarrhea, and vomiting (not bilious vomitus). Impacted fecal material is associated with encopresis and constipation and does not involve bilious vomitus.

140. **D. Inspiratory stridor.**

    Stridor, one of the hallmarks of epiglottitis, is caused by inflammation and swelling of the epiglottis. This, along with the child's tripod position and refusal to lie down most supports the nurse's suspicion of epiglottitis. The child's temperature, sore throat, and tachypnea are also commonly attributed to other conditions such as bronchiolitis, tonsillitis, tracheitis, and pneumonia.

141. D. Work with the case manager to organize a patient care conference.

The best action for the nurse to take is to work with a case manager to organize a patient care conference. A patient care conference would include all clinicians involved in the infant's care, which will include the parents, social worker, and nutritionist. During the conference, the nurse can identify aspects of the infant's care that require parental teaching. It also allows the parents opportunities to meet with all the infant's caregivers in one place, and to ask questions and receive support. Having the social worker provide options for community support, asking the nutritionist to review the infant's nutritional requirements with the parents, and teaching the parents to maintain the infant's pulmonary hygiene are all useful actions for the nurse can take, but each action alone does not accomplish as much as a patient care conference.

142. B. Administration of a bronchodilator.

After securing the client's airway, the nurse would administer albuterol, a bronchodilator that enlarges the lumen of the airway, to facilitate breathing. The nurse would monitor the client's vital signs and contact the healthcare clinician; however, the patient's breathing takes priority. A cardiac monitor may be applied, depending upon the facility's policy.

143. B. Test an elimination diet and assess for decreased symptoms.

Food allergies can be determined by eliminating the suspected food and observe for symptoms. They are best identified by elimination. Suspected foods are reintroduced one at a time and the patient is assessed for return of symptoms if allergic. Skin testing with either a patch or intradermal injection is ineffective for determining food allergies. Serum antibody levels can be measured but are not specific in helping to determine food allergies.

144. B. Restricted diet depending on the amino acid.

Special diet restrictions and synthetic medical foods are the two most successful methods of controlling enzyme deficiencies. Dietary restriction is the primary treatment modality for inborn errors of metabolism. The goal is to control the substrate accumulation by reducing or eliminating carbohydrates, proteins, or both.

145. A. Urine catecholamine metabolites.

Urine catecholamine metabolites identify specific tumor markers used to differentiate a neuroblastoma from other tumors. Complete blood count (CBC) determines abnormal blood loss, anemias, or suggests disorders affecting bone marrow. An ANC measures the numbers of neutrophils. Serum chemistries indicate levels of electrolytes.

146. D. The child will have a pressure dressing where the incision was made.

The parents should be made aware of the expectation of having a pressure dressing over this insertion site to prevent bleeding. This procedure is usually performed with sedation. The parents should also expect the nurse to assess the dressing every 15 minutes, minimally, for the first hour and then twice 30 minutes apart. Children are expected to be scared due to the invasiveness of the procedure and may need distraction. The procedure does not involve the abdomen and a regular diet as tolerated is expected after anesthesia has worn off.

147. A. "My baby will need to be constantly fed and for a long time after the surgery."

Children with congenital heart defects typically have increased nutritional needs related to increased cardiac and respiratory capacities. Infants need highly nutritious milk, breast or sometimes fortified, in a short amount of time, under 20 to 30 minutes. Unfinished milk can be added by gavage if necessary.

148. B. Encourage open communication and discuss tobacco and alcohol use and effects with the child.

Open communication about use of substances and peer pressure facilitates conversation within the family. Forbidding alcohol and tobacco make them more desirable sometimes.

Not allowing the consumption of alcohol or smoking in the house is appropriate but this will more than likely happen outside of the parental home. Adult consumption of the same substances that are forbidden to the children sends conflicting messages.

149. **B. Reposition the infant frequently.**

    Frequent positioning is to decrease pressure in the cranial ventricles and other areas. Urine protein is not a concern for patients diagnosed with hydrocephalus. Less stimulation is beneficial and a rectal temperature is not warranted and every 15 minutes is unnecessary.

150. **C. Assess for the presence of a support system.**

    The mother is stressed and frustrated at not being able to calm the infant. Her statement about not knowing how much more she can stand indicates that the mother/infant dyad is in crisis and the situation could possibly lead to abuse if not addressed. The best intervention is to determine if the mother has a support system; someone who can provide respite for her. The mother may have all the knowledge needed to parent her infant but is just overwhelmed by the inability to calm the infant. There is not enough information to determine whether the infant has any developmental delays. Completing the visit without the mother is not the ideal option even if it gives her a short respite from her infant.

151. **D. "The therapist will use play to encourage your child to express her feelings."**

    Play therapy is used to assist a child in expressing their feelings and emotions when they may not have the ability to express them in words. It will give the clinician insight into what has caused the child's change in behavior and will provide a basis for planning future sessions with the child and parents. Family therapy will likely be part of the child's plan of care, but the clinician will likely want to meet with the child and parents separately first. Group therapy is used with preteen and teenaged groups allowing peers to sharing experiences and focus on relationships. Cognitive behavioral therapy is used to teach children how to change their reactions and negative thought patterns to more positive alternates.

152. **D. Toe touch weight-bearing with crutches is allowed.**

    After surgery, the patient is allowed only toe-touch weight bearing with crutches for at least 6 weeks. Prior to surgery, there is the potential for developing AVN if the slip worsens. A wheelchair would be needed if the patient had a pin placed in both hips. In that case, crutches could not be used, no weight bearing would be allowed, and the wheelchair would be needed for longer than 2 weeks.

153. **B. The child will be admitted for intravenous antibiotics.**

    The most appropriate next step is admission for intravenous antibiotics. In light of the child's symptoms, past history of varicella infection, and the fact that the family denies any trauma to the extremity, there is the strong possibility of osteomyelitis which requires antibiotic therapy. The laboratory result indicates infection and x-ray result suggests osteomyelitis. Based on the information, the child should not be discharged home after receiving an analgesic. Although the child may need an orthopedic consult and to be instructed how to use crutches, the most appropriate next step is admission for IV antibiotics.

154. **A. Ensure the infusion rate is based on mg/kg/minute.**

    IVIG is administered milligrams/kilogram/minute and is always given intravenously. The nurse should monitor for adverse reactions every 15 minutes for the first hour of infusion then every 30 minutes for the remainder of the infusion. If discomfort or pain occurs at the IV site, an ice pack may help to alleviate the discomfort. The infusion need not be discontinued. IVIG should not be piggybacked or mixed with other medications or fluids.

155. **D. Rectal exam.**

A hallmark characteristic of Hirschsprung disease is an empty rectum on exam that is often followed by a forceful bowel movement. The distended abdomen, poor appetite, and infrequent bowel movements are all symptoms of Hirschsprung disease, but the empty rectum is the finding most indicative of the disease.

156. **B. 327 mL.**

Convert the weight in pounds to kilograms: 36 lbs / 2.2 kg = 16.36 kg
16.36 kg × 20 mL = 327.2 mL rounded to 327 mL bolus.

157. **C. Pancreatic enzyme insufficiency.**

Pancreatic enzyme insufficiency results from the production of thick mucus that damages the pancreatic ducts, blocking the enzymes needed for digestion and absorption from entering the digestive tract. This can result in poor weight gain and failure to thrive regardless of the amount of food taken in. Tenacious sputum production affects the respiratory system, causing pneumonia and impaired lung function. Altered electrolyte balance results from excessive sodium loss through the sweat glands. Hypersecretion of gastric acids results in gastroesophageal reflux disease (GERD).

158. **C. Demonstrates ease of breathing.**

The nurse should prioritize the goal related to pulmonary functioning, in this case, how easily the child is able to breathe. Maintaining adequate nutrition, demonstrating adequate coping skills, and exhibiting no signs of infection are all goals important to the plan of care of a child diagnosed with CF but the priority focus should be on the child's ease of breathing.

159. **D. Cyanosis.**

Late signs of respiratory distress include cyanosis, slow respiratory rate (RR), bradycardia, altered mental status. Early signs of respiratory distress include tachypnea, tachycardia, nasal flaring, retractions, agitation, pallor, fatigue.

160. **A. "I'm so happy this condition will get better with age."**

This allergy does not get better with age and is life-long. Shrimp should be avoided because it is a type of shellfish. The parents and family need to understand the importance of knowing food ingredients to avoid allergic reaction, and it can be easier to monitor possible allergy triggers when cooking at home, as opposed to dining at restaurants.

161. **D. Rapid weight gain in a short amount of time.**

A history of rapid weight gain and long-term corticosteroid therapy suggests this child may have Cushing disease, which could be confirmed using an adrenal suppression test. A height increase is not related to Cushing disease. Hirsutism or excessive hair growth can occur. A loss of calcium in the bones (osteoporosis) can occur with long-term corticosteroid use.

162. **B. von Willebrand disease.**

The primary clinical manifestations of von Willebrand disease are bruising and mucous membrane bleeding from the nose, mouth, and gastrointestinal (GI) tract. Bleeding associated with von Willebrand disease may be severe and lead to anemia and shock, but deep bleeding into joints and muscles, like that seen in hemophilia, is rare except with type III von Willebrand disease. Bleeding with hemophilia is usually due to an injury. Chronic iron deficiency anemia does not cause spontaneous bruising and bleeding. Disseminated intravascular coagulation is a secondary condition not a primary one and includes symptoms of bleeding (petechiae/purpura, hematuria, bleeding from IVs).

163. **B. "I see my child squat when we take our morning walks."**

The walking toddler may squat periodically to relieve a hypercyanotic spell. This position serves to improve pulmonary blood flow by increasing systemic vascular resistance. Toddlers are very active and should be moving a lot, rarely out of breath is not a concern. Daily napping is normal.

164. **C. Administer pain medications such as salicylates.**

    Pain control and relief are the highest priorities for the child with rheumatic fever. Log rolling is not necessary with rheumatic fever (indicated with spinal surgery), however, position the child to relieve joint pain, handling carefully. Anti-inflammatory medications such as salicylates are given to relieve joint inflammation pain, and for anti-platelet aggregation, and usually in high doses only for rheumatic fever. Salicylates are more common than narcotic opioids. Patient-controlled anesthesia is not typically used for children. While the use of non-pharmacologic measures is helpful for pain management, medications should be first priority for faster relief for moderate to severe pain.

165. **A. Platelet count.**

    Children scheduled for a tonsillectomy should be monitored for bleeding before and after surgery. The tonsillar area is highly vascular and postoperative bleeding can be a complication. Platelet count, prothrombin time (PT), partial thromboplastin time (PTT), hemoglobin and hematocrit (H/H), white blood cell (WBC) count, and urinalysis will be ordered before surgery. A nurse can recognize risk for bleeding based on the platelet count results. Creatinine level, ESR, and CRP are not related to bleeding.

166. **C. Rigid extension and pronation of the arms and legs.**

    Extension and pronation of the extremities is the definition of this posturing. This positioning is not limited to the fingers, and the extension and pronation is for all four extremities.

167. **C. "My dad says I'm not worth spending money on."**

    The parent's statement negates the child's worth and is a red flag that the child is possibly experiencing emotional and/or physical abuse. Although somatic complaints such as headaches are associated with child abuse, there could be an organic reason for the headaches. The fact that the child feels the sister is the favorite could be the child's perception but not necessarily the reality, and the fact that the child is not allowed to try out for activities could be due to other reasons; therefore, neither statement is the best indicator of abuse and would require additional investigation.

168. **A. Develop a therapeutic relationship with the parents.**

    The nurse should develop a trusting therapeutic relationship with the parents that respect the parents' expertise in their child's needs and care. This will go a long way in ensuring optimum care for the child. It is important for the nurse to maintain a routine close to the child's home routine but ensuring a trusting therapeutic relationship with the parents is the priority. The nurse should encourage parental participation in the child's care and keep them updated on the plan of care. This will happen as a result of the nurse developing a therapeutic relationship with the parents.

169. **A. Treatment will depend on the disease severity and the child's age.**

    LCP is a self-limiting disease involving avascular necrosis (AVN), bone resorption, revascularization, and bone regrowth. It is a process that can take several years to complete. The best description is that treatment depends on the age of the child and the degree of severity when diagnosed. Children 8 years and older may require surgery followed by physical therapy and the use of a walking aid. Younger children tend to fare better and may only require restrictions on strenuous activities and anti-inflammatory medications to alleviate pain and muscle spasms. It is incorrect to state definitively that pain relief and rest are hallmark treatments, that physical therapy is paramount to an optimal outcome, and that the patient will require surgery and will use a walking aid as treatment depends on the stage and severity of disease.

170. **C. The mother's perinatal records.**

The mother's prenatal, perinatal, and intrapartum records will show whether she was screened and/or treated for group B *Streptococcus* (GBS). GBS is the number one cause of sepsis in newborns. This neonate's symptoms strongly suggest sepsis (hypothermia, tachycardia, tachypnea, mild respiratory symptoms, lethargy, and poor feeding). At 2 weeks of age, the neonate would just be starting the immunization schedule. It would be appropriate for the nurse to ask about the family's exposure to illnesses, but the mother's records would provide more insight into the neonate's condition. At 2 weeks post birth, the nurse may not have access yet to the results of the neonate's genetic/metabolic screening.

171. **B. Utilize approved combination vaccines.**

In order to administer several vaccines safely and efficiently, the nurse should administer approved combination vaccines. At 15 months old, a toddler would be scheduled to receive diptheria, tetanus, acellular pertussis (DTap); *Haemophilus influenzae* type b (Hib); pneumococcal conjugate; inactive polio vaccine (IPV); varicella; and measles, mumps, rubella (MMR). The combination vaccines ProQuad (MMR and varicella) and Pentacel (DTaP, Hib, and IPV) can be given to decrease the number of injections the toddler would need. The nurse should not mix single dose vaccines in the same syringe. The nurse may need to administer an injection in more than one extremity, but the best action is to utilize the combination vaccines. Having the parent bring the child back for a second day causes the family undue inconvenience.

172. **C. Renal status.**

Monitoring the newborn's renal status is most important so as to identify any decreases in urinary output which could indicate poor perfusion. Poor perfusion is strongly associated with the development of NEC and is a sign of worsening disease. Assessing nutrition would not be most important in detecting worsening disease. An infant with NEC would be nil per os (NPO) and would be receiving total parenteral nutrition (TPN) to support the nutritional status. Assessing pain is important to the plan of care but monitoring perfusion is most important to detecting worsening disease. Monitoring and assessing skin integrity would be an important part of the plan of care for a newborn that required surgical treatment for NEC.

173. **A. Anemia.**

Meckel's diverticulum is an outpouching of the ileum and is characterized by painless rectal bleeding and stools that are brick or "currant jelly" colored. Excessive bleeding can lead to anemia. Encopresis is incontinence of stool associated with chronic constipation, developmental delays, and a predisposition to the condition. It is not a potential complication of Meckel's diverticulum. Vitamin D deficiency is associated with short bowel syndrome not Meckel's diverticulum. An inguinal hernia is characterized by a herniation of the bowel or other viscera into the inguinal canal and is not a potential complication of Meckel's diverticulum.

174. **B. Avoid administering with milk, antacids, or iron.**

Administering this medication with alkaline substances can reduce its effectiveness. The medication should be administered with meals or snacks, not between meals. Tablets should not be chewed or crushed but should be swallowed whole. If extended-release capsules are prescribed and the patient is unable to swallow them whole, they may be opened, and the contents mixed with an acidic food such as applesauce. The mixture should then be swallowed without chewing and followed with water. If a dose is missed, it should not be taken with the next scheduled dose.

175. A. Observe each parent as they perform the skill on the child.

The best way for the nurse to evaluate the parents' understanding of the teaching is to observe each parent as they perform the skill. This allows the nurse to identify and correct any misconceptions. Providing guidance through each step as the parents perform the skill will not allow the nurse to properly evaluate the parents' understanding of how to perform the skill. Providing written instructions may help to reinforce the teaching but it does not allow the nurse to evaluate the parents' understanding of how to perform the skill. Asking the parents to verbalize their understanding of the teaching does not allow the nurse to evaluate whether the parents can accurately perform the skill.

INDEX

abusive head trauma, 62
acceptance, grieving process, 359
acetaminophen dosing and poisoning, 141–142, 411
acid/base balance, 167–168
acid/base imbalance, 189, 190
acne, 32, 234–236, 253, 254
acquired immune deficiency syndrome (AIDS), 277–279, 283, 284, 285, 286
active immunity, 263, 272
acute adrenal crisis, 210–211, 230
acute lymphoblastic leukemia (ALL), 123–124
acute myelogenous leukemia (AML), 123–124
acute poststreptococcal glomerulonephritis, 168–170
acute renal failure, 399, 425
acute rheumatic fever (ARF), 114–115
acyanotic defect, 104, 118, 120
    atrial septal defect, 104
    coarctation of the aorta, 107
    ventricular septal defect, 106
acyanotic subgroup, 104
Adam's forward bend test, 200
Addison's disease, 211–212
ADHD. *See* attention deficit hyperactivity disorder
adolescent assessment
    cardiovascular assessment, 31
    cognitive development, 32–33
    genitourinary assessment, 31–32
    head, eyes, ears, nose, and throat, 31
    integumentary assessment, 32
    nursing interventions, 33
    physical assessment, 30–31
    psychosocial assessment, 32–33
    psychosocial development, 33
    respiratory assessment, 31
adrenal disorders
    acute adrenal crisis, 210–211
    Addison's disease, 211–212
    chronic adrenocortial insufficiency, 211–212
    congenital adrenal hyperplasia, 213–214
    Cushing syndrome, 212–213
    pheochromocytoma, 214–215
adrenal tumors, 212, 213
advocacy, 370
agoraphobia, 288, 310
AIDS. *See* acquired immune deficiency syndrome
ALL. *See* acute lymphoblastic leukemia
allergic rhinitis, 41–42, 55, 56, 416
allergies, 275–277, 283, 284

Allis sign, 192
allow natural death (AND), 359–360
amblyopia, 58
American Nurses Credentialing Center (ANCC), 4–7
AML. *See* acute myelogenous leukemia
ANCC. *See* American Nurses Credentialing Center
anemia, 16, 123, 409, 414
    aplastic anemia, 125
    beta thalassemia, 125
    iron deficiency anemia, 129–130, 409
    sickle cell anemia, 133, 138, 414
anencephaly, 68
AND. *See* allow natural death
anger, grieving process, 358, 359, 360, 411
anorexia nervosa, 294–296, 312
anterior pituitary gland tumor, 381, 409
antibody protection, 275
antigens, 263, 411
antistreptolysin-O (ASO), 115, 169, 188
anxiety disorders, 287–289, 310
aorta, coarctation of, 107–109
aplastic anemia, 125, 392, 409, 419
appendicitis, 142, 165, 166, 413
ARF. *See* acute rheumatic fever
ASD. *See* autism spectrum disorder
ASDs. *See* atrial septal defects
ASO. *See* antistreptolysin-O
assent, 371
asthma, 82–87, 97, 98, 386, 394, 420, 425
    action plan, 87
    assessment, 83
    classification of asthma severity, 83
    discharge planning, 86–87
    nursing interventions, 83–85
    special considerations, 85
Asthma Action Plan, 87, 97, 98
asthma exacerbation, 386, 394, 413, 420
atopic dermatitis, 275–277, 284
atrial septal defects (ASDs), 104–106
atrophy, 234
attention deficit hyperactivity disorder (ADHD), 290–291, 309, 310, 382, 388, 410, 415
auscultation, respiratory assessment, 81
autism spectrum disorder (ASD), 274, 291–293, 310, 417
Auto-Injector, 284
autonomy, 370, 371, 376, 384, 412
autopsy, 361–362

bacterial diseases vaccines, 264–265
bacterial (septic) meningitis, 67–68, 75, 76
bacterial skin infections, 239–240
　cellulitis, 239
　impetigo, 239–240
bargaining, grieving process, 358–359
Barlow's sign, 192, 206
behavioral and psychosocial conditions
　anxiety disorders, 287–289
　attention deficit hyperactivity disorder, 290–291
　autism spectrum disorder, 291–293
　depression, 293–294
　eating disorders, 294–296
　intentional self-injury, 297
　learning disabilities, 298–299
　neonatal abstinence syndrome, 299–300
　obsessive-compulsive disorder, 301–302
　oppositional defiant disorder and conduct disorder, 302–303
　substance-related disorder, 304–305
　suicidal ideation, 305–306
　Tourette Syndrome, 306–307
behavioral signs, of vision impairment, 72
beneficence, 370, 371, 372
beta thalassemia, 125–126
bilateral conjunctivitis, Kawasaki disease, 114
bilateral myringotomies, 49
biliary atresia, 142–143, 164
bioethics, 370, 371, 377, 378
blood gases, 82
blood pressure
　assessment, school-aged children, 27
　assessment, infants, toddlers, and preschoolers, 16
　pediatric cardiovascular system, 103
body substance isolation (BSI), 284
body surface area (BSA), 236
bone cancer, 126–127
bowel obstruction, 427
BPD. *See* bronchopulmonary dysplasia
brace wearing, 201
brain tumor, 58–59
breastfeeding, 18, 54, 284
brittle bone disease, 199. *See also* osteogenesis imperfecta
bronchiolitis, 88–89
bronchodilator, 84, 98, 428
bronchopulmonary dysplasia (BPD), 87–88, 99, 100, 326, 420
Brudzinski's sign, 58, 67, 76, 424
BSA. *See* body surface area
BSI. *See* body substance isolation
bulimia nervosa, 294–296, 342
Burkholderia cepacia, 93, 94
burns, 236–238, 253, 254, 332, 392, 419
　abuse, 332, 333, 334–335, 339, 388, 414
　assessment, 236–237

nursing interventions, 237–238
nursing process review, 233–234
pediatric anatomy and physiology, 233
total body surface area, 236
water burns, 20

CA-MRSA infection. *See* community-associated methicillin-resistant *Staphylococcus aureus* infection
carbohydrates, foods low in, 412
cardiac arrhythmia, 344, 392, 418
cardiac catheterization, 107, 381, 390, 403, 409, 416, 428
cardiovascular assessment
　adolescents, 31
　school-aged children, 27
cardiovascular conditions, 101
　acute rheumatic fever, 114–115
　atrial septal defect, 104–106
　coarctation of the aorta, 107–109
　congestive heart failure, 110–111
　infective endocarditis, 113
　Kawasaki disease, 114
　pediatric cardiovascular system
　　congenital heart defects, 104
　　focused physical examination, 102–103
　　normal heart, 103
　　physiology, 104
　　relevant history, 101–102
　sepsis, 111–112
　Tetralogy of Fallot, 109–110
　ventricular septal defect, 106–107
cardiovascular perfusion, 397, 423
cardiovascular system, pediatric, 101–104
caregiver, caring for, 362
caring
　for caregiver, 362
　for child who has become an organ donor, 362
cast while bathing, 427
CD. *See* Crohn's disease
celiac disease, 143–144, 164, 165, 166, 383, 386, 410–411, 413
cell-mediated immune response, 275
cellular immunity, 271
cellulitis, 239, 251, 252
central diabetes insipidus, 223
central nervous system functions, 57
cerebral palsy (CP), 60–61, 382, 410
cerebrovascular accident, 424
certification, 3
Certified Pediatric Nurse (CPN), 4, 7
　exam, 4–6
CF. *See* cystic fibrosis
chemical burns, 236, 237, 346
chest radiograph, 82, 93
CHF. *See* congestive heart failure
child abuse, 327–328, 339, 340, 401, 406, 426, 431

child maltreatment and neglect, 327
  child neglect, 328–330
  consequences of, 328
  factitious disorder imposed on another, 330–331
  Munchausen by proxy, 330–331
  physical injury, 331–335
  sexual abuse, 335–337
child neglect, 327, 328–330, 341, 342
Child Well-Being Scale, 329
CHL. *See* conductive hearing loss
chronic adrenocortical insufficiency, 211–212
chronic lung disease (CLD), 394, 420
circumcision, 18, 187, 188, 391, 418
CLEAN Checklist, 329
cleft lip and palate, 144–145, 163, 164, 411
CLD. *See* chronic lung disease
clubbing, 102, 120
CMV. *See* cytomegalovirus
CoA. *See* coarctation of the aorta
coarctation of the aorta (CoA), 107–109
cognitive development
  adolescents, 32–33
  school-aged children, 28–29
cognitive impairments, 382, 410
cold shock, 112
common cold, 45
communication, therapeutic, 222, 232, 293, 326
community-associated methicillin-resistant *Staphylococcus aureus* (CA-MRSA) infection, 401, 427
compulsions, 301, 302
concussion, 31, 62, 354
conduct disorder, 302–303
conductive hearing loss (CHL), 44–45
congenital adrenal hyperplasia, 213–214
  salt-losing, 213, 214
  simple virilizing, 213
congenital aganglionic megacolon, 151–152. *See also* Hirschsprung disease
congenital clubfoot, 202–203
congenital heart defects, 104, 398, 424
congenital hypothyroidism, 224, 225, 229, 230, 232, 397, 423
congenital nasolacrimal duct obstruction, 43
congenital nephrotic syndrome, 178
congested cough, 118
congestive heart failure (CHF), 110–111, 117, 118, 387, 392, 400, 414, 419, 426
conjunctivitis, 42, 401, 426
consciousness, level of, 421, 423
constipation, 145–146
contact dermatitis, 240–241, 251, 252
CP. *See* cerebral palsy
CPN. *See* Certified Pediatric Nurse
critical coarctation, 109
Crohn's disease (CD), 152–155, 389, 415
croup syndromes, 89–91

cryptorchidism, 170
cultural diversity, 356–357
Cushing syndrome, 212–213, 229, 230, 231, 232, 405, 430
cyanosis, 101–102, 430
cyanotic defect, Tetralogy of Fallot, 110
cyanotic subgroup, heart defects, 104
cystic fibrosis (CF), 92–94, 97, 98, 402, 405, 407, 408, 428, 430, 432, 433
cystitis, 182–184
cytomegalovirus (CMV), 44

dacryostenosis, 43
DDH. *See* developmental dysplasia of the hip
death
  after the death, 361
  assessment of physical manifestations, 359
  developmental stages, understanding, and interventions for, 356–357
  process, care needs through, 360–361
  unexpected, 360
dehydration, 164, 171–173, 187, 188, 189, 190, 389, 405, 415, 430
deliberate self-harm, 297
denial, grieving process, 358, 366
depression, 16, 30, 33, 293–294, 404, 429
  stage of grieving process, 359, 360–361
dermatologic conditions, 233–234
  acne, 234–236, 253, 254
  bacterial skin infections, 239–240
    cellulitis, 239
    impetigo, 239–240
  contact dermatitis, 240–241
  diaper rash, 240–241
  pediatric anatomy and physiology, 233
  pediculosis, 244–245
dermis, 233, 252
developmental dysplasia of the hip (DDH), 191–194, 205, 206, 207, 208, 391, 417, 424
diabetes insipidus, 223, 230
diabetic ketoacidosis (DKA), 216, 232, 414
diaper rash, 240–241
diarrhea, 146–147
digitalis, 426
dislocatable hip dysplasia, 191
dislocation hip dysplasia, 191
disruptive mood dysregulation disorder, 294
diurnal enuresis, 173, 174
DKA. *See* diabetic ketoacidosis
DMD. *See* Duchenne muscular dystrophy
DNR. *See* do-not-resuscitate
do-not-resuscitate (DNR), 359–360, 377, 378
doughnut pattern, immersion burn in, 333
Down syndrome, 320–322
Duchenne muscular dystrophy (DMD), 194–195, 385, 412
dyscalcia, 298

dysgraphia, 298
dyslexia, 298
dysplasia, hip, 191
dyspnea, 101

eating disorders, 294–296
eczema, 275–277, 283, 284
educational neglect, 328
effusion, otitis media with, 49
emancipated minors, 369
emergencies
    assessment and stabilization, 343–344
    cardiac arrhythmias, 344
    extremity emergencies, 344–346
    eye injuries, 346
    inhalation injury, 347
    pediatric life-threatening respiratory illnesses, 347
    respiratory emergencies, 348
    shock, 348–349
    trauma emergencies, 349
emotional neglect, 328
encephalocele, 68
endocrine and metabolic conditions, 209–210
    adrenal disorders
        acute adrenal crisis, 210–211
        chronic adrenocortical insufficiency, 211–212
        congenital adrenal hyperplasia, 213–214
        Cushing syndrome, 212–213
        pheochromocytoma, 214–215
    pancreatic disorders
        type 1 diabetes, 216–217
        type 2 diabetes, 218
    parathyroid disorders
        hyperparathyroidism, 220–221
        hypoparathyroidism, 219–220
    pituitary disorders
        diabetes insipidus, 223
        hyperpituitarism, 221–222
        precocious puberty, 222
    thyroid disorders
        hyperthyroidism, 225–226
        hypothyroidism, 224–225
end-of-life care, 355, 356
    after the death, 361
    anticipated progression of disease process, guidance for, 357–358
    caregiver, caring for, 362
    death, assessment of physical manifestations, 359
    death process, care needs through, 360–361
    grieving process, 358–359
    organ donation and autopsy, 361–362
    supporting end-of-life decision-making, 359–360
    unexpected death, 360
end-of-life decision-making, 359–360
Enterobiasis, 260–261
Enterobius vermicularis, 158
enuresis, 173–174, 187, 188

enzyme deficiencies, 403, 428
epidermal necrolysis, 246–247
epidermis, 233
epiglottitis, 91–92, 98, 399, 402, 425, 427
epilepsy, 70–71
epinephrine, 277, 284, 423, 428
    EpiPen®, 277, 283, 284
    EpiPen Jr®, 277, 284
epispadias, 175
epistaxis, 43–44, 55, 56, 387, 414
Erikson's theory of psychosocial development, 29
erythema multiforme major, 246–247
esophageal atresia, 147–148
ethics, 370–373
Eustachian tube, 41, 54, 424
Ewing's sarcoma, 126–127, 139, 140
exam blueprint
    Certified Pediatric Nurse Exam, 4–5
    Pediatric Nursing Certification exam, 5–7
extremity emergencies, 344–346
eye injuries, 346
eyes, ears, nose, and throat conditions, 41
    allergic rhinitis, 41–42
    conjunctivitis, 42
    dacryostenosis, 43
    epistaxis, 43–44
    hearing loss, 44–45
    infectious rhinitis, 45
    laryngomalacia, 45–46
    obstructive sleep apnea syndrome, 46–47
    otitis externa, 47
    otitis media ear infection, 48–49
    otitis media with effusion, 49
    periorbital cellulitis, 50
    pharyngitis, 50–51
    sinusitis, 51
    Streptococcus tonsillitis group A, 51–52

factitious disorder by proxy, 330–331, 339, 340, 382, 410
factitious disorder imposed on another (FDIA), 330–331, 339, 340, 382, 410
Fallot, Tetralogy of, 109–110, 119, 120
FASD. *See* fetal alcohol spectrum disorders
FDIA. *See* factitious disorder imposed on another
fear, death, 360, 366
febrile seizures, 73, 401, 426
feeding pattern, history for cardiovascular assessment, 101
femur fracture, 398, 424
fetal alcohol spectrum disorders (FASD), 313, 315
fetal alcohol syndrome, 313–315, 323, 324
fever of unknown origin, 255–256
fine pincer grasp, 14
fissure, 234
fluid balance, 420
follicle-stimulating hormone (FSH), 222, 296

food allergies, 275–277, 403, 428
formula feed, 18
fragile X syndrome, 315–316, 323, 324
FSH. *See* follicle-stimulating hormone
fungal infection, 241–242, 252
furosemide, 118, 120, 421, 425
futility of care, 373

GABHS. *See* group A beta-hemolytic *Streptococci*
GAD–7. *See* Generalized Anxiety Disorder–7
Galeazzi sign, 192
gastroenteritis, 148–149, 163, 164
gastroesophageal reflux disease, 149–150, 413
gastrointestinal and nutritional conditions
   acetaminophen dosing and poisoning, 141–142
   appendicitis, 142
   biliary atresia, 142–143
   celiac disease, 143–144
   cleft lip and palate, 144–145
   constipation, 145–146
   diarrhea, 146–147
   esophageal atresia and tracheoesophageal fistula, 147–148
   gastroenteritis, 148–149
   gastroesophageal reflux disease, 149–150
   hepatitis, 150–151
   Hirschsprung disease, 151–152
   inflammatory bowel disease, 152–155
   intussusception, 155–156
   Meckel diverticulum, 156
   necrotizing enterocolitis, 157
   pediatric gastrointestinal system, 141
   pinworms, 158
   pyloric stenosis, 158–160
   vomiting, 160
gastrointestinal assessment, school-aged children, 27
gastrointestinal system, pediatric, 141
gastrostomy tube, caring for, 320
GBS. *See* group B *Streptococcus*
GCS score. *See* Glasgow Coma Scale score
generalized anxiety disorder, 287, 310
Generalized Anxiety Disorder–7 (GAD–7), 289
genitourinary assessment
   adolescents, 31–32
   school-aged children, 27
genitourinary, renal, and reproductive conditions
   acid/base balance, 167–168
   acute poststreptococcal glomerulonephritis, 168–170
   cryptorchidism, 170
   dehydration, 171–173
   enuresis, 173–174
   epispadias and hypospadias, 175
   hemolytic uremic syndrome, 176–177
   hydrocele, 177–178
   nephrotic syndrome, 178–179
   pyelonephritis infection, 180–181
   renal system and kidney function, 167
   testicular torsion, 181–182
   urinary tract infection, 182–184
   varicocele, 184–185
genitourinary system, 167
gentamycin, 425
Giardia lamblia, 260–261, 271, 272
Glasgow Coma Scale (GCS) score, 395, 421
Gower sign, 194, 195
grieving process, 358–359
group A beta-hemolytic *Streptococci* (GABHS), 257–258, 271, 272
group B *Streptococcus* (GBS), 257–258, 432

Haemophilus influenzae, 261
   meningitis, 67
   otitis media, 48
   type b (Hib), 91
      epiglottitis, 91, 92, 98
   vaccine schedule, 265
hair loss, 140
HBIG. *See* hepatitis B immunoglobulin
headaches, 61–62, 75, 76
head, eyes, ears, nose, and throat (HEENT) assessment
   adolescents, 31
   school-aged children, 26
head injuries, 62–63, 381, 394, 409, 421
Health Insurance Portability and Accountability Act (HIPAA), 369, 376
hearing loss, 44–45
HEENT assessment. *See* head, eyes, ears, nose, and throat assessment
helminthic infection, 158
hematologic and oncologic conditions
   aplastic anemia, 125
   beta thalassemia, 125–126
   bone cancer, 126–127
   chemotherapy, 131, 136
   hemophilia, 127–128
   hyperbilirubinemia, 128–129
   idiopathic or immune thrombocytopenia, 129
   iron deficiency anemia, 129–130
   leukemias, 123–124
   lymphoma, 130–131
   neuroblastoma, 131–132
   pediatric hematology and oncology, 123
   retinoblastoma, 132–133
   sickle cell disease, 133–134
   von Willebrand factor, 134–135
   Wilms tumor, 135
hemolytic uremic syndrome (HUS), 176–177, 187, 188, 388, 415
hemophilia, 127–128, 137, 138
hepatitis, 150–151, 267
hepatitis A vaccine schedule, 267
hepatitis B immunoglobulin (HBIG), 272

hepatitis B vaccine schedule, 267
Hib. *See Haemophilus influenzae* type b
hip dysplasia, 191–194, 205, 206, 207, 208, 391, 417, 424
HIPAA. *See* Health Insurance Portability and Accountability Act
Hirschsprung disease, 151–152, 164, 405, 430
hirsutism, 230
HIV infection. *See* human immunodeficiency virus infection
HLHS. *See* hypoplastic left heart syndrome
Hodgkin lymphoma, 130, 139, 140
Home Accident Prevention Inventory, 329
HOME Inventory, 329
hospice care, 355–356, 417
human immunodeficiency virus (HIV) infection, 277–279, 283, 284, 285, 286, 381, 391, 393, 409, 417, 420
human papilloma vaccine schedule, 268, 273, 274
humoral immunity, 275
HUS. *See* hemolytic uremic syndrome
hydrocele, 177–178
hydrocephalus, 63–64, 75, 76
hyperbilirubinemia, 128–129, 137, 138
hyperlipidemia, 188
hyperosmolar hyperglycemic syndrome, 218
hyperparathyroidism, 220–221
hyperpituitarism, 221–222, 381, 400, 409, 426
hypersensitivities, 275–277, 283, 284
hyperthyroidism, 225–226, 232
hypertrophic, pyloric stenosis, 158–160
hypervigilance, child's care, 366
hypogammaglobulinemia, 279–280, 283, 284
hypoparathyroidism, 219–220
hypoplastic left heart syndrome (HLHS), 119, 120
hypospadias, 175, 187, 188, 391, 418
hypotension, in sepsis, 112
hypothyroidism, 224–225, 229, 230, 231, 232, 397, 423
hypoxic ischemic encephalopathy, 316–317, 323, 324, 325, 326

IBD. *See* inflammatory bowel disease
idiopathic/immune thrombocytopenia, 129
IE. *See* infective endocarditis
IHP. *See* individualized health plan
IICP. *See* increased intracranial pressure
immune response, 263
immune system, 263
immune thrombocytopenia, 129
immunity, 263
immunizations, 263
    viral diseases and vaccines for prevention
        bacterial diseases vaccines, 264–265
        meningococcal vaccines, 265–266
        pneumococcal vaccines, 266
        viral diseases vaccines, 267–270
immunodeficiency, 275

immunoglobulin, 275, 280, 383, 384, 387, 404, 410, 411, 414, 429
immunologic memory, 263
immunology
    allergies, 275–277, 283, 284
    human immunodeficiency virus infection and acquired immune deficiency syndrome, 277–279
    hypogammaglobulinemia, 279–280
    Severe Combined Immunodeficiency, 280–281
impaired growth, 101
impetigo, 239–240, 251, 252, 389, 393, 415, 416, 420
inactivated vaccines, 263
increased intracranial pressure (IICP), 64–65, 73, 406, 431
individualized health plan (IHP), 30
infancy
    assessment, 11–16
    diagnostics, 16–17
    nursing interventions, 17
    patient and family education, 18–20
infectious diseases
    fever of unknown origin, 255–256
    group A beta-hemolytic *Streptococci,* 257–258
    group B *Streptococcus,* 257–258
    infectious diseases that are not vaccine-preventable, 256–263
    methicillin-resistant *Staphylococcus aureus,* 258–259
    Mycobacterium tuberculosis, 259–260
    parasitic illness, 260–261
    vector-borne illness, 261–262
    viral exanthems, 262–263
infectious gastroenteritis, 163, 164
infectious rhinitis, 45
infective endocarditis (IE), 113
inflammatory bowel disease (IBD), 152–155
influenza vaccine schedule, 268
inhalation injury, 347
inner ear, 41
insect stings and spider bites, 242–244
inspiratory stridor, 427
integumentary assessment, adolescents, 32
intentional self-injury, 297
intermittent nocturnal incontinence, 173–174
intravenous fluid rehydration, 232
intravenous immunoglobulin therapy (IVIG), 280, 284, 387, 404, 414, 429
intussusception, 155–156, 163, 164
iron deficiency anemia, 129–130, 400, 409, 426
irritant contact dermatitis, 240–241
isolation, grieving process, 358
isotretinoin, 235
IVIG. *See* intravenous immunoglobulin therapy

jaundice, 138
justice, 370–371

Kawasaki disease, 114, 117, 118, 400, 426
Kernig's sign, 58, 67, 76
kidney function, 167
kidney infection, 180–181
knee asymmetry, 192
knee-chest position, 110, 120

laryngomalacia, 45–46, 409
laryngotracheobronchitis (LTB), 425
latex allergies, 274, 275
LCP. See Legg–Calvé–Perthes disease
lead, 16, 65–67, 415
lead poisoning/plumbism, 65–67
learning disabilities, 298–299
Legg–Calvé–Perthes disease (LCP), 195–196, 205, 206, 407, 431
lemon glycerin swabs, 136
leukemias, 123–124
leukotriene receptor antagonist, asthma, 84
LH. See luteinizing hormone
lice. See pediculosis
life-limiting conditions, 355
limp, 196
live attenuated vaccines, 263, 420
lower respiratory infection, 383, 411
lower urinary tract infection, 182–184
low-flow supplemental oxygen therapy, 97, 98
LTB. See laryngotracheobronchitis
lumbar puncture, 77, 78
luteinizing hormone (LH), 222, 296
Lyme disease, 261–262
lymphoma, 130–131, 139, 140

macroglossia, 421, 423
macular rash, 234
MBP. See Munchausen syndrome by proxy
McBurney's point, 166
measles–mumps–rubella vaccine schedule, 269, 272, 273, 274, 402, 427
Meckel's diverticulum, 156, 272, 407, 432
medical neglect, 328
meningitis, 67–68
meningocele, spina bifida, 68, 69
meningococcal vaccines, 265–266
metabolic acidosis, 168, 421
metabolic alkalosis, 159, 160, 164, 168
metabolic conditions, endocrine and, 209–210
    adrenal disorders
        acute adrenal crisis, 210–211
        chronic adrenocortial insufficiency, 211–212
        congenital adrenal hyperplasia, 213–214
        Cushing syndrome, 212–213
        pheochromocytoma, 214–215
    pancreatic disorders
        type 1 diabetes, 216–217
        type 2 diabetes, 218

parathyroid disorders
    hyperparathyroidism, 220–221
    hypoparathyroidism, 219–220
pituitary disorders
    diabetes insipidus, 223
    hyperpituitarism, 221–222
    precocious puberty, 222
thyroid disorders
    hyperthyroidism, 225–226
    hypothyroidism, 224–225
metabolic disorders, 384, 411
methicillin-resistant *Staphylococcus aureus,* 240, 258–259, 401, 427
microaspiration, 324
middle ear, 41
mitochondrial disorders, 317–318, 325, 326
morphine sulfate, 254
Munchausen syndrome by proxy (MBP), 330–331, 339, 340, 382, 410
mupirocin calcium cream, 415
murmurs, 103
musculoskeletal assessment, school-aged children, 28
musculoskeletal conditions
    developmental hip dysplasia, 191–194
    Duchenne muscular dystrophy, 194–195
    Legg–Calvé–Perthes disease, 195–196
    nursemaid's elbow, 197
    Osgood-Schlatter disease, 198
    osteogenesis imperfecta, 199
    pediatric musculoskeletal system, 191
    scoliosis, 200–201
    slipped capital femoral epiphysis, 201–202
    talipes equinovarus congenita, 202–203
musculoskeletal system, pediatric, 79, 191
Mycobacterium tuberculosis, 259–260
myelomeningocele, 68, 69, 77, 78, 421

nail clubbing, 102, 110, 120
NAS. See neonatal abstinence syndrome
nasal-pharyngeal washings, 82
nasal vasopressin, 230
nasolacrimal duct obstruction, 43, 53, 54
NEC. See necrotizing enterocolitis
necrotizing enterocolitis (NEC), 157, 407, 432
negative feedback, 209–210
negligence, 372
neonatal abstinence scales, 299
neonatal abstinence syndrome (NAS), 299–300, 311, 312
nephroblastoma, 135
nephrogenic diabetes insipidus, 223
nephrotic syndrome, 178–179
neural tube defects, 68–70. See also spina bifida.
neuroblastoma, 131–132, 137, 138, 403, 428
neurologic conditions
    amblyopia, 58

neurologic conditions (cont.)
  brain tumor, 58–59
  cerebral palsy, 60–61
  febrile seizures, 73
  headaches, 61–62
  head injuries, 62–63
  hydrocephalus, 63–64
  increased intracranial pressure, 64–65, 73
  lead poisoning/plumbism, 65–67
  meningitis, 67–68
  neural tube defects, 68–70
  pediatric neurologic system function
    assessment, 57
    central nervous system functions, 57
    medical treatments, 57–58
    neurologic assessment, 58
    neurologic system, 57
  seizure disorder, 70–71
  sensory impairment
    hearing impairment, 44–45
    visual impairment, 71–72
  spina bifida, 68–70
neurovascular checks, 208
nocturnal enuresis, 173, 174
nonaccidental head trauma, 333, 340
non-Hodgkin lymphoma, 130–131
nonmaleficence, 370–371, 372, 376
nonverbal learning disorder, 298
nosebleed, 43–44, 55, 56
nursemaid's elbow, 197
nursing ethics, 369, 370
nursing, professional responsibilities and ethics in, 369–370, 372, 376
nutrition
  infancy, 12
  preschoolers, 12
  toddlers, 12
nystatin, 241, 252

obesity, type 2 diabetes, 218
obsessions, 301, 302
obsessive-compulsive disorder, 301–302
obstructive sleep apnea syndrome, 46–47
occulta, spina bifida, 68, 69
octreotide acetate, 426
OI. See osteogenesis imperfecta
oncologic conditions, hematologic and
  aplastic anemia, 125
  beta thalassemia, 125–126
  bone cancer, 126–127
  chemotherapy, 131, 136
  hemophilia, 127–128
  hyperbilirubinemia, 128–129
  idiopathic or immune thrombocytopenia, 129
  iron deficiency anemia, 129–130
  leukemias, 123–124
  lymphoma, 130–131
  neuroblastoma, 131–132
  pediatric hematology and oncology, 123
  retinoblastoma, 132–133
  sickle cell disease, 133–134
  von Willebrand factor, 134–135
  Wilms tumor, 135
ophthalmic drops, 42
opisthotonic position, 67
OPO. See organ procurement organization
oppositional defiant disorder, 302–303
oral health, 17
oral rehydration solution (ORS), 173
oral/written language disorder, 298
organ donation, 361–362
organ procurement organization (OPO), 362
ORS. See oral rehydration solution
Ortolani maneuver, 192
Ortolani's sign, 192
Osgood-Schlatter disease, 198
osteochondritis, 198
osteogenesis imperfecta (OI), 199, 388, 415
osteosarcoma, 126–127, 397, 423
otitis externa, 47
otitis media, 48–49, 398, 424
otitis media, with effusion, 49
outer ear, 41
  infection, 47
oxygen delivery systems, asthma, 82

PANDAS. See Pediatric Autoimmune Neuropsychiatric Disorder Associated with Streptococcus
PANS. See Pediatric Acute-Onset Neuropsychiatric Syndrome
palliative care, 355, 390, 395, 413, 417, 422, 426
  after the death, 361
  anticipated progression of disease process, guidance for, 357–358
  caregiver, caring for, 362
  death, assessment of physical manifestations, 359
  death process, care needs through, 360–361
  grieving process, 358–359
  organ donation and autopsy, 361–362
  supporting end-of-life decision-making, 359–360
  unexpected death, 360
palmar grasp, 14
pancreatic disorders
  type 1 diabetes, 216–217
  type 2 diabetes, 218
pancreatic enzyme insufficiency, 430
panic disorder, 288
papular rash, 234
paralytic polio, 422
parasitic illness, 260–261
parathyroid disorders
  hyperparathyroidism, 220–221
  hypoparathyroidism, 219–220

passive immunity, 263, 271, 272
paternalism, 372
patient-controlled analgesia (PCA) pump, 206
Pavlik harness, 193–194, 207, 208, 391, 417
PCA pump. *See* patient-controlled analgesia pump
peak flow meter, 85–86
PED-BC™. *See* Pediatric Nurse - Board Certified
Pediatric Acute-Onset Neuropsychiatric Syndrome (PANS), 301
Pediatric Autoimmune Neuropsychiatric Disorder Associated with Streptococcus (PANDAS), 301
pediatric cardiovascular system
   congenital heart defects, 104
   focused physical examination, 102–103
   normal heart, 103
   physiology, 104
   relevant history, 101–102
pediatric gastrointestinal system, 141
pediatric musculoskeletal system, 79, 191
Pediatric Nurse - Board Certified (PED-BC™), 4
   exam, 5–7
Pediatric Nursing Certification Board (PNCB®), 4–5
pediculosis, 244–245
percussion, respiratory assessment, 81
periorbital cellulitis, 50
Perthes. *See* Legg–Calvé–Perthes disease
Pfizer-BioNTech COVID-19 vaccine, 267
pharyngitis, 50–51
pheochromocytoma, 214–215, 229, 230
phobias, 287, 288
physical assessment, adolescents, 30–31
physical injury, child maltreatment, 331–335
physical neglect, 328
pinworms, 158, 165, 166
pituitary disorders
   diabetes insipidus, 223
   hyperpituitarism, 221–222
   precocious puberty, 222
pituitary tumors, 213
plaque, 234
plumbism, 65–67, 419
PNCB®. *See* Pediatric Nursing Certification Board
pneumococcal vaccines, 266
Pneumocystis jiroveci pneumonia, 278, 279, 285, 286
poisonings
   assessment and stabilization, 343–344
   cardiac arrhythmias, 344
   gastrointestinal decontamination, 354
   inhalation injury, 347
Polanksy's Childhood Level of Living Scale, 329
polio vaccine schedule, 267–268
polycythemia, 102, 120, 123
polysaccharide vaccine, 263, 266
positive feedback, 210
post-tonsillectomy, 392, 419
potassium, 421
precocious puberty, 32, 222

premature infant medical disorders, 318–320
preschoolers
   assessment, 11–16
   diagnostics, 16–17
   nursing interventions, 17
   patient and family education, 18–20
pressure gradient, 103
pressure ulcers, 245
primary enuresis, 173
primary idiopathic nephrotic syndrome, 178–179
privacy, adolescent assessment, 30
professional responsibilities
   bioethics, 370–373
   in nursing, 369–370
   nursing ethics, 370
Professional Standards in Pediatric Nursing, 369
psychosocial assessment
   adolescents, 32–33
   school-aged children, 28–30
psychosocial development
   adolescents, 33
   school-aged children, 29–30
puberty, 27, 28, 30, 31–32
pulmonary function tests, asthma, 82
pulmonary stenosis, 109
pulse oximetry, 81–82
   pediatric cardiovascular system, 103
pustule, 234
pyelonephritis infection, 180–181
pyloric stenosis, 158–160, 163, 164

quality-of-life assessment, 372

radial head subluxation, 197
radiation burns, 236
radiation therapy, 127, 139, 140, 395, 421
rales, respiratory assessment, 81
recombinant vaccine, 263
renal system, 167
respect for autonomy, individual rights, 370–371
respiratory acidosis, 168, 190, 413
respiratory alkalosis, 168
respiratory assessment
   adolescents, 31
   school-aged children, 27
respiratory complications, 423
respiratory conditions
   asthma, 82–87
      assessment, 83
      classification of asthma severity, 83
      diagnostics, 83
      discharge planning, 86–87
      nursing interventions, 83–85
      special considerations, 85
   bronchiolitis, 88–89
   bronchopulmonary dysplasia, 87–88
   croup syndromes, 89–91

respiratory conditions (*cont.*)
  cystic fibrosis, 92–94
  epiglottitis, 91–92
  pediatric musculoskeletal system, 79
  respiratory assessment parameters
    initial assessment, 80
    oxygen delivery systems, 82
    physical assessment, 80–81
    respiratory dysfunction, diagnostics for, 81–82
respiratory distress syndrome, 94–95
respiratory dysfunction, diagnostics for, 81–82
respiratory emergencies, 348
respiratory stridor, 412
respiratory syncytial viral (RSV) infection, 82, 326, 397, 423
retinoblastoma, 132–133, 139, 140
rheumatic fever, 114–115, 117, 118, 272, 406, 431
rhonchi, respiratory assessment, 81
right lower quadrant (RLQ) pain, 166, 206
RLQ pain. *See* right lower quadrant pain
rotavirus 5 (RV5) vaccine, 163, 164, 269, 274
routine tonsillectomy, 384, 412
RSV infection. *See* respiratory syncytial viral infection
RV5 vaccine. *See* rotavirus 5 vaccine

salicylates, 431
Salmonella, 260–261
salt-losing congenital adrenal hyperplasia, 213, 214
SCA. *See* sickle cell anemia
scabies, 245–246
scalding liquid burns, 236
scale, 234
scar, 234
SCARED. *See* Screen for Child Anxiety Related Disorders
scarlet fever, 51, 53, 54, 425
SCFE. *See* slipped capital femoral epiphysis
school-aged children, 25
  cardiovascular assessment, 27
  cognitive development, 28–29
  diagnostics, 30
  gastrointestinal assessment, 27
  genitourinary assessment, 27
  head, eyes, ears, nose, and throat, 26
  musculoskeletal assessment, 28
  nursing interventions, 30
  physical assessment, 25
  psychosocial assessment, 28
  psychosocial development, 29–30
  respiratory assessment, 27
SCID. *See* Severe Combined Immunodeficiency
scoliosis, 200–201, 205, 206, 207, 208, 422
Screen for Child Anxiety Related Disorders (SCARED), 289
Shaken Baby Syndrome. *See* abusive head trauma
secondary enuresis, 173

secondary nephrotic syndrome, 178
seizure disorder, 70–71, 75, 76, 385, 411, 412
selective mutism, 287
self-care, 362
self-determination, 370, 375, 376
sensorineural hearing loss (SNHL), 44, 45, 55, 56
separation anxiety disorder, 287
sepsis, 111–112
septicemia, 111–112
serous otitis media, 48
serum ferritin, 426
serum osmolarity, 171
Severe Combined Immunodeficiency (SCID), 280–281, 285, 286
sexual abuse, 335–337, 341, 342
shock, 348–349, 394, 400, 421, 426
short bowel syndrome, 391, 396, 418, 422
sickle cell anemia (SCA), 133, 137, 138
sickle cell disease, 133–134
sickle cell trait, 133
sickling, complications of, 133
simple face mask, 98
simple virilizing congenital adrenal hyperplasia, 213
sinusitis, 51
skeletal survey, 334, 340
skin assessment, newborn, 233–234
skin color, 80, 416
skull fractures, 62
SLE. *See* systemic lupus erythematosus
slipped capital femoral epiphysis (SCFE), 201–202, 206, 207, 208, 404, 429
SNHL. *See* sensorineural hearing loss
social anxiety disorder, 288
social justice theory, 376
soft tissue injury, 62, 332
spacers, asthma, 84
spasmodic laryngitis, 391, 418
special developmental needs, 313, 322
  fetal alcohol syndrome, 313–315
  fragile X syndrome, 315–316
  hypoxic ischemic encephalopathy, 316–317
  mitochondrial disorders, 317–318
  premature infant medical disorders, 318–320
  Trisomy 21, 320–322
specific reading comprehension deficit, 298
speech and communication, 421
speech therapy, 164
spina bifida, 68–70. *See also* neural tube defects
spiritual needs, 361
squatting, 102, 412
Staphylococcus aureus, 239, 240, 252, 258–259, 401, 415, 427
steeple sign, 90, 99, 100
sternal precautions, 106
steroids, asthma, 84

Stevens–Johnson syndrome, 246–247
strep throat, 51–52, 257–258, 272
Streptococcus tonsillitis, 51–52, 53, 54
Streptococcus tonsillitis group A, 51–52
study plan, pediatric nurse certification, 8
subcutaneous tissue, 233
subluxation, hip dysplasia, 191, 197
substance abuse. *See* substance-related disorder
substance-related disorder, 304–305
sudden abdominal pain, 155, 164
suicidal ideation, 305–306
sweat chloride test, 82, 93
systemic lupus erythematosus (SLE), 402, 427

tachycardia, 103, 344, 409, 419
tachypnea, 101, 118, 230
talipes equinovarus congenita, 202–203
Tanner stages, 27, 31–32, 33, 35, 36
    and cognitive development, 32–33
TB. *See* tuberculosis
TBSA. *See* total body surface area
tense fontanelle, 419
testicular torsion, 181–182
Tetralogy of Fallot, 109–110, 119, 120
thalassemia intermedia, 125
thalassemia major, 125, 126
thalassemia minor, 125
thalassemia trait, 125, 126
thermal burns, 236
thyroid disorders
    hyperthyroidism, 225–226, 232
    hypothyroidism, 224–225, 229, 230, 231, 232, 397, 423
thyroid-stimulating hormone (TSH), 210
tinea infections, 241–242
tissue destruction, 236
toddlers
    assessment, 11–16
    diagnostics, 16–17
    nursing interventions, 17
    patient and family education, 18–20
tonsillectomy, 46, 47, 52, 384, 392, 406, 412, 419, 431
total body surface area (TBSA), 236
total parenteral nutrition (TPN), 418
Tourette Syndrome (TS), 306–307
TPN. *See* total parenteral nutrition
tracheoesophageal fistula, 147–148
tracheostomy, 319, 325, 326
tracheostomy securement device change, 319
tracheostomy tube, suction of, 319
trauma emergencies, 349
tremors, 299, 312
Trendelenburg sign, 206
Trisomy 21, 320–322, 323, 324
Trousseau sign, 219, 229, 230

TS. *See* Tourette Syndrome
TSH. *See* thyroid-stimulating hormone
tuberculosis (TB), 17, 255–256, 259–260
Turner syndrome, 119, 120
tympanostomy tubes, 49, 53, 54
type 1 diabetes, 216–217, 387, 414
type 2 diabetes, 218

UC. *See* ulcerative colitis
ulcer, 234
ulcerative colitis (UC), 152–155
umbilical cord, 18, 299
undescended testes, 170
unexpected death, 360
universal precautions (UP), 284
UP. *See* universal precautions
urinary tract infection (UTI), 182–184, 386, 413
urine catecholamine metabolites, 428
urticaria, 138
UTI. *See* urinary tract infection

vaccine schedule meningitis B, 265–266
vaccine schedule pneumococcal conjugate, 266
vaccine schedule pneumococcal polysaccharide, 266
vagus nerve stimulator (VNS), 385, 412
values, 370
VAR vaccine schedule. *See* varicella vaccine schedule
varicella (VAR) vaccine schedule, 270
varicocele, 184–185
VCUG. *See* voiding cystourethrogram
vector-borne illness, 261–262
ventricular septal defect (VSD), 106–107, 118
ventricular shunt malfunction, 392, 419
ventriculoperitoneal shunt, 75, 76
vesicular rash, 234, 252
viral cause, hepatitis, 148–149
viral exanthems, 262–263
viral (aseptic) meningitis, 67
vision, diagnostics for infants, toddlers, and preschoolers, 17
VNS. *See* vagus nerve stimulator
voiding cystourethrogram (VCUG), 180, 386, 413
volume overload, 106
vomiting, 160
von Willebrand disease, 134–135, 406, 430
von Willebrand factor (VWF), 134–135
VSD. *See* ventricular septal defect
VWF. *See* von Willebrand factor

warm shock, 112, 120
Wilms tumor, 135, 139, 140
wish fulfillment, 361
withdrawal, 360–361
WITHDRAWAL acronym, 300
withholding of care, 378

Wong-Baker FACES Pain scale, 411
wounds, 233–234, 248–249
  burns, 236–238
  dermatologic conditions, 239–241
  fungal infections, 241–242
  insect stings and spider bites, 242–244
  pediatric anatomy and physiology, 233
  pressure ulcers, 245
  scabies, 245–246

Zika, 261–262